The Economics of New Health Technologies

Incentives, Organization, and Financing

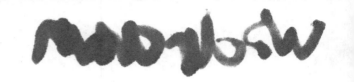

The Economics of New Health Technologies
Incentives, Organization, and Financing

Edited by

Joan Costa-Font

LSE Health and European Institute;
London School of Economics and Political Science,
London, UK

Christophe Courbage

International Association for the Study of Insurance
Economics (The Geneva Association),
Geneva, Switzerland

Alistair McGuire

LSE Health;
London School of Economics and Political Science,
London, UK

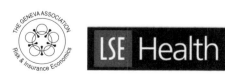

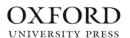

OXFORD
UNIVERSITY PRESS

OXFORD

UNIVERSITY PRESS

Great Clarendon Street, Oxford ox2 6DP

Oxford University Press is a department of the University of Oxford.
It furthers the University's objective of excellence in research, scholarship,
and education by publishing worldwide in

Oxford New York

Auckland Cape Town Dar es Salaam Hong Kong Karachi
Kuala Lumpur Madrid Melbourne Mexico City Nairobi
New Delhi Shanghai Taipei Toronto

With offices in

Argentina Austria Brazil Chile Czech Republic France Greece
Guatemala Hungary Italy Japan Poland Portugal Singapore
South Korea Switzerland Thailand Turkey Ukraine Vietnam

Oxford is a registered trade mark of Oxford University Press
in the UK and in certain other countries

Published in the United States
by Oxford University Press Inc., New York

© Oxford University Press, 2009

British Library Cataloguing in Publication Data

Data available

Library of Congress Cataloging in Publication Data

Data available

Typeset in Minion by Cepha Imaging Private Ltd., Banglore, India
Printed in Great Britain
on acid-free paper by the
MPG Books Group, Bodmin and King's Lynn

ISBN 978-0-19-955068-5 (Pbk.)

10 9 8 7 6 5 4 3 2 1

Contents

Part 4 **Innovation, social demand, and valuation**

Part 5 **Incentives, mechanisms, and processes**

Preface

Innovation is an essential process of change that affects the dynamics of welfare in modern societies. In the area of health care, innovation directly impacts on welfare through improving people's health and targeting specific needs. However, the rate at which societies introduce new technologies varies widely and is not independent of the various incentives in place in different health sectors. Incentives to the introduction of new technologies are both organizational and monetary, as well as implicit and explicit, for example, impacting through reimbursement schemes and the design of patents. Given the importance of health insurance and third-party payments, both at a general state level and at the individual's level, the influence of financial incentives on innovation appears to be an important question that calls for new theoretical and empirical examination. Moreover, the dynamics involved in analysing innovation uptake and diffusion also complicates examination of the level of welfare achieved. This book attempts to pursue the analysis of these different determinants in the process of technology innovation. It differs from existing books in that it covers the impact of innovation in health care from a number of different disciplinary perspectives, discussing some of the key issues that are currently being researched in the literature.

Technological change in health care has not only led to huge improvements in health services and the health status of populations, it has also been a major driver of health care expenditure. Although offering remarkable benefits, changes in technology are not free and often entail significant financial, as well as physical or social risks. These costs and benefits need to be balanced out within the wider health care sector environment of government regulations, insurance contracts, and reimbursement schemes, and individuals' decisions to use and consume certain technologies. With this in mind, this book aims to address the following important objectives:

- to provide a detailed definition of technological change as applied to the health sector;
- to identify drivers of innovation in several health care areas;
- to present the existing mechanisms and processes that ensure efficient development and use of medical technologies;
- to analyse the impact of advances in medical technology on health, health care expenditure, and health insurance.

The book is mostly based on contributions from a seminar organized in Geneva in October 2007 under the auspice of the Foundation Brocher, and supported by the Geneva Association and the LSE Health (London School of Economics and Political Science). It is composed of 17 contributions from various experts in their respective fields.

The books commences, first, with a section that contains an introductory chapter by Alistair McGuire and Victoria Serra. This chapter positions the debate of technology change in health care in the context of health systems reform. It introduces readers to definitions of technological change and innovation, and their impact in driving health system change and output (expenditures). It summarizes an aspect of the literature and contains important insights that need to be accounted for when examining health care technological change and expenditure trends.

Following this introduction, the next section deals with the role of incentives, governance, and institutions as they influence health care technology. This section begins with a chapter by Davide Consoli, Andrew McMeekin, J. Stan Metcalfe, Andrea Mina, and Ronnie Ramlogan that examines the role of process in innovation, which is often disregarded. They analyse an interesting evolutionary perspective and present empirical evidence from an example of intra-ocular lens and the treatment of glaucoma. This chapter focuses on systems of innovation, arguing that generation and delivery of new medical practices is dependent on the creation of sophisticated innovation systems that rely on the specialization, diversification, and co-ordination of activities that are complementary to health care institutions.

Chapter 3 by Nick Bosanquet, emphasizes the heterogeneity of innovation in health care, and discusses the importance of governance and risk assessment. In particular, he suggests that current trends are dominated by a process of switching from what he regards as 'big ticket' technology and provider-capture to a scenario of 'small ticket' technology, arguing that this switch is supported by appropriate clinical and financial structures. The chapter proposes ways through which this switch can take place through the introduction of payment by results and offers examples of experiences where incentives exhibit successful 'small ticket' innovation.

In the following chapter Victoria Serra-Sastre and Alistair McGuire then discuss the role of technology diffusion in the area of pharmaceutical treatments. This chapter is an up-to-date literature review of the main determinants of technology diffusion, including a discussion of the social, economic, and institutional constraints that enable pharmaceuticals to reach their targeted market.

The third section of this book deals with contributions addressing the links between technological change and health insurance.

The paper by Mark Pauly and Adam Isen explores the extent to which the linking mechanism between growing real income and growing medical spending is affected by health insurance. They strongly suspect that the design of health insurance may facilitate, but can also distort the pattern of technology adoption. They hypothesize that changes in health insurance in individual countries and variations in health insurance across countries might be expected to influence the pace, shape, and cost of technological change. In particular, they derive economic models of the relationship between insurance, and the demand for and supply of new technology in a market-based setting with private supply of both medical care and insurance. The authors take specific account of the key role that the physician's advice, judgment, and action must play in both interesting patients in new technology and supporting higher demands for it.

The chapter by Peter Zweifel nicely complements the previous one. It argues that there is a dual causal link between technological change and insurance. On the one hand, technological change often presents new opportunities, but also challenges to insurers. However, what has been rarely recognized is that insurance may also induce technological change, in the guise of both product and process innovation. The existence of health insurance serves to bias the mix between the two in favour of product innovation. Thus, the bias in favour of cost-increasing product innovation in health care may explain why technological innovation in medicine is viewed as a mixed blessing by many.

Chapter 7, by Marin Gemmill, Victoria Serra-Sastre, and Joan Costa-Font, empirically investigates the effect of health insurance coverage on the use of relatively new prescription drugs in the USA. The authors focus the analysis on statins, a class of lipid-lowering drugs that were considered a major breakthrough after a number of important clinical trials were published. To examine various aspects of adoption they explore two dependent variables: the probability of statin uptake and the number of statins consumed adjusted by the defined daily dose. Their findings suggest that insurance is an important determinant of positive statin use and the number of statins purchased. Interestingly, statin use is highest among those with public insurance coverage only, and those with both public and private insurance coverage, even after adjusting for other important determinants, such as health status.

Chapter 8, by Lilia Filipova and Michael Hoy, addresses the complex issue of the use of genetic advances by health insurance. Technical innovation in medical care in general generates a great deal of interest and controversy. Of particular and special interest, relative to other forms of technical innovation in the economy, is the role of insurance markets (or public insurance) in influencing the adoption of medical innovations. An additional important factor in the context of genetic advances, such as the development of new genetic tests, is the impact of regulations prohibiting insurers from using test results directly as relevant factors in the design and pricing of insurance contracts. Such regulations, of varying force, have been adopted throughout much of Europe. The authors discuss how such regulations may affect the way that genetic advances affect the adoption of genetic tests and related health care strategies, and what impact this could have on both insurers and consumers.

Part IV covers various topics under the label of innovation, social demand, and valuation.

The first chapter of this section, by Roland Eisen and Yasemin Ilgin, deals with the link between ageing and pharmaceutical innovation. In particular, the authors ask whether elderly people spend more on pharmaceuticals as an easy treatment option, or whether the pharmaceutical industry reacts to this trend of 'population greying' by directing research and development of new pharmaceuticals in this direction. They first outline a general way in which the process of innovation might be conceptualized, stressing the importance of 'induced' innovations. Then they develop their main hypothesis with empirical investigation, namely that, as the proportion of elderly in a population rises, not only does the share of pharmaceutical expenditure rises, but also the share of pharmaceutical R&D devoted to this part of the population. With the help of a simple econometric model they test this hypothesis and present some new results.

The following chapter, by Manuel García-Goñi and Paul Windrum, aims at obtaining a better knowledge of health innovations, their key drivers, and dynamics. The authors focus on the interaction between two agents—health service providers and patients. The case study presented in this chapter highlights the importance of modifying the quantity and quality of the health information provided to patients, and the way in which that information is provided. With that aim, they have selected a case study consisting of the substitution of one educational programme for diabetes patients for a new one. Their study provides a number of important insights into the real impact of the interaction between health providers and patients on long-term health status. This work therefore presents a new approach to understanding health service innovations, through the education and information provided to chronic patients in the public sector.

Chapter 11, by Nicola Pangher, describes the nature of revolutionary new health technologies, and its potential application and innovation in health care delivery. It focuses on the challenges that these technologies pose for both business and the health care system. The chapter is especially interesting as its reveals that as soon as a new technology is available on the market, the 'right' to the best existing treatment, escaping in many cases all the evidence-based guidelines, acts as a push for technology inception.

The following chapter, by Joshua Graff Zivin, Matthew Neidell, and Lauri Feldman, discusses the introduction of uncertainty and irreversibility in cost-effectiveness analysis to determine optimal funding and resource allocation for medical technologies, research, and treatment.

Chapter 13, by Adam Oliver and Corinna Sorenson, reviews some of the concerns raised against the use of economic evaluation in the decision-making process, from a wide range of disciplinary and stakeholder perspectives. The authors also offer some reflections on the National Institute for Health and Clinical Excellence (NICE) as a user of health economic evaluation to assess whether health care interventions ought to be made available in the National Health Service (NHS) in England and Wales.

The final section of the book contains four chapters, and looks at incentives, mechanisms, and processes.

Chapter 14, by Joan Rovira, discusses what instruments should be used to confer individuals with incentives to develop new treatments for existing conditions, especially in the field of pharmaceuticals. The author provides an insightful chapter on the meaning and characterization of pharmaceutical innovation, and how it is related to well-being and other social goals, concluding with thoughts on the best way to promote such products and reimburse innivation. This chapter challenges the role of patent protection, whilst discussing alternatives.

Frank R. Lichtenberg, in the following chapter, attempts to examine the contribution of innovation to the health system by looking at its effects in the long-term care sector. Particularly, he empirically examines whether medical innovation has reduced the age-adjusted nursing home residence rate. The study also estimates the costs that innovation brings to the integrated care-cure system through the impact on nursing home care costs.

An area where innovation has strong potential impact on the health system lies in information technologies. Given that the health sector is well known to exhibit important informational asymmetries, the accessibility of information through the Internet can have an influence on the search for health information. Joan Costa-Font, Caroline

Rudissill, and Elias Mossialos contribute to this debate by discussing the effect of health information and providing empirical evidence from a European cross-sectional database on the determinants of higher demands for health arising from Internet use. The evidence tests some theoretical frameworks on how individuals learn and update their knowledge for health purposes, drawing from European data.

This final section concludes with a chapter by Hristina Petkova, which considers how new knowledge generated by advances in science can be assimilated into public health care systems, allowing quicker integration of new technology into routine care. An example is drawn from maturity-onset diabetes of the young (MODY) study applied to two very different health care systems: Germany and the UK. The author shows that differences in the organization, funding, and delivery of care generally can affect genetic innovation. The degree of institutional take-up of testing for MODY as a single gene disorder with highly differential diagnosis and established clinical implications for alternative treatment, shows strong association with the general pattern of the health care structures. The implementation trajectories for MODY diagnosis in the two countries diverge at several points, from research expertise and pattern of provision, to diffusion channels in mainstream service.

We believe that each of these chapters is able to summarize an important issue concerning the innovation debate and contributes, in its own way, to a better understanding of the role innovation has both at the macro-level, and at the delivery (meso-) and micro-level in the health care sector. The effectiveness of innovation in improving peoples' welfare depends on its diffusion and inception by the relevant agents in the health and health production process. Therefore, policy-makers at the system level, as well as regulators who decide upon the institutional frameworks, together with managers, technicians, consumers, and patients are all involved in this whole process of technology change. These multifaceted interactions are well covered in this book.

We hope this book will appeal to all those working in the field of heath and health care, together with health economists and policy analysts, as well as practitioners and policy-makers, academics and practitioners in management, social policy, and technology, along with researchers and interested readers. The book has mainly pedagogic goals, and is aimed at those studying economics, social science, management science, science innovation, or technology, and especially those working or interested in the pharmaceutical industry, medical devices, and generally in health-related industries.

Contributors

Nick Bosanquet,
Imperial College,
London, UK

Davide Consoli,
Manchester Institute of Innovation
Research (MIoIR),
Manchester Business School,
Manchester, UK

Joan Costa-Font,
LSE Health, and European Institute,
London School of Economics and
Political Science,
London, UK

Roland Eisen,
Department of Economics,
University of Frankfurt,
Frankfurt, Germany

Lauri Feldman,
Columbia College,
Chicago, USA

Lilia Filipova,
University of Augsburg,
Augsburg, Germany

Manuel García-Goñi,
Departamento de Economia
Aplicada II,
Universidad Complutense de Madrid,
Madrid, Spain

Marin Gemmill,
LSE Health, London School of
Economics, London, UK

Joshua Graff Zivin,
School of International Relations and
Pacific Studies,
University of California,
San Diego, USA

Michael Hoy,
Department of Economics,
University of Guelph,
Guelph, Canada

Yasemin Ilgin,
Institute of European Health Policy and
Social Law (ineges),
Goethe University Frankfurt am Main,
Frankfurt, Germany

Adam Isen,
Business and Public Policy
Department,
Wharton School,
University of Pennsylvania,
Philadelphia, USA

Frank R. Lichtenberg,
Columbia University, New York, USA
and National Bureau of Economic
Research, Cambridge, MA

Alistair McGuire,
LSE Health, London School
of Economics,
London, UK

Andrew McMeekin,
Manchester Institute of Innovation
Research (MIoIR),
Manchester Business School,
Manchester, UK

J. Stan Metcalfe,
Manchester Institute of Innovation
Research (MIoIR),
Manchester Business School,
and Centre for Business Research,
University of Cambridge, UK

Andrea Mina,
Centre for Business Research,
University of Cambridge
Cambridge, UK

Elias Mossialos,
LSE Health, London School of
Economics,
London, UK

Matthew Neidell,
Department of Health Policy and
Management,
Columbia University,
New York, USA

Adam Oliver,
LSE Health, London School of
Economics,
London, UK

Nicola Pangher,
ITALTBS SpA,
Trieste, Italy

Mark V. Pauly,
Health Care Systems Department,
Wharton School,
University of Pennsylvania,
Pennsylvania, USA

Hristina Petkova,
EGENIS, ESRC Centre for Genomics
in Society,
University of Exeter,
Exeter, UK; King's College London,
London, UK

Ronnie Ramlogan,
Manchester Institute of Innovation
Research (MIoIR),
Manchester Business School,
Manchester, UK

Joan Rovira,
University of Barcelona,
Barcelona, Spain

Caroline Rudisill,
LSE Health, London School of
Economics,
London, UK

Victoria Serra-Sastre,
LSE Health, London School of
Economics,
London, UK

Corinna Sorenson,
LSE Health, London School of
Economics,
London, UK

Paul Windrum,
Manchester Metropolitan University
Business School (MMUBS),
Center for International Business and
Innovation (CIBI),
Manchester, UK

Peter Zweifel,
University of Zurich,
Zurich, Switzerland

Part 1

Introduction

Chapter 1

What do we know about the role of health care technology in driving health care expenditure growth?

Alistair McGuire and Victoria Serra-Sastre

Introduction

While there has been a long standing interest in the level of health care expenditure and, in particular, its relationship to GDP there has, until relatively recently, been little active interest in the growth of health care expenditure. There is a considerable literature on the determinants of the level of health care expenditure (see Gerdtham and Jonsson 2000) with an associated literature that highlights the role of third party payment systems and moral hazards as driving the level of such expenditure. This literature does not consider a major component of health care expenditure growth that is the focus of this paper – health care technology. In considering technology as a driver of health care expenditure, this chapter will provide a short overview of the literature on this topic, discuss certain trends in health care expenditure growth, then summarize conceptual definitions of technological change as a means of highlighting what is known empirically about the role technology plays in driving health care expenditure, as well as considering the role that various health system characteristics have on the uptake and diffusion of health care technology. If health care technology is indeed a major driver of health expenditure then it is important to recognize that future expenditure on medical research, which induces technological change, is liable to increase levels of expenditure. This is liable to be the case even if effective health technology assessment (HTA) programmes are put in place, as generally HTA considers technologies after a certain level of diffusion has already taken place. Indeed, one reason for a continuing expectation that technology will drive health expenditure rests on the increasing share of R&D expenditures, which are being appropriated by the health sector across a number of countries. For example, between 1995 and 2001 state-funded health R&D rose by an average of 9 per cent per annum in the OECD countries. This chapter begins with a brief overview of the literature on the factors influencing health care expenditure growth to ensure that a focus on health care technology is legitimate, before turning to the other aspects of interest raised above.[1]

Background

Burton Weisbrod (1991) was among the first to consider the dynamic role of health care technology in driving expenditure. He noted that the post-war era had seen significant rises in the level of health care expenditure across a number of countries with different health care systems and, in focusing his attention on the USA, concluded that, while moral hazard might be a plausible influence on rising expenditure levels, there might be a common factor across health care sectors that explained this common trend in health care expenditure growth across a number of countries. His common denominator was health care technology, but he hypothesized a two-way causal relationship between the changing characteristic of health care insurance from reimbursement based on 'costs incurred' to one that was somewhat independent of the actual costs incurred, through HMO or DRG type systems with the reimbursement based on average treatment costs of case type, which allowed a certain openness in the funding system, but also provided incentives for health care providers to pursue cost-increasing health care technologies. At the same time this cost-increasing technology faced the consumer with an incentive to broaden their insurance coverage, as such technology results in either the average cost of treatment increasing for the individual, or the variance of the cost of certain treatments increasing, or both. With both the average cost and variance increasing as new technology is taken up, the individual consumer has a strong incentive to demand higher insurance coverage against unpredictable higher cost items. The coupling of the changing characteristics of insurance and the increasing demand for insurance provided a conceptual mechanism to support the argument that technology was a major driver of health care expenditure growth.

It was Joseph Newhouse (1992) who took up the mantle of exploring precisely how important health care technology might be in driving health expenditures. Newhouse, again with a focus on the USA, pointed out that health care expenditure growth in that country had been approximately 4 per cent per annum for over five decades. He subsequently set out to identify a range of potential drivers underlying expenditure growth, both on the demand side (e.g. demographic ageing, insurance demand, income growth) and supply side factors (e.g. supplier-induced demand and productivity differentials). He then attempted to quantify the influence of each of these arguing, with some conviction, that none of these factors independently could account for more than a small part of the growth in health care expenditure. With regards to ageing he raised the issue left to a number of others to empirically detail that while the population demo-graphy was ageing this had a limited effect on the growth of health care expenditure, as most expenditure at the individual level occurred in the last few years of life. In other words, as Peter Zweifel and colleagues have noted 'per capita

---

[1]   There is remarkably little purely theoretical literature on the impact of health care technology on the sector. For a recent example of how this might be developed see Miraldo (2007).

(health care expenditure) is not necessary affected by the ageing of the population due to an increase in life expectancy. Rather, an increase in the share of expenditure to the elderly seems to shift the bulk of HCE to higher age ...' (Zweifel *et al.* 1999, p. 493). There is now considerable agreement that ageing in and of itself does not contribute in a major manner to increasing the rate of growth of health care expenditure (Seshamani 2004).

Newhouse then went on to discuss the role of prices and used evidence from the RAND health insurance experiment to note that with an price estimated elasticity around –0.2 to –0.33 the movement from average to zero co-insurance rates would not explain more than a small proportion of the rise in total health expenditure. Note that this static mechanism does not necessarily run counter to Weisbrod's contention as the latter's argument is more dynamic in nature. Similarly, taking an elasticity of income, Newhouse suggests that rising incomes could not explain more than a small proportion (0.25 per cent) of the growth in health care expenditures. On the supply side, he also dismisses supplier inducement given the lack of empirical evidence on its' role in expenditure growth. He acknowledges that, if the health care sector experiences slower productivity gains than other parts of the economy, in line with Baumol's original thesis that service industries find it more difficult to increase productivity, then this could cause rising relative prices, which when coupled with inelasticity of demand would then result in higher expenditure. However, again it is suggested that this could only ever be a small component of health care expenditure growth.

In summary, Newhouse contends that any combination of the above could only account for around 50 per cent, at the very most, of growth in health care expenditures in the USA over the previous five decades. He concludes that the growth in health care expenditure must therefore be driven by another factor, which he proposes is health care technology.[2] Similar analysis by the US Congressional Budget Office (2008) also concludes that approximately 50 per cent of the rise in US health expenditure was attributable to the introduction of new health care technology. The arguments are so generic and the empirical evidence used so transferable that this general conclusion can be held to extend to other OECD countries. Indeed, similar calculations have been undertaken by the Australian Productivity Commission (2005) to arrive at essentially the same conclusion.

This study examines the growth in Australian health care expenditure by breaking down expenditure growth into a number of components, then determining the residual growth in expenditures, which is, as with the Newhouse study, attributed to health care technology. Specifically, the study considers:

$$\Delta E = \sum_{i=1}^{n} \varepsilon_i g_i + R$$

where ΔE is the average annual growth rate of expenditure, ε_I is the elasticity of the ith growth factor, g_i is the average annual growth rate of the ith growth factor and R is the

---

2 Okunade and Murthy (2002) use R&D expenditure as a proxy for technological change and confirm Newhouse's original hypothesis using co-integrating regression techniques, which establish a long-term relationship between expenditure on R&D and health care expenditure.

residual average annual growth rate, which is attributed to technology. The growth factors that are included are:

♦ demographic change, where again the actual ageing of the population is held to have minimal impact;

♦ the movement in the relative price of health care, where it is acknowledged that, because of the normal difficulties faced in indexing quality improvements derived from improved technology, there may be an indirect influence of technological change on health care expenditure coming through these relative price movements;

♦ income, again a minimal influence;

♦ the proportion of individuals with private insurance, where once again moral hazard arguments are applied, but again with minimal force.

Under a range of assumptions the study finds that the residual growth attributable to technological changes influence on expenditure growth varies between approximately 17 to just over 55 per cent.

Pita Barros (1998) has noted further that, while there remains a substantial variation in the level of health care expenditure per capita across OECD countries, this dispersion fell between the 1960s and the 1970s, and has remained somewhat constant since. As he notes, if medical technology spreads across countries then, notwithstanding the impact of relative health care prices, expenditure growth in countries with lower levels of health care will witness faster growth as they catch up over time. Indeed, his results appear to support this convergence and the inference that health care technology is both driving health care expenditures generally and also leading to faster growth in countries that originally had lower levels of expenditure. In his regression results, again interpreting the residual effect as being reflective of the role of health care technology in explaining health care expenditure growth, Barros finds technological change explains around 30 per cent of the increase in health care expenditure.

Technological change is therefore a prime culprit in explaining health care expenditure growth empirically, but the mechanisms through which it operates appear not to be well understood, judging by the reliance in most studies on the interpretation of the residual to define the effect. Before turning to discuss the mechanism it is useful to conceptually define technological change.

What is meant by technological change?

It is actually of some import when discussing technological change to be rather precise when defining the analytical notion that is being studied. This is important, not least, because a number of different empirical representations may be used to capture the effect of technological change. Two aspects of technological change are particularly pertinent. The first is that, in theory, technological change could be associated with a new formulation of the transformation of inputs into output(s). As such, new technology defines a new production function and, therefore, is associated with embodied technical change. Thus, technical change that requires change of the factor input is referred to as embodied technical change. Yet both conceptually and empirically, this is not how technological change is commonly formulated. Secondly, although there is a dynamic element involved in technological change the precise interaction of time and technological change is rarely studied; and this observation extends to the consideration of the uptake and diffusion of new technology. In particular, there is a recognition that technological advance requires some interaction with time. A specific concern here relates to the use of a time variable or a time trend to indicate technological change. Such specification can, at most, only ever be an approximation, as it relies on the technical change being disembodied. That is, the technical change does not require new factor inputs or a significant change in the fundamental production process; an example of disembodied technical change often given is organizational change. Alternatively, disembodied technical change is sometimes characterized as depending on a learning rate; thus, the learning-by-doing mechanism that leads to improved volume output relations would provide an example of disembodied technical change. Noting that the production function describes the shape and positions of isoquants, it is important to recognize that even disembodied technical change can impact on both the shape, referred to as factor-augmenting technical change, or position, through influence on the expansion path of production, which may or may not be homogenous.

All such problems have led to the empirical examination of technological change being associated with a number of conceptual approximations. Three such approximations are discussed below. First, derived from the notion that technological change is associated with changes in the relative price of inputs in the production function analysis may be carried forward through examination of production function responses to these relative price changes. Secondly, derived from the notion that technological change is a dynamic process, analysis is sometimes carried forward through the identification of a time variable, which is held to encapsulate the impact of technological change through shifts in the production function. Thirdly, direct measures focused on the rate of technical change have been developed, based on considering the rate of change in output relative to the rate of change of observed inputs use, and factor and output prices. Such measures are based on the calculation of index numbers, which reflect the rate of technological change over time. It is instructive to say a bit more about each within the context of health care and giving empirical examples of these three effects: we do so below.

Technological change and isoquant analysis: relative price responses

To the extent that health care inputs can be defined in bundles, for example, different drugs bundled to form the input 'medical management' and different procedures bundled as 'surgery', the introduction of new technology can be considered through examination of the change in relative input prices induced by the technology changing the nature of the bundles. This is possible through examination of isoquants and the alteration of the production function induced by relative price changes. The influence of any new technology is limited through aggregation and examined through aggregate relative price effects. It may, however, help to explain the mechanism through which a new health care technology with lower unit costs can result in higher total health care expenditure. Consider Figure 1.1, which represents the normal textbook example of initial cost equilibrium and a resulting equilibrium after the unit cost of surgery has fallen as a result of a new technology being added to the surgery bundle.

The unit cost of surgery falls so there is a substitution effect (movement $x_1 - s$) and output effect as there is a re-alignment of the production process as the relative prices of inputs have changed with the same expenditure further output can be gained (movement 1–2), and a profit/surplus effect, as with the change in input prices the marginal cost condition, which determines the profit/surplus maximizing point has changed (movement 2–3). Note that this final movement has resulted in increased expenditure by a further parallel movement in the isocost curve after the substitution and output effect have been accounted for. The first two effects are standard (and analogous to the substitution and income effects witnessed with indifference curve responses to relative output price changes). The third, profits/surplus effect, is less straightforward and is dependent on the production response to the change in input utilization. The change in the input utilization itself depends on the impact that the change in relative input price and usage has on the marginal cost of production, as it is the interaction between marginal cost and marginal revenue, which determines profit/surplus maximizing output. The impact of relative input price changes on marginal cost itself depends on the underlying production function. The overall impact can be ascertained by considering the effect of a change in output (y) on the derived demand for a factor input (x_i) assuming the cost function is continuous. Applying Shepherd's lemma and recognizing that cross-partial derivatives are independent of the order of differentiation, we have:

$$\frac{\delta x_i(w,y)}{\delta y} = \frac{\delta^2 c(w,y)}{\delta w_i \delta y} = \frac{\delta^2 c(w,y)}{\delta y \delta w_i} = \frac{\delta[\delta c(w,y)/\delta y]}{\delta w_i}$$

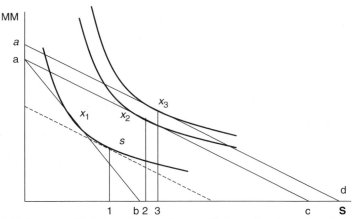

Fig. 1.1 Initial cost equilibrium and a resulting equilibrium after the unit cost of surgery has fallen as a result of a new technology being added to the surgery bundle.

where w is input price and c is total cost. This shows that the change in marginal cost caused by a change in input price (w_i) equals the response of the ith input to changes in output with input prices held constant, and can be positive or negative. If the sign is negative the ith input is said to be regressive (or inferior), if it is positive the ith input is said to be normal. In fact, if all inputs are normal marginal cost must increase with input prices (w_i), which will always be the case if the production function is homothetic.

In Figure 1.2 we have the same scenario as in Figure 1.1, but the production function is shaped such that the relatively inexpensive input, surgery in this case, is 'inferior' and the use of this input falls as output increases. A corollary is easily seen where one might consider the price of an input rising, think of the relative cost of medicines increasing, and yet more of this expensive input is used given the form of the production process. The same mechanism may therefore be applied to a rise in relative prices for one of the inputs. Note, therefore, that it is possible, dependent on the form of the production function, and on whether the input is normal or inferior, for a budget expansion to be rational even if the price of an input rises. If marginal costs decrease there may be a rational budget expansion, even following a rise in the price of input depending on the underlying production function. Folland *et al.* (2003) use similar analysis, but rely on output quality changes to show how technological change may increase expenditure even if, by inference, the unit cost of the new technology is lower than the old.

Culter and Huckman (2003) in a seminal work consider the empirical impact of the substitution effect induced by relative price changes across two types of surgery, coronary bypass surgery (CABG) and percutaneous transluminal coronary angioplasty (PTCA) , where the latter leads to a fall in the input price of treatment. In this way,

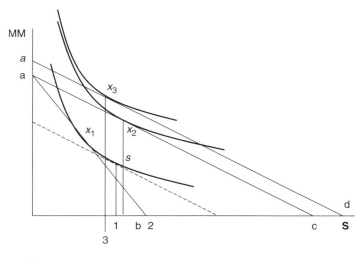

Fig. 1.2 Equilibrium when the new technology increases marginal cost

their analysis is an empirical extension of the analytics outlined above. They estimate the following relatively straightforward empirical specification:

$$\left(\frac{CABG}{Pop}\right)_{it} = \alpha_i + \delta_t + \beta_1\left(\frac{PTCA}{Pop}\right)_{it} + \beta_T\left(\left(\frac{PTCA}{Pop}\right)_{it} xYEAR_{it}\right) + \gamma X_{it} + \varepsilon_i$$

where the dependent variable, the CABG rate per 1000 population aged 45 and over, is regressed against county fixed effects (α_1), year fixed effects, (δ_τ) the PTCA rate per 1000 population aged 45 and over, an interaction term of the PTCA rate per 1000 population aged 45 and over, with $YEAR_{it}$, a vector of indicators of 3-year periods, and a vector of demographic controls (X_{it}), including the percentage of a counties population that falls into each of three age categories: under 45, 45–64, and over 65, and the rate of total hospital discharges per 100,000 population to control for shifts in overall hospitalization rate. They also include the different form of payment mechanism (Medicare, Medicaid and HMO) as a co-founder.

The coefficients of interest are represented by β_1 and the vector β_T. The sign on these coefficients reflects whether PTCA acts as a substitute (negative sign) or complement (positive sign). By using time-varying coefficients β_T the degree of substitution between these procedures is allowed to change as PTCA matures. This specification is run in levels and, through differencing the variables CABG, PTCA, and total discharges only, is considered with respect to trends in the growth rate. The latter is referred to by Cutler and Huckman as a 'changes' specification. To be precise the levels equation considers the impact of the new technology (PTCA) on the old (CABG) through the coefficient β_1,while the trend is captured in the levels specification by the coefficient vector β_T, which incorporates the time-varying component. The 'changes' specification, therefore, picks up the trend in the rates of change over time. At this point Cutler and Huckman note that unobservable factors correlated with both CABG and PTCA may bias the coefficient vector β_T, but argue that on the basis of the bias being constant over time the coefficient estimated in the 'changes' specification will purge this bias. Their results suggest that over time PTCA substitutes for CABG in around 25–35 per cent of incremental surgery. They argue that, while substitution is extensive there is also a patient expansion effect that dominates the substitution effect and accounts for around 65–75 per cent of incremental PTCA, which may be thought of as a combination of both the output and profit/surplus maximizing effect noted above. That is, the patient expansion effect may be thought of as more output being achievable with the same budget being applied, but additionally and importantly, as it leads to budget expansion, the surplus maximizing level of output is able to increase (assuming the surgical input is normal) as the marginal cost of production falls, and an increase in output and expenditure becomes rational.

A number of criticisms may be levelled at this work. First, there is concern that the bias may not be constant over time, particularly if medical management forms part of the omitted variable problem, as it does in the Cutler and Huckman work. Secondly, sequential endogeniety is clearly operating with past levels of CABG clearly affecting future levels of PTCA (or vice versa). Finally, the lack of control for stationarity in their analysis of time series data may be questioned. That said, follow-up work by

McGuire *et al.* (forthcoming), which corrected for these methodological issues in a similar analysis of technological change associated with the replacement of CABG by PTCA in UK hospitals found supporting evidence that a similar mechanism of substitution dominated by patient population expansion was at work and that the quantifiable level of substitution was around 30 per cent. Again, the conclusion is that the vast majority of the lower unit cost technology, PTCA, is introduced to expand the surgical patient population causing health care expenditure growth.

Technological change identified through a time variable

Of course, as noted above the previous analytical representation of the impact of technological change is somewhat limited as it aggregates the new technology into the existing production function through changes in aggregate input bundles. Given that the specific comparison is across two forms of surgical intervention, this is less of a limitation in this particular case, although similar unit costs for each procedure and expected outcomes are assumed to apply to all forms of PTCA and CABG undertaken in the reviewed studies. A different manner of representing technological change is through a *shift* in the production function as identified through the influence of time (t). This may be represented in the following manner, assuming that output is a function of inputs and time $[y = f(x,t)]$; technological change is then measured by how output changes as time elapses with the input bundle held constant. In other words, the rate of technological change is defined, assuming this function is continuous, as $T(x,t) = [\delta \ln f(x,t)]/\delta t$. As the concept of technological change associated with this approach is not embodied in any specific input bundle, it is referred to as a disembodied technological change. The assumptions underlying this approach are, however, not innocuous as noted above in the discussion of embodied and disembodied technological change. The approach assumes disembodied technological change and that the production function does not require new inputs, although changes in the shape and position of the isoquant may, of course, be incorporated econometrically in the definition of confounding variables, assuming that the production functions holds the same basic form over time.

This is the methodological approach adopted by the Technological Change in Health Care (TECH) research network, which considered the advance of new technology, (CABG, PTCA, and catheterization) aimed at treating acute myocardial infarction across 17 countries (TECH 2001). The econometric specification of the TECH investigation was based on individual patient level data and considered the rates of uptake of different procedures through a time variable when considering the different specific technologies. The results of this approach were reported in a qualitative fashion, but as based on the coefficient of the time trend variable from a regression analysis allowing for confounders. The analysis uses the estimates to classify the various countries into a combination of early or late take-up, and high or low diffusion patterns, relying on descriptive analysis and inference to show that there was considerable variation in the use of new technology in this area of health care across these countries. It ought to be noted that the econometric specification upon which this analysis was founded is neutral with respect to other inputs in the production function; that is there was no consideration of the role of medical or other staffing inputs, or with regards to the interaction with medical inputs. As such, the specification is heuristic with an assumption that technological change does not require new inputs and that the production function maintains the same basic form as time elapses. Notwithstanding these limitations the study shows that there are wide variations in the uptake and diffusion of new surgical procedures across countries, although three patterns of diffusion were characterized; in the study, the USA, Japan, and possibly France, exhibited fast uptake with quick diffusion; Australia, Canada, Italy, Singapore and Taiwan (and France for some procedures) exhibited intermediate uptake and diffusion patterns; most of the Scandinavian countries and the UK showed patterns of late uptake and slow diffusion. Interestingly, and noting that there was less evidence proffered, there was little systematic difference in the uptake and diffusion of low-cost pharmaceuticals across countries, although high-cost drugs exhibited similar patterns to those found with the intensive procedures.

Technological change and index movements

Finally, a third, direct approach aimed at estimating the rate of technical change could be based on the calculation of indices. Here, the measurement follows through an assumption that input utilization changes through time. Again, a general statement of the approach can be based on the functional relationship between output, input and time $[y = f(x,t)]$. Total differentiation with respect to time gives:

$$\frac{\partial y}{\partial t} = \sum_i \frac{\partial f}{\partial x_i} \frac{dx_i}{dt} + \frac{\partial f}{\partial t},$$

which on dividing through by y gives:

$$\frac{d \ln y}{dt} = \sum_i \varepsilon_i \frac{d \ln x_i}{dt} + T(x,t),$$

where ε_i are the output elasticity. Assuming profit/surplus maximization the output elasticity equal the input shares in total revenue, we have:

$$\frac{d \ln y}{dt} = \sum_i \frac{w_i x_i}{py} \frac{d \ln x_i}{dt} + T(x,t),$$

which on re-arrangement gives:

$$T(x,t) = \frac{d \ln y}{dt} - \sum_i \frac{w_i x_i}{py} \frac{d \ln x_i}{dt}.$$

In other words, $T(x,t)$ can be measured by subtracting from the rate of change output over time the change in a weighted sum of input utilization rates of change. The second term in this expression is the Divisia input index. Use of observed data over different time periods gives rise to an approximation such as:

$$T(x,t) = \ln y_t - \ln y_{t-1} - \sum_i \frac{1}{2} [v_{it} + v_{i,t-1}][\ln x_{it} - \ln x_{i,t-1}],$$

where y_t is output at time t, x_{it} is input i utilized at time t and v_{it} is the ratio of the cost of input I at time t to revenue at time t. The third term in this expression is the Tornqvist approximation to the Divisia index.

This general approach has been used to a great extent recently to consider technical progress as distinct from technical change. The definitional difference being that technical progress can be taken to define the relative effectiveness of different factor input bundles, while technological change defines the impact on the production function of a change in underlying technology. A number of studies have attempted to measure the impact of technical progress as it impacts on specific diseases through creating price indices for treatments, which account for the changing nature of these treatments over time. Thus, Skitovsky (1985) collected itemized cost (charge) data on a range of diseases to calculate and compare the average treatment costs for these diseases over time, finding that treatment costs had risen in some areas and declined in others. However, a general criticism of this work was that the treatment outcomes delivered had also varied and a number of studies have since reconsidered disease-specific treatment costs, while attempting to control for changes in outcome. Cutler *et al.* (1999), Cutler and McClellan (2001), and Frank *et al.* (2004) have all considered the productivity of disease specific treatments by comparing treatment costs relative to outcomes, either through analysing changes in costs and outcomes in specific population cohorts over time, or by considering the changes in treatment effectiveness over time and comparing with cost changes through analysis of administration data bases. Generally, and regardless of the methodology adopted or treatment considered, these studies have highlighted that technological change in health care has improved treatment outcomes by a degree that more than justifies the cost increases associated with the introduction of the improved technology. To date, however, attention has not focused on the rate of change of technical progress over time, although this would be a relatively straightforward extension of such work.

Health care technology and diffusion

Against this conceptual background, it is worthwhile investigating the relatively sparse related literature that relates to the explicit investigation of the mechanisms through which health care technology diffuses. The introduction of new technology clearly takes time to reach peak demand and there is a small, recent literature that explicitly considers the mechanics of this diffusion process. Later chapters consider the diffusion of particular technologies, especially medicines at a particular level of aggregation; therefore, consideration is confined here to general enquiry.

In fact, there is little theoretical or empirical analysis of diffusion to date. Escarce (1996) is an early example of an empirical testing of the role of informational externalities, essentially the role of information communicated to other physicians by early adopters of a new health care technology. Using a logistic curve to characterize observed adoption as a means of representing diffusion, as first suggested by Griliches (1957), Escarce considers the diffusion of laparoscopic cholecystecomy in the USA to examine differences in physician characteristics with respect to adoption. While finding a logistic curve fits the data relatively well, he does not find payment structure, as defined by managed care and fee-for-service, to have an influence on uptake.

This contrasts with the findings that follow from the work on the uptake of technology in the area of coronary heart disease by the TECH group referred to in 'Technological change identified through a time variable' in a further analysis that considered the role of country-specific regulation on the diffusion of CABG, PTCA, and catheterization across 16 countries (Beck *et al.* forthcoming). Using regression analysis the impact of different type of health care delivery system, regulatory structure, and payment structure were analysed. Health systems characterized as public contract and classified as reimbursement systems tended to have:

♦ higher adoption rates than public integrated systems;

♦ the central funding of investment was negatively correlated with adoption;

♦ GDP per capita was seen to have a strong role in initial adoption, but the effect of income levels weakened over time as did the impact of institutional characteristics.

Conclusions

It can be concluded that there is much to be done on the conceptual and empirical role of health care technology as a means of explaining health expenditure increases. Note that the basic conceptual approaches taken to defend the hypothesis that technological change does determine health expenditure increases and to quantify the degree of technological change taking place over time, either within a given health care system or a range of systems, remain somewhat naïve. The main methodological approach adopted to support the expenditure driver hypothesis is based on an examination of a residual after attempting to control for other influences on expenditure growth. Whilst this does present calculable estimates of the role that 'technological change' plays, it provides no explanation on the mechanism(s) through which technology influences expenditure.

On this latter point, there have been very few attempts to quantify the impact of technological change on expenditure or to make explicit the mechanism(s) through which technological change occurs. As shown through the examples discussed, the literature is dominated by either examination of isoquants or defining disembodied technical change through discrete terms, using either time variables or indices. Neither approach is perfect, nor are both used only as a means of making econometric or quantitative estimation tractable. The specification of input levels over time, as in the Cutler and Huckman analysis, leads to examination of changes in factor proportions through which the isoquant can be estimated. This time series approach requires specification of functional form and is also only useful in the *ex post* analysis of technical change, i.e. once it has been incorporated into the production process for some time. The second, more direct approach is incapable of yielding information on the isoquant and only offers measurement through approximation if examination is based on time trend movements. A fruitful extension of the direct measurement approach would be the construction of indexes of technical change. Again, such indexes would require assumption, being most easily constructed under assumptions of constant returns to scale and factor neutrality. While this would be a straightforward extension of the explosion of work undertaken on productivity indices for specific diseases that has been undertaken recently, there is not a single example of such specific analysis in the literature to date.

References

Australian Productivity Commission (2005). *Impacts of advances in medical technology in Australia*. Research Report. Melbourne, Productivity Commission.

Bech M, Christiansen T, Dunham K, Lauridsen J, Lyttkens CH, McDonald K, McGuire A and the TECH Investigators (forthcoming 2009). The influence of economic incentives and regulatory factors on the adoption of treatment technologies: A case study of technologies used to treat heart attacks. *Health Economics,* Published Online: Oct 28 2008.

Cutler DM and Huckman RS (2003). Technological development and medical productivity: The diffusion of angioplasty in New York state. *Journal of Health Economics*, **22,** 187–217.

Cutler DM and McClellan M (2001). Is technological change in medicine worth it? *Health Affairs*, **20,** 11–29.

Cutler DM, McClellan M and Newhouse JP (1999). The costs and benefits of intensive treatment for cardiovascular disease. In: J E Triplett, ed. *Measuring the prices of medical treatments.*Washington, DC, Brookings Institution Press.

Folland S, Goodman AC and Stano M (2003). *The economics of health and health care*. Harlow, Prentice Hall.

Gerdtham U-G and Jönsson B (2000). International comparisons of health expenditure: theory, data and econometric analysis. In: AJ Culyer and JP Newhouse, eds. *Handbook of health economics*. Amsterdam, Elsevier.

Griliches Z (1957). Hybrid corn: An exploration in the economics of technological change. *Econometrica*, **25,** 501–22.

McGuire A, Raikou M and Windmeier F (2009). Technology diffusion and health care productivity: Angioplasty in the UK. LSE Discussion Paper.

Miraldo M (2007) *Hospital Financing and the Development and Adoption of New Technologies*, working papers 026cherp. York, Centre for Health Economics, University of York.

Newhouse JP (1992). Medical care costs: How much welfare loss? *Journal of Economic Perspectives*, **6,** 3–21.

Okunade AA and Murthy VNR (2002). Technology as a 'major driver' of health care costs: a cointegration analysis of the Newhouse conjecture. *Journal of Health Economics*, **21,** 147–59.

Pita Barros P (1998). The black box of health care expenditure growth determinants. *Health Economics*, **7,** 533–44.

Seshamani M, Gray AM (2004). A longitudinal study of the effects of age and time to death on hospital costs. *Journal of Health Economics*, **23,** 217–35.

Skitovsky A (1985). Changes in the cost of treatment of selected illnesses. *Medical Care*, **23,** 1345–57.

TECH (2001). Technological change around the world: evidence from heart attack care. *Health Affairs*, **20,** 25–42.

Weisbrod BA (1991). The health care quadrilemma: An essay on technological change, insurance, quality of care, and cost containment. *Journal of Economic Literature*, **29,** 523–52.

Zweifel P, Felder S and Meiers M (1999) Ageing of population and health care expenditure: A red herring. *Health Economics*, **8,** 485–96.

Part 2

Innovation, diffusion, and technology change

Chapter 2

The process of health care innovation: problem sequences, systems, and symbiosis

Davide Consoli, Andrew McMeekin, J. Stan Metcalfe, Andrea Mina, and Ronnie Ramlogan

Introduction

> Nothing better describes the modern medical environment than the vision of the struggle for survival conjured up by Darwin's *Origin of Species* (1859): a competitive arena in which adaptation produces niches in which some flourish, develop, innovate or adapt while other thinkers and practices fall by the wayside; nothing is pre-ordained in terms of fulfilment of some overriding transcendental scheme.
>
> (Porter 1997, p 527)

Just as it is commonplace among economists to link long-term increases in material standards of living with innovation and the growth of new knowledge, so it is the case that medical practice has been transformed to yield major improvements in the treatment of human diseases and pathologies, and this rate of improvement appears to have accelerated in the past 40 or so years. We shall explore this theme by drawing on the idea that the generation and delivery of new medical practices is dependent on the creation of sophisticated innovation systems that transcend public and private spheres of activity. As the epigraph indicates, we follow an evolutionary perspective on this problem in the sense that the development of medical practice is a variation cum selection process, generating alternative solutions to treat medical conditions and selecting across those alternative rival methods.

There are many ways to approach the study of innovation, but the general line we pursue here is that innovations in medical practice are solutions to perceived problems in patient care, but that not all problems have solutions within the prevailing state of knowledge, while those that generate workable solutions are often of very differing efficacy. The reasons as to why progress is so uneven merit close study and are, in part, tied to the unevenness in the growth of our scientific understanding of disease but not in all cases (Nelson 2005). So the interesting question is why the development of medical practice is so uneven within areas of disease and over time, and how this relates to unevenness in the underlying conditions of innovation across countries.

The consequence of following this view is that we direct attention away from single innovations and instead focus upon the sequences of innovation that are associated with particular medical problem sequences. Thus, the most important kinds of innovation are associated with the creation of a new design space within which problems can be defined and solutions sought. Trajectories of innovations are created within this design space as practice, and are used to identify new problems and stimulate the search for desirable forms of improvements.

Before turning to these issues, it is worth highlighting that health innovation triggers a paradox for the extant systems and their management, for their financing and organization, and for the search for solutions to issues connected with human well-being. This paradox is essentially a matter of the stability and order required to efficiently deliver current medical services in contrast with the disruptive effects that innovation necessarily places on that order. Accordingly, several dimensions contribute to this paradox.

Of highest significance is the fact that the concept of innovation in medicine covers an immense range of possibilities, and that the diversity so engendered is a serious barrier to analysis and understanding. At the most general level, the overall design of health care systems continues to be debated, with controversy over issues such as different models of finance, and the relative roles of insurance- and tax-based systems, degrees of central control of resource allocation and the merits of market and planning approaches. However, these are not our concern, despite their importance not only to health care delivery, but to the health innovation process itself.[1] Rather, our focus is upon the rather precise innovations in relation to the treatment of specific conditions normally associated with new drugs, devices, and diagnostics. These are usually well defined and it is not difficult to trace the range of actors involved. Some of these innovations fit within existing modes of practice; in this sense they are incremental, but others can have more radical effects on the organization of systems of health care delivery and may even lead to new types of sub-specializations in medicine. As will be shown in subsequent sections, this concerns both innovations in the therapeutic domain, e.g. the intra-ocular lens (IOL), but also the diagnostic domain, e.g. the case of glaucoma. The position we take here is that it is the innovations in medical procedure are the foundation of long-term improvements in health care and that, while organizational innovations can be very important, the impact of organization is most severely felt on the environment within which basic medical innovations can occur.

Further complications arise from the fact that the sharp conceptual distinction made by Schumpeter between invention, innovation, and diffusion is not sustainable once we focus on the processes involved, for they are marked by multiple feedbacks and interdependencies. In the context of medical innovation, this implies that the alluring sequence of laboratory bench to patient bedside model is simply another,

---

[1] The evolution of managed care in the USA, the organization, governance and funding of tertiary and primary care in the UK are very complex examples of innovation in modes of service delivery that defy simple explanation.

flawed example of a linear innovation model that we – together with several eminent scholars – reject.

Two other aspects of the complexity of medical innovation processes need brief mention before we move to more substantive issues. The first is that it is characteristic of medical innovation processes that they engage with public and private sectors within medicine and health care. The delivery of medical service, the production of medical knowledge, and the generation of drugs, devices, and diagnostic equipment straddle the public and private divide and engage profit and non-profit organizations. The incentive systems and resource allocation processes that shape innovation differ sharply across this divide, and so the intertwining of the two spheres is an essential element in medical innovation and a source of much of the complexity that surrounds it. Following on this is the proposition that medical innovation is a systemic process, which is distributed across multiple actors and organizations to engage the recombination of very different kinds of knowledge over extended periods of time. Secondly, and related to the latter, it is particularly important to take account of the location of medical innovation process within modern capitalism, itself a complex evolving system, and the role of innovation-led competition – or creative destruction as Schumpeter called it – in this form of economic organization. The characteristics of medical innovation processes as we account for them, i.e. systemic, problem-led over extended periods of time, and driven by the growth of knowledge, provide also an important elucidation on the nature of the aforementioned paradox, namely that any innovation is a solution to problems and its emergence serves only to identify further problems.

However, the required systems are 'open' and this raises the paradox again, for open systems are quite unpredictable in terms of what they might create. The reality is that innovation is about the creative destruction of practice; it impinges upon the delivery of existing products and services, and is disruptive with respect to those products and services. Gains to the new are losses to the established way of managing and doing things – not only financial losses, but also losses in human capital and experience, and professional and social position.

There is a final dimension of the foregoing paradox, perhaps one that goes right to the heart of our main topic of interest. Usually, we imagine that innovations are efficiency and/or effectiveness enhancing, otherwise there is no incentive for rational decision makers to adopt them. In economic terms, for example, the canonical model of innovation is that the 'new' sustains a higher level of efficiency than the 'old', within the environment in which they are first introduced. However, the efficiency gain is quite compatible with an innovation accounting for an increased share of total economic expenditure, so there is no necessary paradox in the 'cost containment' controversy that advances in medical technology lead to demands for greater health care budgets. Our conjecture on the relation between medical innovation and medical expenditures is of interest for three reasons.

Firstly, the positive feedbacks that innovation generates. The story of the intra-ocular lens, which is presented later in this chapter, is a perfect case in point. As medical advances lead citizens to longer active lives, they also generate a range of maladies associated with ageing, which demand solutions and generate expectations on their availability.

Medical progress, together with improvements in clinical organization expands the market for medical technology so that – insofar as lives are extended – demand for treating diseases associated with ageing follows as a necessary consequence of success.

Secondly, many innovations are commonly associated with the idea of cost-savings, but in medicine, in particular, this productivity notion has to be adjusted for corresponding changes in the quality of outcomes over the whole intervention cycle from the patient presenting to final discharge. Innovations like the IOL, nowadays a common procedure in ophthalmic surgery, make available what was previously impossible, and so the private costs of pain and disability can now be born in the public sphere. The effects of such radically new procedures are improvements in efficiency (previously the cost of the procedure was infinitely high) together with increased areas of medical demand. Such impossibilities rendered actual, whether drugs, devices or diagnostics necessarily have the effect of expanding resource costs by generating a net increase in the number of medical services that are available even though costs per patient may have declined. Matters are rendered more complex by the labour intensive nature of medical delivery systems in general, including, as we should, the costs of training health care practitioners. The labour deemed necessary for the humane treatment of patients and that required to record and track medical information on patients renders medical services particularly suspect to cost increases. Despite efforts to rationalize the delivery of medical services, the record of productivity improvement is not impressive with the effect that the relative price of medical services tends to increase over time, even with a fixed basket of treatments.

Thirdly, the problematic aspects of this kind of successful innovation are very much weighed by the fact that the resources available to fund healthcare engage political processes rather than market processes alone. This is true of the European system whether tax or social insurance financed and of the USA system where, despite the greater reliance on private insurance, an aging population brings more citizens within the net of Medicare. Here, it is worth noting that differences in the proportion of GDP spent on health in advanced economies is largely due to differences in non-public funding.

In concluding this introduction, our aim is to bring together these threads, and point to the idea that the policy objective should be to foster and order the development of an open system of medical innovation, capable of sustaining and co-ordinating a rich and necessarily unpredictable set of innovation related experiments.

Medical innovation as a long-term learning process

No one will doubt the importance of innovation in improving the treatment of a wide range of diseases through the transformation of medical practice. Innovations have been fundamental drivers of change in healthcare delivery, in some cases eliminating diseases that were formally of high incidence (e.g. polio, measles) in others enabling treatments that have offered solutions to previously untreatable conditions – as in cardiology with the innovation of coronary bypass surgery (CABG) and percutaneous transluminal coronary angioplasty (PTCA). It is an impressive record, yet that record is very uneven, in the case of some cancers and glaucoma, for example, there has been very little progress. If medical innovations are the answer to particular problems, then the problems are very varied and very different in their resistance to a solution.

The innovation management and health policy literatures present several analyses of medical devices markets, and provide numerous opportunities for deepening our understanding of the micro-dynamics of invention, innovation, and diffusion of medical technologies. Although many important insights have been gained and a number of characteristics of the medical device sector have been profiled, we argue that relatively little effort has been put hitherto into disentangling the mechanisms through which progress in medicine takes place and the general properties of health innovation processes. A number of flaws emerge across different strands of research, namely the structure and dynamics of innovation in medicine are often assumed, instead of being analysed. They tend to be taken in isolation from the broader framework of socio-economic systems, or are rather narrowly defined as the process of discovery of new drugs and devices. Put succinctly, the way medical innovation processes are portrayed in the literature often appears to be disconnected from a careful assessment of the systemic processes through which health services enabled by new technologies are delivered (Consoli and Mina 2007). Apart from a few notable exceptions, scholars of innovation, who are arguably best equipped to capture the *systemic* and *dynamic* aspects of health innovation processes, seem to have and left the debate to health economists, health policy and health management scholars. One of the purposes of this essay is to address such a gap and to explore new avenues.

Innovation processes are typically non-linear and progress relies on mechanisms of feedback between research, development, and practice. The main reason why feedback from clinical practice is so important is the radical uncertainty associated with new treatment options (Geljins and Rosenberg 1994). Whether these enable the achievement of new goals or provide more efficient tools to solve known problems, the reaction of the body, like in all complex systems, cannot be predicted in any reliable way (Geljins *et al.* 1998). As a consequence, advancement in the treatment of diseases has much in common with trial-and-error learning typical of engineering-based innovation processes where incremental improvements and eventual drawbacks are discovered only through actual use of the new techniques (Constant 1980; Vincenti 1991).

Feedback from practice also means that the involvement of users (von Hippel 1976, 1988) has been identified as a fairly robust regularity of innovation in medical devices. Expert users are not simply sources of information, since they know the medical need to be satisfied; they know the need and at the same time articulate plausible ways to satisfy it. In this sense, they are genuine sources of invention and capable of generating innovation when they possess entrepreneurial motivation and skills that are necessary to turn new ideas into business (Roberts 1989). The literature is rich in anecdotal, as well as more systematic examples of this.[2]

---

[2] Among others, Roberts and Hauptman (1985) provided evidence from a dataset of biomedical firms located in the US State of Massachusetts, de Vet and Scott (1992) from Californian suppliers

Both the reliance of manufacturers on users and the latter's activities across academic and commercial domains also suggest that innovation in medical devices originates rather systematically at the interface of different institutional settings (Blume 1992) and involves above all, university departments, academic medical centres, general hospitals, firms, and regulators. It is across their boundaries that scientific and technological learning occurs, and technology transfers take place. The main avenues for technology transfer are extensively discussed in Campbell *et al.* (2004), who – net of communication flows between innovators and regulators – broadly identify three main paths: (i) general dissemination of knowledge; (ii) university–industry relationships and (iii) commercialization activities. The first encompass education and training for practitioners, the organization of dedicated conferences and meetings, and publication activities. The second include university profits from contracts, consulting fees, and other research support generated by trading research expertise. The third accounts for the activities of university technology transfer offices and university patenting.[3]

With respect to all three types of technology transfer processes, research hospitals and, more generally, research foundations/institutes where clinical services are also delivered are especially important institutions. On the one hand, they tend to be teaching institutions and to form integral parts of academic institutions. In this sense, they are the prime mechanisms for the intergenerational diffusion of knowledge, whose tacit components are often predominant in the field of medicine. On the other hand, research hospitals provide the organizational links between basic science, mostly produced in universities, with experimental phases of research where firms are involved as partners in the development of prototypes (be they drugs or devices) or as suppliers of products that must be tested in clinical trials in order to receive market approval. In this case, firms often act as sponsors for the trials. These are expected to provide unbiased evidence of the safety and comparative advantage of the innovations on which the decision of the regulators to approve their introduction in the market place will depend.

Another important – and often neglected – aspect of the nature of the innovative process in medicine is the role of diffusion not only its own right as the process through which new treatments reach an increasing number of patients, but also as the context in which such innovations are modified, adapted, improved, and better understood. Gelijns *et al.* (1998) argue that 'innovation is a learning process that takes place over time, and a fundamental aspect of learning is the reduction of uncertainty' (p. 694). Uncertainty, they argue, results from the complexity of the human system, which poses severe limits to the possibility of predicting the effects of new procedures.

---

of medical devices, Shaw (1986) from a sample of UK firms and Biemans from a subset of Dwutch medical device companies (1991).

[3] As is widely discussed in the literature, although there is still disagreement on the long-term risks versus benefits of these decisions, investments by universities in applied research aimed to patenting has increased dramatically after the implementation of the Bayh-Dole act in the US or of Bay-Dole types of policy intervention in other countries. With respect to this issue in the specific field of medical innovation, see Gelijns and Rosenberg (1999) and Zinner (2001).

The typically narrow target of clinical trials, and the heterogeneity of the patients recruited to test new drugs and new devices in early phases of development add to the difficulty of finding in the short run unexpected benefits associated with new treatments. As a consequence, the experience gathered in clinical practice and the resulting post-innovation improvements of experimental techniques can hardly be overstated.[4]

Furthermore, communities of practice (Brown and Duguid 1991) are important loci for the development of new knowledge, and it is often at this level that new problems emanate and are identified. It is through the performance of clinical practice that particular 'glitches' and potential solutions become apparent. These cannot be independent of the organizational and institutional bases of relevant networks of individuals. As a consequence, scientific and technological knowledge co-evolve with the social networks in which the process is embedded. Not only, in fact, is knowledge distributed within communities, but also distributed across communities linked through a variety of formal and informal mechanisms of exchange. The advancement of medical knowledge relies of continuous feedbacks between science and technology, and the nature and intensity of interaction across communities at different points in time are of great importance to the emergence, growth, and transformation of medical micro-innovation systems.

In seeking to understand these innovation processes more fully, it may help to distinguish, in traditional fashion, four important general influences on the rate and direction of innovation, namely: the opportunities to innovate, the resources necessary to innovate, the distribution of incentives to innovate and, indeed, to resist innovation, and, finally, the capabilities to innovate. As to opportunities these are closely tied to the specific medical problems and the background understandings in terms of science and technology as to what is possible, recognizing that opportunities in one area may be the unintended consequences of improvements in unrelated areas. The knowledge base on which medical innovation opportunities depend is very broad. Advances in genetics and the fundamental knowledge of cell processes represent one end of a spectrum in which medical interventions are shaped by basic scientific knowledge, while at the other extreme are almost pure examples of procedures that constitute medical engineering of human body processes, of which the artificial hip and the intra-ocular lens are pre-eminent examples. In many of these cases, theory is not available to predict the effects of the procedure, the test is a simple one of practical efficacy, and so there is a close correlation between practice and the growth of knowledge about the procedure. Resources are, of course, a key issue, not simply to develop the possible invention, but to turn it into practice, which may require capital investment in devices, and will almost certainly require investments in training clinicians

---

[4] Also, as Gelijns and Rosenberg (1994) recall, innovations may not come from biomedical research in the first place, but from other fields (i.e. ultrasound, laser, magnetic resonance) and the development of medical devices is especially dependent on a number of technological competences that are not core to medical sciences (i.e. optical engineering) and nevertheless cannot be understood if not in association with i) the surgical practice in which they are utilized and ii) the broader contest of their approval, marketing and distribution.

and other staff in a new procedure. Incentives too are complex, and range from the profits anticipated by medical supply companies to the professional status sought by scientists and clinicians. Capabilities to manage the process of innovation are also complex to unravel. A useful distinction is between those that engage with the internal processes of an innovating organization and those that relate to its ability to create an external organization to draw on the support of other actors in the innovation process. Both dimensions of management matter as does the ability to integrate internal and external dimensions of the innovation process (Henderson 1994). Innovations may succeed or fail in relation to issues arising in any one or more of these dimensions. Each of these elements is an important aspect of the innovation process with different degrees of malleability in terms of policy to influence innovation. Thus, the standard policy of providing tax breaks for company R&D or innovation subsidies to particular projects are policy tools that influence resources and incentives at the R&D margin, but have little or no direct effect on innovation opportunities or capabilities to manage the innovation process.

However, this four-fold schema does not capture in our view the most important issues, which fall instead into three groups: (i) in relation to the evolution of problem sequences; (ii) in relation to the systemic aspects of the innovation process; and (iii) in relation to the positive feedback between diffusion-based experience and the development of an innovation.

Problem sequences

The starting point here is the perception that an innovation is a proposed solution to a problem, a problem in relation to the production of some particular good or service. An entrepreneurial conjecture has been created that the particular way of solving a medical problem can be achieved differently. An entrepreneurial conjecture is thus a statement of disagreement about current practice, a view that a medical activity can be conducted in new ways. To articulate that conjecture is to change knowledge and understanding, so the essence of enterprise and the entrepreneurial function is to de-correlate the understanding that guides existing practice. It is because innovation challenges the current state of understanding that there is a close connection between innovation and the development of knowledge.

Let us begin by restating the notion that innovations are rarely, if ever, uniquely circumscribed events and outcomes. They are better seen as trajectories of improvement *sequences* in which procedures are progressively refined and extended in their scope of application. Furthermore, by extending the range of application and improving practice, solutions to medical problems challenge the boundaries of scientific understanding and thus contribute to reshape them. Our conjecture is that such a process consists in the exploration of an *emergent design space*, unfolding in a largely path-dependent fashion within bounds set by the changing perceptions of the problem (Metcalfe *et al.* 2005).

Accordingly, the accumulation of medical knowledge occurs along *trajectories of change* that emerge over time in the search for better and better solutions to clinical problems (Metcalfe *et al.* 2005; Mina *et al.* 2007; Consoli and Ramlogan 2008). Such trajectories emerge in the form of sequences of innovative ideas, reflect coherent directions of change, and signal the cumulativeness of research activities whose results build on previous knowledge. These involve specific configurations (for example, technical designs) embodying ways of combining knowledge which become formal and informal standards (Utterback 1994) in the search for solutions to problems. Moreover, the associated devices, diagnostics, and drugs are only the signatures of knowledge and practice, and as one innovation problem is solved so others range into view and form new foci for innovative effort within the broad objective to improve the efficacy of the overarching procedure. All innovation is an exploration of the unknown; it is a discovery process that is neither random nor completely canalized. Progress means finding new problems and the solutions to these problems may lie in different domains of knowledge and communities of practice. The emergence of trajectories (Dosi 1988) also implies that evolution of knowledge is not random. At the same time the direction of progress can very rarely be seen *ex ante*, which means that there can be little determinism in the process through which trajectories of change take form. Research paradigms thus understood emerge through complex processes and out of the highly distributed activities of practitioners who carry different experiences and competences and, at the same time, fuel different visions.

Moreover, the power of theoretical understanding in relation to medical problems is often severely circumscribed, and limits on deductive analysis mean that practice and experience play a major role in shaping the growth of knowledge in many medical fields. Medicine is not alone in this, but much of its practice is more akin to art than science, much of what is achieved is effectively engineering on life processes. The idea of problem sequence then maps into innovation sequences. An initial innovation opens up the conception of a new design space that is exploited by a series or trajectory of innovation at times competitive at times complementary. Each innovation is a shift in the problem sequence a growth of knowledge. Innovation sequences can halt, the problems being beyond knowledge and imagination, awaiting some breakthrough perhaps in a quite unrelated body of knowledge to restore momentum to the innovation process. Thus, one can readily identify the importance of extra medical developments in knowledge, such as lasers and electronics, which bear significantly upon improved opportunities for diagnosis in several areas, glaucoma among them.

The second dimension of organization is of increasing importance the nature of the innovation system in which the problem sequence evolves.

The systemic approach

Innovation in medicine is systemic, that is to say it is a distributed process whereby problems are solved and created by the engagement of multiple actors within multiple organizations guided by multiple incentive systems. This perspective emphasizes the importance of the division of labour in providing the resources and capabilities to create and maintain a system to respond to emerging opportunities and constraints.

The notion of innovation systems initially emerged as a framework for understanding: (i) the distribution and co-ordination of innovation activities across multiple and heterogeneous actors; and, (ii) the importance of institutions in shaping innovation. Early studies focused on national systems (Freeman 1988; Lundvall 1988; Nelson 1988), emphasizing the country-specific institutions that might account for variations in innovation performance between nations. Later studies defined their system boundaries according to specific technologies (Carlsson 2002) or sectors (Malerba 2002). These approaches assume no geographical boundary to the system, but emphasize respectively, the role of institutions specific to either technology or sector. Each of the three approaches has its merits, but one of the features of unfolding innovation sequences is that their *scale* and *scope* can often be emergent properties (Coombs *et al* 2003). Over time, the organizational arrangements and institutional framing of an innovation sequence transect geographical boundaries and build bridges between different sectors and hitherto unconnected technological domains.

Much has been written about the concept of national innovation systems and certainly medicine is organized, financed, and regulated in different ways in different countries. These national domains are important, not least because they are the frame in which policy that impinges on medical innovation is organized. However, frequently this literature falls into two traps: it confuses innovation with invention, and it confuses the notions of innovation ecology and of innovation system.

What a systems perspective allows is a distinction to be made between 'medical innovation ecologies', the set of individuals usually working within organizations who are the repositories and generators of new knowledge, and the 'system making' connections between the components that ensure the flow of information whether in general or directed at a specific purpose. In relation to medicine the individuals include clinicians, scientists, and technologists, managers, and regulators working in organizations as diverse as hospitals, university and firm laboratories, medical bureaucracies and public bodies. Included in this ecology are those organizations that store and retrieve information, as well as those that manage the general flow of information in multiple formats. They exhibit collectively a division of labour that is characteristic of the production of knowledge and this is reflected, for example, within and between the universities, and public and private research activities that are major components in any modern knowledge ecology. Ecologies are typically national in scope, with subnational degrees of variation, which reflect rules of law and language, funding regimes, business practice, and the social and political regulation of business (Carlsson 1997; Carlsson *et al.* 2002; Cooke *et al.* 2002). However, and quite crucially, any innovation ecology is the basis for a system, but it is not a system of itself until subsets of the actors are connected with the intention of promoting innovation. Furthermore, the purpose of the connections is to combine multiple sources of knowledge and innovative capability through the flow of information. Thus, barriers to information flow, barriers to converting information flow into knowledge, lack of appropriate sources of the requisite information all fit under the umbrella of imperfectly connecting ecologies into systems.

The logic of this view is that innovation systems are constructed to solve 'local' innovation problems (Antonelli 2001, 2005) and that they are constructed around the medical problems that shape innovation not only the problems that shape the growth of science and technology. Moreover, since the solution of one problem typically leads to different and new problems we would expect that as the problems evolve so the actors in the system, and their pattern of interconnection must also evolve and while ecologies are more permanent the systems are more transient. Thus, there is a close connection between the notion of trajectories of technological solutions within a particular technological paradigm, the evolving problem sequence, and the dynamic notion of an innovation system (Dosi 1982).

Thereby actors are guided by different incentive systems – of profit and shareholder value, of the relief of suffering, of professional advancement, of medical ethics and regulatory norm, of administrative efficacy – and these different sets of incentives do not naturally guide the innovation problem in the same direction. The fact that innovation disrupts existing practice adds to the incentive incompatibilities for it adds uncertainty and, thus, non-computability to the administrative task, it diminishes the profitability of rival existing patterns of practice, and it may render obsolete human capital and long followed habits and procedures. Innovations are dangerous and so are innovators. Thus, for example, it is not difficult to find evidence of the open hostility of medical practitioners to innovations that challenge the status quo.

Regulation, of course, plays a major role in framing innovation system and shaping the outcomes of these innovation processes, whether of the national formal kind as with the FDA or NICE or more subtly through the professional norms that are applied to determine what is a solvable problem and what is an appropriate solution. At one level it protects the population of patients and reduces the problems of unanticipated consequence that have occasionally amounted to disasters for medicine; at another level it can give a procedure a credibility that reduces uncertainty about its effects so stabilizing the market for some device or drug. As a *quid pro quo* regulation imposes constraints on the exploration of the relevant design space, and necessarily extends the time for an innovation sequence to develop and be tested through experience. Even such a seemingly trivial step as taking a process from batch scale to commercial scale may lead to the denial of regulatory approval.[5]

Hence, while there are national, medical innovation ecologies of hospitals, universities, regulators, and firms, it is not at all obvious that these constitute a national medical innovation system in the sense usually meant. A system requires connections and the connections are typically formed for the purpose of solving problems. Depending upon the problems in hand, there will be multiple local innovation systems supported by the relevant ecology, reflecting the problem sequences in hand, the location of the actors at the leading edges of technological advance, particular links with the science base, and the specific uses towards which the intended innovations are directed. Moreover, it follows naturally that the connections and actors can, and increasingly do in medicine, spread across national boundaries. Medical science has always been international in its dissemination practices. Furthermore, it is commonplace to find medical supply firms collaborating with overseas suppliers or customers, to find them drawing on the skills of foreign universities or even setting up R&D facilities in overseas markets. Indeed, it leads to the idea that global competition for resources in the

---

5 The Wall St Journal (10/08/07), reports the difficulties faced by Genzyme Corp. which produces a drug for Pompe disease, a rare and sometimes fatal enzyme disorder. The company has been denied FDA approval for a scaled up plant to produce commercial quantities of the drug because it cannot to be proved that the plant produces the same drug as produced by the small scale, laboratory methods on which the case for initial approval was based.

formation of innovation systems is a central feature of the modern capitalist dynamic in which information is an international commodity.

The immediate consequence of this perspective is that local innovation systems are dynamic. The evolution of problems leads to the corresponding evolution of the innovation systems, as new problems draw upon new bodies of knowledge for their solution. If systems are formed around problems, and are then localized, very diverse in their nature and dynamic, they will involve necessarily different sets of actors to respond to the changes in the nature of the problem.

Diffusion and the growth of knowledge

The overarching proposition that emerges from the foregoing discussion is that the growth of knowledge and its application within changing design spaces fuel the dynamics of health innovation systems. Let us elaborate on this point. In the perspective presented here knowledge has two dominant features: it has a systemic structure, and it is provisional and open to challenge, that is to say, it is the outcome of a distributed dynamic process (Leijonhufvud 2000). Accordingly, the trajectory of innovation in any particular field of medicine depends on the construction of mechanisms for the co-ordination of complementary bodies of knowing, be they scientific research, the activity of communities of practitioners, the design of regulation, the delivery of patient care, or the market process (Metcalfe *et al* 2005; Mina *et al* 2007; Consoli and Ramlogan 2008). Under this perspective, problem-finding and problem-solving are open-ended and complementary processes in that the search for solutions is directed by the interpretative system through which problems have been defined (Loasby 1998).

In the context of experimental sciences like medicine, this implies that refutation stimulates new search, but also that the effectiveness of this is contingent on how much consensus can be gathered on the boundaries of the problem. As Loasby (2003) makes clear, consensus is best reached when the boundaries of the search space are narrowed to a manageable degree. Thus, scientific conjectures and empirical experiences tend to be organized and channelled through communities, or networks of knowledge. In a nutshell, knowledge growth is an uncertain process that depends on the organization of search efforts, and on the selection of appropriate degrees of openness and closure for the emerging system of understanding.

Allied to this is the idea that the reliance of medical knowledge upon clinical practice implies strong interdependencies between innovation and the diffusion of medical technologies. The reason is that the ramifications of innovative procedures are only fully realized over the long-term and through extensive information feed-back gathered in a systematic way from the dispersed adoption decisions of clinicians. It is through trial-and-error adoption processes that problems are identified and become the basis for readjustments in the focus of inventive effort, so that practice and the specifics of devices and drugs can be said to co-evolve. In fact, while it is essential to recognize that the characteristics of innovative technologies are important determinants of their diffusion patterns, it is equally important to emphasize that it is in the process of diffusion that technologies evolve as new insights are generated for further innovation. In other words, the framework that enables and constrains adoption decisions is fundamental not only as a set of conditions that determines who benefits from new treatments and to what extent, but also as a platform for further techno-logical advance. Hence, the evolution of medical technologies jointly depends on the activity of innovative suppliers and on that of those organizations – medical research centres and hospitals above all – where the associated new clinical services are delivered.[6]

These three dimensions of the medical innovation process, namely, extended prob-lem sequences, distributed innovation systems, and the interdependence between practice and the growth of knowledge can be illustrated through the results of two case studies of medical innovation. In one, the intra-ocular lens, innovation opened up a design space that has led to a sequence of successful innovations solving the problem of cataract. In the other, the diagnosis and treatment of glaucoma, the design space of problems has not generated a successful closure.

The intra-ocular lens

The innovation of the intra-ocular lens (IOL) has radically transformed the concep-tion, design and delivery of a major medical service, the removal of cataracts com-bined with their replacement by a functioning lens. The IOL is the solution to a pressing medical condition, age-related cataracts, which affect over half the popula-tion of people over 50 – the fastest growing population cohort in the OECD countries. Cataracts, the clouding of the eye's crystalline lens, are the most frequent cause of defective vision in later life. The restriction of the passage of light is progressive and results in blurred vision, colour distortion and glare disability in the presence of bright light. 'Couching' cataracts (pushing the clouded lens out of the line of sight) was a traditional operation practised in the 18th century by itinerant 'oculists', and eye sur-gery was one of the first fields of specialism as medicine took its modern form in the 19th century. Before WWII the standard surgical 'cure' was removal of the lens; a suc-cessful operation meant that light could now pass to the retina but without being focused as a clear image (the condition known as aphakia). The only corrective meth-od was to use 'pebble glasses', thick and unwieldy spectacle lenses that gave poor post-operative vision, magnifying and distorting images (Kaufman 1980). The risk of infection and of collateral operative damage meant that this was a procedure of the last resort for most patients. To describe this operation as an ordeal in which defective vision is replaced by defective vision seems entirely appropriate (Linebarger *et al.* 1999). Yet by the end of the 20th century the IOL had become the standard comple-ment to cataract surgery, which itself had become one of the most frequently per-formed outpatient operations in the advanced industrial world (Linebarger *et al.* 1999). A major survey of the histopathology of IOLs opines that, 'lens implantation is among the safest major procedures in modern surgery' (Apple *et al.* 1984).

---

[6] Also, hospital administrators, payers, insurers and regulators are increasingly influencing the rate and direction of medical innovation by explicitly identifying priority needs and re-defining modes of financing that incentivize the emergence and diffusion of cost-reducing technological solutions in the face of escalating health expenditures (Newhouse 1992).

The solution to this problem involved the creation of a new innovation design space as a result of the work of Harold Ridley, an eminent eye surgeon who worked at Moorfields hospital in London. Ridley's innovation, introduced in 1949 and based on his own inventive efforts, has brought great benefit to countless patients, and has greatly increased the efficiency and effectiveness with which the clinical procedure is carried out. It has been achieved by the creativity of many 'imitating' clinician inventors combined with the development of a trans-national medical–industrial complex that has changed radically the innovation system in this field of ophthalmic medicine. The particular invention and innovation systems have co-evolved with the changing innovation problem. A procedure originally based around pioneering 'hero-surgeons' deploying 'craft technique', has evolved into a 'routine, quasi factory' procedure capable of being effected in a local medical centre by clinician nursing staff and supplied with high quality lenses from competing companies. This is, indeed, a fundamental transformation of a service activity and its skill base has lead to new specialisms within the field of ophthalmology.

Of all the developments that have transformed Ridley's innovation and operative method into a mass procedure, by far the most important has been the adoption of phakoemulsification techniques for cataract extraction. The originator of this technology was Charles Kelman, a Professor of Clinical Ophthalmology in the USA (New York). He experimented for many years using the high frequency energy of a vibrating needle to fragment a cataract, which could then be sucked clear of the eye through a much smaller incision (2–3 mm) than that traditionally associated with the prevailing technique (c. 7 mm). Improvements followed quickly and the first crude machines were made available commercially in 1970, signalling the shift in the locus of leading edge of commercial cataract innovation to the USA.[7] Obviously, it is pointless to make a small incision with the phako technique to remove the cataract, if one has to make subsequently a larger incision to insert a conventional rigid or semi-rigid PMMA lens. So the new method opened up a new set of problems that stimulated the development of foldable lenses.

Most remarkably, phakoemulsification has led to cataract extraction becoming routine and has raised the prospect of cataracts being removed by trained nursing staff. The bottleneck represented by the delicate skill of the surgeon was to a degree replaced by standardized, mechanized, and replicable practice, and the economics of the procedure transformed as the operation became possible as an ambulatory procedure performed in a few hours.

Radical effects on the delivery of health services have followed from the introduction of IOLs. For the patient, an operation that formerly required months of incapacity is now recovered from in a matter of hours. For health services, there has been an enormous increase in capital and labour productivity associated with the increased patient throughput and the ambulatory nature of the modern procedures. Corresponding to these surface effects have been major changes in the education and training processes

---

[7] They were manufactured by a company called Cavitron Surgical Systems, long since disappeared from the record.

for nurses and clinicians. However, not all the methods proved to be successful initially, and in many cases lenses have had to be removed or, in extreme cases, eyesight has been lost. As with many medical procedures, the experimental costs are necessarily born by the patients. Cataract surgery is a branch of human engineering that is not based on a predictive science that covers the case of every patient as if they each present identical problems to be solved. Moreover, the risks of any procedure raise questions about the efficacy of regulatory procedures, whether by the community of practitioners or by the State.

As with any substantial innovation, it challenged established interests and perceptions of appropriate medical practice, and the nature of the professional hostility to this innovation is an intriguing aspect of the story and it is not entirely irrational. Ridley's IOL was a double innovation in terms of conception and surgical procedure. It was a radical alternative to established practise and it challenged an established viewpoint that cataract extraction was the best that could be achieved. As a new technique, it placed great demands on the skill of the surgeon and created major risks during and after the operation. This is not a distortion of the situation for it took another 30–40 years before all the design, manufacture, and surgical problems were solved. That, of itself, is a measure of how radical was Ridley's invention. Correspondingly, important complementary technologies that Ridley and his immediate supporters could turn to, in order to find solutions and counter the barrage of criticisms were not available, so adding to the uncertainty surrounding the innovation.

Cataract surgery is not a theoretically-grounded science, theory does not predict how an individual patient will respond to any method, so it is not entirely unreasonable that experience should dominate the world-view of its practitioners or that professional reaction is conservative. Another factor is important here. A medical innovator will know that his technique will involve risks for the immediate patient that may only become clear over an extended horizon. In putting the development of the technique above the interests of the immediate patient, the innovator is invoking an abstract notion of patient welfare in general. When the technique is established, others will benefit, but the moral dilemma is clear, the cost of progress for many may be born directly by individual patients. This is precisely the dilemma that the rules and norms of the profession are meant to deal with and these rules, as accumulated social capital sunk in the profession, will constrain and channel the acceptance of new methods to make life difficult for innovators. Equally, no account can properly ignore the many patients willing to endure the risks of a new and experimental treatment, and so benefit future generations.

Thus, we find the eminent Duke-Elder, in the 1959 edition of his authoritative 11-volume text, noting that the novelty and difficulty of the technique had led to few surgeons using it (Vol. 11, p. 289). There is no reason to doubt that this negative assessment was generally held within the ophthalmological community of the time. Indeed, by then, Ridley, fearful of legal action against his method, was close to abandoning the implantation of IOLs. What is significant is that Ridley's innovation did ultimately sweep the world. Yet in the mid-1960s it appeared to be a dead end, and it is doubtful if he or anyone else could foresee the steps that would transform the invention into a widely adopted innovation. How and why did this transformation take place? To answer this question we have to explain how the implantation of IOLs progressed from a local method practiced in multiple ways by different surgeons, to a virtually uniform, universally applied technique. Part of the answer is provided by the emergence of a community of IOL practitioners. This group of enthusiast surgeons formed the basis of a series of highly localized micro-innovation systems, introducing new variants on a trial-and-error basis, and communicating the outcomes in the professional literature, at conferences and in visits to their respective medical centres. Such communities are vital to the formation of standards and they form the institutional framework in which trial-and-error experimentation is translated into accepted norms of practice. Thus, an emerging community is an important part of the development mechanism and underpins a normal process through which individual knowledge comes to be more highly correlated and is built into a body of shared understanding.

Important though these aspects are, they are not what we want to emphasize. For Ridley and his immediate followers and imitators were 'hero-surgeons' working in clinical contexts, governed by the selection processes of instituted practices and resource allocation in publicly-funded health services in Europe. By the 1980s the locus of innovation and development had shifted to a medical–industrial complex dominated by five or six trans-national companies located in the USA. These companies, as a matter of policy, build very close working relations with the present generation of ophthalmic clinicians and fund a great deal of the R&D activity. What they have created in the search for competitive advantage is a new kind of innovation system. In so doing, they join together the processes of selection and development on which the growth of this particular activity depends. This takes us to an interesting perspective on the emergence and development of systems of innovation; namely, that innovation systems are not natural givens, they have to be constructed and they are constructed around specific innovation problems. In the process, the system and the problem co-evolve. At the national level there are sets of knowledge accumulating, storing and transmitting capabilities, in universities, hospitals, and research institutes. In medicine, these capabilities are connected by a range of informal and formal, national and international practitioner networks.

However, these constellations of capabilities do not constitute an innovation system; they are at best an invention system. To translate latent capabilities into an innovation system requires the activities of for profit firms, focused upon specific classes of innovation problem. Firms play the key role in constructing an innovation system, making the connections between different actors to focus attention on the solution to problems they define, and articulating and combining together the multiple bands of knowledge required for innovation. In its combinatorial role the firm is a unique organization within innovation systems. Thus, the development system for a particular class of problems is not there naturally, it is assembled within the competitive process and competition leads to connection, and connection to collaboration. It is not simply that the innovation processes are distributed across multiple agencies and actors, it is much more that they are embedded in different selection processes, market and non-market, and that the associated very specific innovation system constitutes the external organization of the firms. By virtue of this link with the competitive process we are dealing with rival innovation systems as fluid as the competitive processes that underpin them. Connections are made and broken as commercial advantage dictates. Such systems are certainly not monolithic, they are created, grow, stabilize, and decline, and they involve, as in the IOL case, a subtle and changing interaction between public capability and private action. However, that is the exactly the point, the link between competition and innovation is multi-faceted. Innovation creates diversity and diversity, in true evolutionary fashion, makes competition feasible.

The case of glaucoma

Glaucoma provides a quite different perspective on the nature of medical innovation in that the problem has not as yet proved amenable to a solution sequence, rather it has developed a series of innovations in diagnostic procedures and devices that are of considerable importance. Indeed, with each new diagnostic procedure the evidence that followed led to greater refinement of the problem and an awareness of the multiple dimensions of the condition.

Glaucoma is a chronic disease of the optic nerve which, if untreated, eventually causes blindness.[8] Global prevalence of the disease is estimated at 50–70 million, of which 7–8 million finally suffer total blindness (Source: Glaucoma Foundation[9]). Damage caused by glaucoma can be slowed or arrested, but not reversed: patients affected by glaucoma experience progressive impairment of visual field as damage to the optic nerve advances.[10] Despite an abundance of theories in textbooks and specialized literature, the pathogenesis and the development of this disease have not been clearly identified.[11] The chase for this 'silent thief of sight' goes back well over 150 years, a period in which many research routes have been attempted (Albert and Edwards 1996). Progress in diagnostics has brought about various techniques to detect the onset of glaucoma, but the connection between the degenerative process in the structure of the eye and loss of vision has not been fully clarified. If anything, more and more accurate research has reinforced the notion that glaucoma is a complex disease, and that ophthalmology has still a limited grasp of the connections among the wide range of causes and symptoms.

Our outline of major advances in both ophthalmologic research and practice focuses on two phases of scientific exploration and underpinning diagnostics. The first (1870–1950s) is characterized by learning-by-doing, a lack of standardization, and a spurt in variety of techniques and devices. This phase is dominated by the establishment of

---

8   Indeed, there is a connection between the two cases, in that the insertion of an IOL is a solution to one specific type of glaucoma.

9   http://www.glaucomafoundation.org/

10   The optic nerve plays a fundamental role as it connects the eye to the brain.

11   A comprehensive, yet accessible also to non-practitioners, overview of the state-of-the-art in research on glaucoma can be found in the authoritative article by Quigley (2004). See also Consoli *et al* (2005).

a scientific paradigm whose limitations would only become clear eighty years later. The second phase (1960–2000s) heralds a reorganization of knowledge characterized by the specification of clear(er) standards and a tentative classification of the various manifestations of the disease (Duke-Elder 1959).

In the early stage of research on glaucoma, most of the attention was concentrated on the fabric of the eye, in particular the iris, which controls light levels inside the eye (similar to the aperture on a camera) and is the tissue at the centre of which the pupil is found. In this area circulates aqueous humor, which has an important role in that it bathes external parts the eye, namely the lens and the cornea. The pressure of such fluid, called intra-ocular pressure (IOP), regulates the nourishment of the optic nerve, which is in the inner part of the eye. It is well known that elevated pressure can obstruct the microcirculation of blood and, in turn, if blood does not properly nourish the optic nerve some of its tissues die, causing an excavation, known as 'cupping'.

The prevailing scientific understanding of glaucoma at the end of the 1800s was based on the notion that a congested appearance of the eye, a typical glaucoma symptom, depended on abnormal levels of IOP. This, in turn, defined the paradigm of understanding, and the design space of both therapeutic and diagnostic techniques. Early therapies such as incisional surgery of the eye and, subsequently, *ad hoc* drugs were designed explicitly to lower abnormal pressure. Unfortunately, however, both practices were only partially successful among patients and often to different degrees. With the limited therapeutic success, it soon came to be believed within the scientific community that the concept behind IOP-lowering techniques rested upon faulty scientific foundations. This is a point that Nelson (2005) has repeatedly stressed: the ability to provide solutions to medical problems does not always imply a sound understanding of the diseases. Most often, practical and scientific understanding proceeds unevenly.

The guiding heuristic for the design of diagnostic tools for glaucoma was a combination of eye-visualization and pressure measurement. The standard instrumentation in an ophthalmologist's studio in the first half of the 1900s included direct and indirect techniques (Consoli *et al.* 2005). Among the former were visualization tools such as the *ophthalmoscope* (to observe the optic nerve), the *funduscope* (to examine the back of the retina through a dilated pupil), and the *gonioscope*, a variation of the former two techniques used to scrutiny the anterior chamber of the eye. These were used together with the *tonometer*, an instrument to measure eye pressure, which featured two basic variants (e.g. indentation and applanation). Direct techniques seek to provide an objective assessment of the structural feature of the eye. Indirect ones, such as *perimetery*, instead are based on the collaboration of the patients who is required to report on perceived alterations of the visual field. This kind of technique has scientific importance in that it revealed that visual field loss manifests itself with gradual intensity and, thus, that glaucoma is a progressive disease with diverse incidence among patients. The basic design of most of such instruments changed after the 1960s following the assimilation of modern technologies at root of sophisticated techniques for digital imaging (i.e. scanning laser ophthalmoscope, scanning laser polarimetry) and digital measurement (i.e. electronic indentation tonometer).

Beginning in the 1960s, the scientific notion that IOP was uniquely associated with glaucoma had been strongly criticized and gave way to a different approach to its study. Within the prevailing paradigm, glaucoma is understood as a family of diseases whose pathogenesis follows different routes according to structural features of the eye, and whose incidence affects patients to a different degree because of the co-existence of other pathologies such as a heart condition or diabetes (Drance 1997; Walton 1997). Accordingly, the second phase of scientific research on glaucoma features a strong emphasis towards differentiation of the design space by opening up new research avenues in line with the changing perception of the nature of the disease. Recent research has focused on the characteristics of the degenerative process that is observed on the optic nerve. While it is widely accepted within the scientific community that loss of vision is attributable to this, there is no definitive explanation for the causative factors or for its progression. Remarkable advances in diagnostics have been achieved through the expansion of the knowledge base; thus, with the adoption and development of lasers and computers, as well as the juxtaposition of basic sciences, such as microbiology.

Interestingly enough, although the unitary association between IOP and glaucoma has been challenged for some 50 years, treatment is still largely based on the variants of the IOP-lowering axiom with the recent addition of laser surgery. This is so because elevated intra-ocular pressure remains the most easily treatable factor. In fact, greater specialization in pharmacotherapy has brought about a spur of alternatives like selective and non-selective β-blockers and inhibitors. As a consequence, prescribed regimens have now evolved into patient-specific combinations of these medications. New research is seeking to operationalize improved understanding on the aetiology of glaucoma and to generate therapies for those cases that cannot be treated with IOP-lowering techniques. The field of gene therapy holds great promises and is expected to trigger significant advances, although the practical implementation of this type of treatment is still in its infancy. Again, it seems clear that advancements in basic research (i.e. genetics) proceed unevenly with respect to practical applications that may be implemented.

Summing up, scientific progress in glaucoma indicates that, despite many advances, key questions about this disease still loom large: can glaucoma be detected with certainty? Can it be cured? If so, how can a cure be created? Such, we surmise, is the nature of progress when the problem is inaccurately specified or too complex to understand given the prevailing knowledge base.

Our conjecture is that when the boundaries of existing knowledge have all been explored and the paradigm is still not capable of offering a solution, the paradigm itself becomes a problem and a wider reformulation of the scientific endeavour becomes necessary.[12] Following Hayek's (1952) insight, Brian Loasby (2001: 403) argues that the development of new knowledge builds upon a system of 'imperfectly-specified connec-

---

[12] Echoing the warnings of Mokyr (1998) and Loasby (2001), the evolutionary view of this paper is not based on a mechanism of Neo-Darwinian blind selection, but rather on guided selection. The variation we deal with is the result of specific choices in search of a solution to a problem.

tions'. Every system of understanding is founded on the specification of a problem, but at the same time every problem must be necessarily open to redefinition whenever new knowledge changes the contours of that problem. The counterpart to this is a perfectly connected system, which is closed because the contours of the problem do not change over time. If a system has to be able to produce the twists and the shifts that are necessary to correct a paradigm of understanding, like in medicine, then we should expect to observe some 'weak' form of path dependence (David 2001). This interpretative view sits well with the idea that progress in medicine is a journey that departs from and ends in the province of practice. That is to say, a wrong paradigm is likely to produce (partially) ineffective solutions in the diagnostic or in the therapeutic sphere, but in so doing it also urges the need for a change of perspective, which is a prerequisite of novelty. Our qualitative analysis shows that the timing of the emergence of new conjectures and the complementarities that they require in order to be accepted in an established system are crucial. Because these processes unfold at different times, the appearance of a 'better' explanation can be hampered by lack of fitness with respect to the environment, whereby appropriate institutions or complementarities of the kind discussed above are not in place. As Mokyr put it (1998: 126) 'knowledge can be active or dormant, depending on whether it maps onto [the set of feasible techniques], regardless of how widely it is accepted'.

Conclusion

Our general conclusion about the medical innovation process is that the growth of knowledge is punctuated by specialization, diversification, and co-ordination. Such a process is driven by complementarities that are not a natural given, but rather the result of specific efforts to create the capabilities that are necessary to fuel development (Rosenberg 1982). This highlights the role of institutions that facilitate co-ordination across forms of specialization. In both our case studies, teaching hospitals represent an important institutional innovation that has fostered systematic connections between basic science and medical practice, and has *de facto* reconfigured the interaction between laboratory and the clinic. Finally, we note that diversity within a body of scientific research is likely to generate variety also in the mechanisms underpinning knowledge production. It has been shown that as medical knowledge becomes more complex its organization is progressively distributed and cuts across traditional boundaries, such as the traditional public–private divide. Although our primary focus has been the epistemic dimension, the importance of other realms cannot be underestimated, especially the division of labour among research, patient care, and regulation. This seems to indicate a promising research avenue focused on how distributed invention and innovation processes are formed, how they are co-ordinated, and how they change over time.

More generally, there appear to be three lessons to be drawn from the above. The first is the length of time it takes to fully realize an innovation sequence. As we have seen in the IOL case, there is not a single innovation, but rather a field of design that leads to many complementary innovations – *a trajectory of change*. In exploiting this trajectory the relation between industry and medical practice is a vital element in the post-innovation improvement process. Secondly, many medical innovations do not fall within the definition of science-based innovations other than in a loose sense; rather, they are often constituted by conceptually simple engineering devices made complex by the sensitive nature of the medium in which it is implanted. Neither IOL, PTCA, nor the artificial hip, for example, originated out of basic medical research, but rather were led by inventive surgeons and clinicians seeking solutions to immediate patient problems. Thirdly, the innovations in devices and practices often need to be sustained and complemented by changes in delivery systems for the spread of technology leading to important examples of new divisions of labour and skilled specialisms within the field of medicine.

References

Albert MD and Edwards DD (1996).*The history of ophthalmology*. Cambridge, Blackwell Science.

Antonelli C (2001). *The microeconomics of technological systems*. Oxford, Oxford University Press.

Antonelli C (2005). Models of knowledge and systems of governance. *Journal of Institutional Economics*, **1**, 51–73.

Apple DJ, Mamalis M, *et al.* (1984). Complications of intraocular lenses: A historical and histopathalogical review. *Surveys of Ophthalmology*, **29**, 1–54.

Blume S (1992). *Insight and industry: On the dynamics of technological change in medicine*. Boston, MIT Press.

Brown JS, Duguid P (1991). Organizational learning and communities of practice: towards a unified view of making, learning and innovation. *Organizational Science*, **2**, 40–57.

Campbell EG, Powers JB, Blumenthal D and Biles B (2004). Inside the triple helix: technology transfer and commercialization in the life sciences, *Health Affairs*, **23**, 64–76.

Carlsson B, ed. (2002). *New technological systems in the bio industries – An international study*, Boston, Kluwer Academic Publishers.

Carlsson B, Jacobsson S, Holmen M and Rickne A (2002). Innovation systems: analytical and methodological issues. *Research Policy*, **31**, 233–45.

Consoli D and Mina A (2009). An evolutionary perspective on health innovation systems, *Journal of Evolutionary Economics* (forthcoming).

Consoli DA, McMeekin A, Ramlogan R, Mina A, Tampubolon G and Metcalfe JS (2005). *Progress in medicine: Structure and evolution of know-how for the treatment of glaucoma*. CRIC Discussion Paper Series No. 72, University of Manchester.

Consoli D and Ramlogan R (2008). Out of sight: problem sequences and epistemic boundaries of medical know-how on glaucoma. *Journal of Evolutionary Economics*, **18**, 31–56.

Constant EW (1980). *The origins of the turbo jet revolution*, Baltimore, Johns Hopkins University Press.

Cooke P, Uranga MG and Extebarria G (1997). Regional innovation systems: Institutional and organizational dimensions. *Research Policy*, **26**, 475–91.

Coombs R, Harvey M and Tether BS (2003). Analysing distributed processes of provision and innovation. *Industrial and Corporate Change*, **12**, 1125–55.

David PA (2001). Path dependence, its critics and the quest for historical economics. In: P Garrouste and S Ioannides, eds. *Evolution and path dependence in economic ideas: Past and present*. Cheltenham, Edward Elgar.

de Vet JM and Scott AJ (1992). The southern Californian medical device industry: Innovation, new firm formation, and location. *Research Policy*, **21**, 145–61.

Dosi G (1982). Technological paradigms and technological trajectories: a suggested interpretation of the determinants and directions of technical change. *Research Policy*, **11**, 147–62.

Dosi G (1988). The nature of the innovative process. In: G Dosi, C Freeman, R Nelson G Silverberg and L Soete, eds. *Technical change and economic theory*, London, Pinter.

Drance SM (1997). The changing concept of glaucoma in the 20th century. In: EM Van Buskirk and M B Shields, eds. *100 years of progress in glaucoma*, Lippincott–Raven.

Duke-Elder S (1959). *System of ophthalmology*. London, Henry Kimpton.

Freeman C (1988). Japan: A new national system of innovation? In: G Dosi, C Freeman, R Nelson, G Silverberg and L Soete, eds. *Technical change and economic theory*, pp.330–48. London, Pinter Publishers.

Gelijns AC and Rosenberg N (1994). The dynamics of technological change in medicine. *Health Affairs*, **13**, 28–46.

Gelijns A and Rosenberg N (1999). Diagnostic devices: An analysis of comparative advantages. In: D Mowery and R Nelson, eds. *Sources of industrial leadership*. Cambridge, Cambridge University Press.

Hayek FA (1952). *The sensory order*. London. Routledge.

Henderson R (1994). The evolution of integrative capability: innovation in cardiovascular drug discovery. *Industrial and Corporate Change*, **3**, 607–30.

Kaufman HE (1980). The correction of aphakia. *American Journal of Ophthalmology*, **89**, 1–10.

Leijonhufvud A (2000). *Macroeconomic instability and co-ordination: Selected essays of Axel Leijonhufvud*. Cheltenhan Northampton, Edward Elgar.

Linebarger EL, Hardten DR, *et al.* (1999). Phacoemulsification and modern cataract surgery. *Surveys of Ophthalmology*, **44**, 123–47.

Loasby BJ. (1998). The organization of capabilities. *Journal of Economic Behaviour and Organization* **35**, 139–60.

Loasby BJ (1999).*Knowledge institutions and evolution in economics*, The Graz Schumpeter Lectures. London, Routledge.

Loasby BJ (2001). Time, knowledge and evolutionary dynamics: why connections matter. *Journal of Evolutionary Economics*, **11**, 393–412.

Loasby BJ (2003). Closed models and open systems. *Journal of Economic Methodology,* **10**, 285–306.

Lundvall B (1988). Innovation as an interactive process from user producer interaction to the national system of innovation. In: G Dosi, C Freeman, R Nelson, G Silverberg and L Soete, eds. *Technical change and economic theory*, pp. 349–69. London: Pinter Publishers.

Malerba F (2002). Sectoral systems of innovation and production. *Research Policy*, **31**, 247–64.

Metcalfe JS, James A and Mina A (2005). Emergent innovation systems and the delivery of clinical services: the case of intra-ocular lenses. *Research Policy*, **34**, 1283–304.

Mina A, Ramlogan R, Tampubolon G and Metcalfe JS (2007). Mapping evolutionary trajectories: applications to the growth and transformation of medical knowledge. *Research Policy*, **36**, 789–806.

Mokyr J (1998). Induced technical innovation and medical history. *Journal of Evolutionary Economics*, **8**, 119–37.

Nelson R (1988). Institutions supporting technical change in the United States. In: G Dosi, C Freeman, R Nelson, G Silverberg and L Soete, eds. *Technical change and economic theory*, pp.312–29. London, Pinter Publishers.

Nelson RR (2005). Physical and social technologies, and their evolution. In: RR Nelson, ed. *Technology, institutions, and economic growth*. Harvard University Press.

Newhouse JP (1992). Medical care costs: how much welfare loss? *Journal of Economic Perspectives*, **6**(3), 3–21.

Porter R (1997). The greatest benefit to mankind: a medical history of humanity. New York, W.W. Norton and Company.

Quigley HA (2004). *New paradigms in the mechanisms and management of glaucoma. Eye*, The Doyne Lecture. Available online at: http://dx.doi.org/10.1038/sj.eye.6701746

Roberts EB (1989). The personality and motivations of technological entrepreneurs, *Journal of Engineering and Technology Management*, **6**, 5–23.

Roberts EB and Hauptmann O (1986). The process of technology transfer to the new biomedical and pharmaceutical firm. *Research Policy*, **15**, 107–19.

Rosenberg N (1982). *Inside the black box: Technology and economics*. Cambridge, Cambridge University Press.

Utterback J (1994). *Mastering the dynamics of innovation*. Boston, Harvard Business School Press.

Vincenti W (1991). *What engineers know and how they know it*. Cambridge, Cambridge University Press.

von Hippel E (1976). The dominant role of users in the scientific instrument innovation process. *Research Policy*, **5**(3), 212–39.

von Hippel E (1988) *The sources of innovation*. Oxford, Oxford University Press.

Walton DS (1997). The development of glaucomas: 100 years of progress: 1896–1996. In: EM Van Buskirk and MB Shields, eds. *100 years of progress in glaucoma*. Lippincott–Raven.

Zinner DE (2001). Medical R&D at the turn of the millennium. *Health Affairs*, **20**(5), 202–9.

Chapter 3

Technology: scientific force or power force?

Nick Bosanquet

Introduction

Technology is often presented for healthcare as an extraneous variable, a *deus ex machina*, that can be used to explain the continuing rise in health care costs. The pioneering work of Ann Scitovsky introduced the concepts of cost-reducing and cost-increasing technology (Skitovsky, 1985), yet these have not been widely used. The general consensus seems to be that most technology raises total expenditure, either through higher unit costs or through raising the volume of procedures. Recent events seem to have born out Schwartz's forecast in 1994 that health services were on the brink of a period of rapid technological change and the consensus is that the change has cost a great deal (Schwartz 1994).

The aim of this chapter is to explore another model of how technology is determined. In fact, the changes in technology that have actually happened have been more diverse than was envisaged in 1994. Alongside the 'big ticket' technology projected by Schwartz, a 'small ticket' technology has grown up, which is much more available outside large hospitals in clinics, doctor's surgeries, or pharmacies. This opens a range of choices for health policy on the design of new types of local services. Investment is no longer just about investment in hospitals. Health systems face a choice of valuing different combinations of big ticket and new, more local technology for prevention and care. The rise of small ticket technology opens up a range of very different investment opportunities from those available in the past four decades.

Background

The future development of technology will not be determined only by impersonal forces of science, demography and changing disease patterns from outside the health service – it will depend on whether health services can develop a creative and flexible response to new problems. The new feature of the last decade has been the very strong gains from using competition and choice in a number of countries, and the effect this has had on the range of technology used. The coming of new technology has been linked to the development of competition and pluralism. The moves to competition have been particularly significant in insurance-based Bismarck systems, where it is possible for the funder to be independent of the provider (Health Consumer

Powerhouse 2008). The internal market has worked better in such systems than it has in the more centralized tax-funded systems. Can health care grasp the opportunity to use new kinds of small ticket technology and new approaches to patient care involving much better communication? The issue goes far beyond technology. The future of health services depends on whether health agencies can break away from old patterns, and unleash the forces of innovation and quality improvement that are there in health services.

Technology is usually presented as a given emerging from outside the health system. Both corporations and universities have some interest in the romantic view of technology – that it emerges from the heroic and selfless quest for innovation. Innovation emerges from pure research, science, and technology, all of which are dynamic, but dynamic because of the intellectual quest, rather than because of commercial considerations.

By another perspective, technology is not just the product of pure technical factors, the technological investments made reflect the interplay of professional forces and interests. In markets driven by consumers, the tendency is for the market to expand and cheapen technology. The outlook is very different when public sector producers control the funding. The technology developed will have few if any financial or market constraints.

The main drivers in this technology environment are:

♦ The incentive to develop technology with high capital costs and which requires highly-qualified staff to operate and interpret the results. In mass markets technology becomes simpler and usable by a wide range of users. In health care this was rarely the case.

♦ Clinical governance standards that mandate the use of expensive technology.

♦ Risk assessment that stresses the gains to the use of high tech equipment.

♦ Low levels of capacity use, which are brought about, in part, by the limited availability of specialist staff. High capital and labour costs also reduce the customer's ability to pay.

Big ticket technology tends to create a toxic combination of long waiting times with low levels of capacity use. Typically, the utilization rate on public sector MRI scanners is about half of that on privately owned ones. There have been proposals for making more use of leasing to ensure that health services are not tying up funds in 'frozen capital' (Siemens 2006). This may help in reducing capital costs, but the problems of securing cost-effective operation remain.

Big ticket technology has led, in the past, to rising costs and longer queues. This is essentially because it uses scarce resources in staffing, which are always bound to be in short supply. The term 'provider' capture has been widely used and it presence widely suspected, but it has rarely been given any specific content. It could mean, however, that provider/professional utility led to investment in big ticket technology and its associated large hospitals that, in turn, helped to generate rising costs and access problems, with the general result that as the 'market' expands supply price rises. There is no sign of the developments found in markets where supply and demand have a virtuous circle by which more demand stimulates cost-reducing innovation.

The shortage leads, in fact, to higher entry barriers by raising the entry price. The entry problems may increase further through an arms race between local or regional centres to compete in big ticket technology – so that to the problems of rising cost may be added those of low levels of capacity utilization. These are typical impacts within the UK system. Within the USA, spending on imaging rose 20 per cent a year between 1999 and 2006. Scans per 1000 insured persons rose from 85 to 234 in the USA since 1999 (Whelan 2008). Pittsburgh has more MRI machines than Canada. The scan may not only incur direct cost, it may lead to much higher additional spending on further tests and even surgical operations. Now concerns about radiation exposure through the over-use of scans are finally leading to reductions in the use of scans: but only 18 per cent of requests are being rejected. A high level of over-use is now permanently funded and restrictions will tend to fade over time.

The new development in the last 10 years has been the emergence of more technology for primary care and local pharmacies. This provides an instructive contrast to big ticket technology for secondary care. There are a variety of new local diagnostics and treatment including:

+ cholesterol testing;
+ diabetes monitors;
+ nicotine replacement therapies;
+ IT/communication systems;
+ new methods of treating venous ulcers with Doppler assessment and the four layer bandage.

To these low-cost developments can be added the effects of IT in making the results of big ticket technology more available outside the hospital. Thus, PACS systems are transmitting X-ray pictures and MRI scan results so that they can be used and stored in clinics and doctor's surgeries. These new tools offer much more diagnostic and treatment capability in primary care. There is, in effect, disputed territory between hospitals and clinics where services could go either way. The hospital may broaden what it does in out-reach clinics and in out-patient services, or local physicians and nurse practitioners may expand the range of services through polyclinics, expanded primary care – or nurse-led clinics of which WALMART are starting 3000 in the US.

Such developments were predicted in Regina Herzlinger's powerful work *Market Driven Health Care*, which was published in 1997. She saw America and other developed nations as being at the start of a healthcare revolution:

> These dramatic developments in medical technology enable the decentralization of powerful therapeutic, diagnostic and monitoring services. Services available only at vast, costly, hard to reach hospitals will instead be provided by inexpensive, easy-to-access clinics, physicians' offices, ambulances, and helicopters. The most important feature of this newly formed landscape will be better health for all of us.

Ten years on, most of Europe, indeed most of the developed world, is still waiting. The degree of progress has shown some variability between systems and between specialities, but overall the level of progress has been far short of substantial. The vast majority of patients are still being treated in the old fragmented and hospital-based systems.

Health care in Europe remains a state-funded industry, which continues to roll on with obsolete services, while investing very little in new innovative ones. In fact, the continued spending on obsolete services compresses the margin available for spending on new services. This braking effect on innovation is reinforced by the impact of health technology: assessment that sets much higher standards for new therapies and programmes than for the time served and obsolescent. Health spending is in a rut kept there by the main economic incentive, which is all too often to extract the maximum benefit from producer subsidy, rather than to provide the services chosen by consumers.

In summary, spending on innovative programmes on care pathways E health, telehealth, and new accessible services can be estimated at 5–7 per cent in the UK and Germany, 1–3 per cent in France and Italy, and up to 20 per cent in Scandinavia. Where they do exist the new services tend to be dependent on demonstration projects often time limited and on special sources of funds such as EU grants. Some of these projects may be quite successful, but they are not career enhancing nor is their diffusion at all rapid even if they do succeed.

International evidence

We turn now to explore some of the areas where progress has taken place progress again the odds. What seem to be the main reasons or determinant factors behind choices where this new technology is taken up? Key variables could include the degree of competition in a health system. Where there is stronger competition, it would seem likely to generate incentives to use cost-reducing or quality-improving technology. Competition also creates pressures to increase output, which will create space for the adoption of new technology.

Health services that have moved towards greater pluralism have been the leaders in using small ticket technology. In Scandinavia there has been strong local autonomy though the county responsibility for commissioning services. Hospitals and primary care doctors have shown great drive for investing for IT systems. Doctors in Denmark now have the most advanced use of IT of any doctors. In Sweden, patient choice has lowered waiting times to a few weeks with patients free to move to alternatively-funded providers. In Finland, public health programmes have turned North Karelia round from one of the unhealthiest regions in Europe to one of the best. Finland has the lowest proportion of GDP (7–8 per cent 2005) of any developed country, but other countries in Scandinavia have shown that it is possible to provide a service with excellent access and outcomes for 8–9 per cent of GDP (OECD 2004).These systems have shown much success in developing care programmes. For example, 77.8 per cent of diabetics in Sweden had retinal examinations in the past year compared with 65.6 per cent in the US and 49.0 per cent in Germany. In Spain, the Netherlands, and Australia funding has been mixed, as well as provision. Again, there has been more rapid development of new services. In Spain, Sanitas (the private insurance group owned by the British Mutual Association BUPA) has been a significant investor in E health. In Australia, 45 hospitals in Victoria are linked in a hospital at home scheme. There have been successful national strategies for prevention of skin cancer in a land of eternal sunshine. In the Netherlands, competing insurance funds have to give potential members metrics about their performance. In the UK, new providers have been attracted to provide wider choice in elective treatments, but there are signs that the reform programme is faltering, with strong incentives to public providers to block out competition.

The second key variable affecting the extent of use of small ticket technology would be the extent to which there is a strong primary care role in the health system. Primary care doctors are much more likely to use small ticket technology in diagnosis and care programmes. Health systems can be divided into those with a strong primary care base, as against those with direct access to specialist care and fee-for-service. As Table 3.1 shows the spending levels for the first type of system, at 8–9 per cent of GDP, are well below those for the second type, at 10–12 per cent. Yet all studies of population health, treatment outcomes and patient access show that the first type of system delivers results which are at least as good and in many dimensions better than the second. The use of small ticket technology will grow along with the deepening of activities in primary care. Where primary care doctors carry out more initial assessments and offer more services they are much more likely to use this technology. In contrast when activities are shifted into the secondary sector this will involve use of big ticket technology. Small ticket technology will also show variable use with the different roles of pharmacies and opticians. Where there is a more access and a wider range of services pharmacies and optician practices will be able to expand use of this technology.

Recent research on Kaiser Permanente, sponsored by the Department of Health itself, has confirmed that the first type of system in a regional context can, indeed, deliver very effective results. The original research showed that, on an adjusted PPP basis, the NHS spent $1784 per head, while Kaiser Permanente spent $1984 per head (Feachem et al. 2002). These results were fully adjusted for differences in the age composition of patients and in the differences in the range of services provided by the

Table 3.1 Growth of expenditure on health 1990–2005 – health spending as a percentage of GDP

	1990	2005
Primary care-led systems:		
Denmark	8.5	9.1
Finland	7.8	7.5
Netherlands	8.0	9.2
New Zealand	6.9	9.0
Spain	6.7	8.2
Sweden	8.2	9.1
United Kingdom	6.0	8.3
Fee for service-led systems		
Belgium	7.4	10.3
France	8.6	11.1
Germany	8.5	10.7
Switzerland	8.5	11.6
United States	11.9	15.3

Source: OECD Health Data (2007).

two systems. Yet, later comparisons sponsored by the Department of Health showed that: 'For the 11 causes selected for study, total bed use in the NHS is three-and-a-half times that of Kaiser's standardized rate …'[1] (Ham *et al.* 2003).

The level of spending generated in the first system reflects the costs of providing certain services involving primary care access, referral and protocol-driven secondary care. If this system is associated with higher levels of spending, this implies either higher costs than could be prudently managed or higher levels of activity. There is good international evidence that high levels of health spending are often associated with the flat of the curve – with waste and low quality in care. Detailed criticisms have been made, for example, of the low standard of cancer care in Germany and the poor quality of prescribing in France. A recent OECD summary concluded that:

> While richer countries tend to spend more on health, there is still great variation in spending among countries with comparable incomes. Even more importantly the highest spending systems are not necessarily the ones that do best in meeting performance goals[2]

> (OECD 2004)

Canada supplies a particularly strong example of how funding without reform may lead to an increase in waiting times and greater access problems. Between 1993 and 2003, average waiting times rose 70 per cent over a period when real spending per head rose 21 per cent, in constant 1995 dollars, from \$1836 to \$2223. Thus, higher levels of spending are often taken to conceal problems of low productivity.

Differences in the use of the low ticket technology are also disease specific. There has been particular success in improving services in coronary heart disease, an area of care that has shown very significant improvements in outcome – for example, in the UK, a 40 per cent reduction in premature deaths among males over the past decade.

In coronary heart disease, a new care pathway has emerged linking prevention, treatment of high risk groups with stents, early access to day treatment through better diagnostics and angioplasty, then rehabilitation. The care pathway show gains in innovation through the use of statins, stents, and precautionary home monitoring and telemedicine. In stroke prevention, COPD, and asthma, better primary care IT makes it possible to deliver nurse-led local programmes for high risk groups.

Six primary care practices in Runcorn Cheshire UK covered 64,000 patients. They set up a shared programme to identify patients with high levels of cholesterol. This identified 3300 patients who were assessed by practice nurses and treated with statins. An evaluation showered that in the first year there were 27 fewer deaths and these gains have continued in subsequent years at a cost of £470 per QALY (Colin-Thome 2002). In the UK, the National Service Framework for Coronary Heart Disease (CHD) has been highly successful in providing a focus for service developments.

Across Europe there are signs that the use of care pathways in diabetes may be having highly positive effects on diabetes care, with greater emphasis on prevention and on the use of nurse practitioners to design programmes for patients. In Germany there is

---

[1] Low not small.

[2] COPD Chronic Obstructive Pulmonary Disease, IT Information Technology.

an innovative course run jointly by healthcare Academy Rheine and Roehampton University in the UK (J Huber, personal communication 2008). Other specialties, such as cancer services, are some way behind CHD and diabetes in development of more integrated services (DoH 2007).

There is some greater appreciation of the gains to competition and change. It is clear that use of new technology happens much more rapidly in open systems. In a growing industry there is a cluster of firms that compete for customers. The process of competition is essential for stimulating and speeding up innovation. The drive of these firms in raising output and reducing price in existing product areas makes it essential for firms to develop new products. Their drive to expansion also creates human capital and networks that make it easier for all firms to change and expand. None of these positive conditions exist where there is a monopoly. Instead, there is great interest in blocking any increase in output and minimizing investment in new technology. The traditional case against monopoly was defined in terms of higher prices and static output. We should now focus more on the effect of monopoly slowing down the process of change.

Technology futures

Overall change has come with desperate slowness. The forces of resistance include fear, self-interest, and shortage of working capital. There is fear of change and lack of confidence in new methods, and there is also fear of loss of control. Health services are still run on baronial system. Self-interest is in a continuing automatic flow of funds. Most health providers get paid for doing more of what they did yesterday and new services often carry lower reimbursement, as well as the greater effort and risk required to provide them. Shortage of working capital comes about through the fact that most health systems do not have depreciation systems or reserves to finance change and upgrade technology. In the NHS, the replacement of equipment is often postponed until breakdown and each new technology has to be the subject of special requisition. The path of the innovator has been seen as hard one ever since Machiavelli, but it is particularly hard in health services.

What could be the levers that would make for more rapid change over the next 10 years? The revolution has not gone away and there are powerful patient groups now pressing for change. There is also stronger evidence from other areas of the economy, such as airlines and banking, that digital technology can be crucial in improving service and containing cost.

Health service change and the increased use of IT should be seen in terms of disease-specific strategies. The main focus for change has been on waiting time for elective surgery, but it now needs to shift to care programmes for specific conditions – many of them longer-term medical conditions. As clinical specialization has become more complex and specific, IT has become more generic. Health professionals are certainly affected by more external scrutiny and more competition. This could be a powerful lever for change if professionals begin to see that better communication and use of care pathways is essential to their security and professional futures.

Systems that have developed primary care have found themselves with headroom of 2 per cent or more of GDP compared with those where there is direct access to secondary care. The health systems that deliver access for less than 10 per cent of GDP – Scandinavia, Netherlands, Spain, and Australia – all have strong and developed primary care.

Change has to link to professional concerns about the quality of care. Change alone can deliver on the metrics required to meet professional concerns. It can also be a key resource in helping people to manage time. Most doctors worldwide are faced with a reality of longer working hours and pressure to meet new standards in improving the care of desperately sick patients.

The reality is that improved survival has created a host of new problems in continuity of care for many patients. The increase in medical specialization has made it more difficult to plan care programmes and to involve patients, and there are many more team members with an interest in patients. Add to this that care is no longer be delivered by lifetime professionals who were on duty for 80 h, but by a changing and often inexperienced work force, and you have a recipe for great confusion and disappointment – the day-to-day experience of many patients and staff in health systems worldwide.

Unlocking the full potential of small ticket technology

The key challenge is how to redefine healthcare as a communications programme. At present, healthcare is a series of fragmented activities, where there is every interest in keeping ownership of the fragments. If we get across to professionals that healthcare is a communications and decision programme in which they are trying to pull together a vast amount of disparate information, that will be real change.

Change can be a key resource to managers in linking financial and clinical priorities and programmes. The change to payment by results has begun to have positive effects in many health systems. Many hospital and primary care centres have to earn their income as individual enterprises. They are no longer getting an income automatically in generous annual budgets. Each euro or pound sterling has to be earned through an invoice for service. New technology is the only way in which managers can get this kind of financial information. Across Europe there is a huge challenge in linking financial information with information on clinical activity.

New technology could be the way forward for where services are in great need of redesign. There are few services where communication is more fragmented at present than cancer services. Managers are beginning to struggle with a new paradigm involving prevention, screening, referral, rapid diagnosis, minimally-invasive surgery or active chemo/radiotherapy, and then care pathways for risk management and palliative care. Each stage has effects on other stages. Thus, expansion of screening may generate false positives, which delay treatment for other patients, but in principle this new paradigm offers great hope for improving services against a background of increasing potential for effective treatment, rising patient numbers, and constricted funding (Bosanquet and Sikora 2006).

In the UK, numbers of patients with cancer will increase by 30 per cent over the next 10 years and patients will, in principle, be able to benefit from more complex treatments. Cancer will become a longer-term illness, which will in itself raise treatment costs. There will be new pressures to develop new services in ambulatory and home care. Already much chemotherapy can be delivered at home. In England in 2007, £4.8 bn was being spent on cancer services and, of this, £1.5 bn was spent on patient treatment, with 100,000 emergency admissions a year. The challenge of redesigning service is a massive one, and can only be achieved though use of new technology and E health.

Across Europe health indicators in obesity and activity are worsening, with an additional special problem in the UK of rising levels of drinking especially among teenagers and young people. There is an urgent requirement for new programmes to increase communication and motivation in public health. E health, and new technology can also be presented as the only way of achieving some catch-up in neglected or unpopular services. In the UK there are serious gaps in stroke care, chronic lung disease, and in assistance with deafness and hearing problems.

Stroke is the leading case of adult disability, and just behind CHD and cancer as a cause of mortality. According to a recent National Audit Office Report, 50 per cent of patients do not receive the proper rehabilitation needed to make a proper recovery in the crucial months following a stroke. Many do not receive simple information about their condition and recovery (National Audit Office 2005).

In chronic lung disease (COPD) there are 900,000 people who have been diagnosed. A recent Healthcare Commission Report found that 'In some areas, services provided to people with COPD do not meet existing clinical guidelines and there wide variations in standards of care across the country. In addition, many people with COPD come from communities with high levels of deprivation and often experience difficulty in gaining access to appropriate services. 'The rate of mortality for respiratory disease in the UK is almost double the European average (Healthcare Commission 2006).

Change and E health have to be seen as the only way that health funders are going to be able to make progress to improve services for neglected groups of patients in the community. It is highly unlikely this can be come through the development of further hospital services. The next phase of healthcare could promise real progress in a number of areas in new therapies, and in better results for patients. It also promises to be a time of much greater funding restriction. The Herzlinger revolution has been held off, but is now compelling as, in fact, the only way in which services can gain investment and develop the flexibility to meet new needs.

Conclusion

Technology is then a battle ground between competing models of health care. Primary care technology is low cost and accessible. Secondary care technology is exclusive and expensive. Often there is little information on value and effectiveness but such methods become some of the must dos set by lead clinicians and professional organizations. Such technology as used at present is part of the pull towards specialization and concentration of services on few sites. These choices in technology structure the supplier markets. They lead to a situation in which a few firms dominate a global industry – indeed, concentration in such products as scanners has increased in the past decade.

These changes bring new opportunities for companies involved in health insurance. Innovation becomes more important for health services and more local. Higher patient expectations of new services will test the capability of tax funded services to deliver an expanding range of new services. Health insurance can develop a complementary role to state funded services in offering more scope for innovation. It can use advantages of greater flexibility and greater ability to generate investment in a timely fashion. They can also show greater priority in communicating with patients and clients. Health insurance can develop relationships with a new generation of young people who have less faith in centralized state funded services. They are close to other service activities which use the new small ticket technologies and can use this advantage to develop new activities. The coming of small ticket technology gives extra force to the case for competition and pluralism.

References

Bosanquet N and Sikora K (2006). *The economics of cancer care*. Cambridge, Cambridge University Press.

Colin-Thome D (2002). *Ischaemic heart disease in Runcorn*. Runcorn, Runcorn Primary Care Group.

Department of Health (2007). *Cancer Reform Strategy*. London, DoH.

Feachem R, Sekhri N and White K (2002). Getting more for their dollar:a comparison of the NHS with California's Kaiser Permanente. *British Medical Journal*, **324**, 135–43.

Ham C, York N, Sutch S and Shaw R (2003) Hospital bed Utilisation in the NHS, Kaiser Permanente and the US Medicare programme:analysis of routine data. *British Medical Journal*, **327**, 1257.

Health Consumer Powerhouse (2008). *Euro Health Consumer Index*. Brussels, HCP.

Healthcare Commission (2006). *Clearing the air: A national study of chronic obstructive pulmonary disease*. London, Healthcare Commission, London.

Herzlinger R (1997). *Market driven health care*. Reading, Addison-Wesley.

National Audit Office (2005). *Reducing brain damage. Faster access to better stroke care*. London, NAO.

OECD (2004). *Towards high performing health systems*. Paris, OECD.

Schwartz WB (1994). In the pipeline: A wave of valuable medical technology. *Health Affairs*, **13**, 70–9.

Scitovsky A (1985). Changes in the cost of treatment of selected illnesses 1971–81. *Medical Care*, **23**, 1245–57.

Siemens (2006). *Healthcare affordability—The global challenge*. Munich, Siemens Financial Services.

Whelan D (2008). Cranking up the volume. *Forbes*, 25 February 2008.

Chapter 4

Diffusion of health technologies: evidence from the pharmaceutical sector

Victoria Serra-Sastre and Alistair McGuire

Introduction

> In health care, invention is hard, but dissemination is even harder
>
> (Berwick 2003)

The introduction of new technologies in the economy is generally assumed to provide competitive advantages to the adopters, under the assumption that these innovations are superior to the existing ones. Diffusion of new technologies in the general economic context has been extensively analysed and there is comprehensive empirical evidence from various sectors. The analysis of the diffusion process of medical innovations in the health care market remains preliminary and the understanding of the mechanisms underlying this process is in its infancy. In this chapter we will to summarise the evidence on the diffusion of new pharmaceuticals. Two questions immediately arise: Why is diffusion a major issue of concern within the health care market? In particular, why is diffusion of new pharmaceuticals relevant?

Increasing health expenditure in developed countries over the last decades has been one of the major issues on the agenda of governments and this has lead to the expansion of cost containment policies. Health care expenditure growth has been increasing faster than the annual growth of GDP over the last few decades. In countries such as the UK and USA, with different health care service markets, medical expenditure has increased at an annual rate of 4–5.5 per cent, respectively, over the recent past, well above their GDP growth figures of 2.3 and 3 per cent, respectively. Given the continuing increase in medical expenditure, there has been a growing interest among scholars in determining the factors explaining this continuous increase in costs. Factors such as population ageing, expansion of insurance coverage or increased per capita income have been typically argued to be contributors to the increase in health expenditure. However, it is accepted among economists that they account for only a small proportion of the growth, and technological change has been identified as the single most important factor in explaining the increase in medical expenditure (Aaron 1991; Newhouse 1992, 1993; Fuchs 1996).

The expansion of health care costs led to the development and introduction of new forms of third-party reimbursement payment systems, aimed at the cost containment of medical spending (Weisbrod 1991). In identifying technology advances as responsible for the bulk of medical cost growth, these new types of reimbursement scheme, mainly an evolution from retrospective to prospective payment systems, are likely to modify the incentives in the use of new technologies, especially as innovations tend to have higher total costs of implementation compared with existing technologies. Changes in payment systems through the implementation of cost-containment policies will also have implications in terms of the signals given to the several stakeholders taking part in the market. For instance, the change in reimbursement policies may suggest investment in a portfolio of research and development activities orientated to the type of innovation that is likely to be quickly and easily adopted. Thus, although the diffusion process is concerned with the spread of an innovation over time, ultimately this may have influences on the health insurance market and the development of new technologies (Weisbrod 1991).

Among the different medical technologies in the health care market pharmaceuticals are of particular interest, not only because they represent a sector with fast innovation rates, but also because pharmaceutical expenditure accounts for a considerable portion of the health care expenditure. Spending in pharmaceutical accounts for a mean share of the GDP of 1.2 per cent in OECD countries (Jacobzone 2000). Pharmaceutical expenditure as a percentage of total health spending ranged between 11.7 and 22.4 per cent in 2000, as shown in Table 4.1. Pharmaceutical expenditure has been growing over the last decades in the majority of OECD countries, and even countries where the pharmaceutical bill is not excessive in absolute terms have experienced an increase in the share of total health care expenditure over time.

Advances in medical care open new treatment possibilities for existing and new patients, and therefore there are two possible mechanisms at work, which lead to increasing health expenditure (Cutler and Huckman 2003). On the one hand, there will be a substitution effect in that patients using the incumbent technology will switch to the new treatment, assuming lower unit costs characterise this new technology.

Table 4.1 Total expenditure of pharmaceuticals as a percentage of total health care expenditure

	1980	1985	1990	1995	2000
Australia	8.0	8.1	9.0	11.2	13.5
Canada	8.5	9.6	11.5	13.8	15.9
France	16.0	16.2	16.9	17.6	20.3
Germany	13.4	13.8	14.3	12.8	13.6
Portugal	19.9	25.4	24.9	23.6	22.4
Spain	21.0	20.3	17.8	19.2	21.3
Sweden	6.5	7.0	8.0	12.3	13.8
United Kingdom	12.8	14.1	13.5	15.3	
United States	9.0	8.9	9.1	8.9	11.7

Source: OECD Health Data.

Nevertheless, within the pharmaceutical market drugs tend to be introduced at higher prices (unit costs), as a profit incentive to maintain R&D within the sector, and it is likely that new pharmaceuticals will increase expenditure in the short term reflecting this higher unit cost. Note that such substitution is not based on the classical reduction of resource inputs used in the production function, but in the substitution of one type of input by a new and innovative input in the production process. However, in the long-run this may turn into cost savings derived from the (assumed) higher effectiveness of the innovation in reducing disease morbidity and mortality. On the other hand, there could be an increase in total costs with the use of the innovation by patients that previously were not eligible for treatment (in any particular disease area) with the old technology giving place to the so-called expansion effect associated with the new technology.

The combination of the substitution and expansion effects obviously leads to an increase in the demand for the new technology and, subsequently, an overall increase in absolute terms of the quantity of services provided with the final balance being determined by the magnitude of each of these effects. However, note that the change in demand prices will also determine the size of the contribution that the new technology has with respect to treatment cost increases. Thus, in addition to quantity impacts that operate through the substitution and expansion mechanism, there is another channel through which health care expenditure increase could operate, input price. Generally, new technologies have a higher cost and the overall contribution of technology quantity as a driver of medical spending growth will be also operating through the impact on marginal cost imposed by higher technology price.

Tables 4.2 and 4.3 show the growth of pharmaceutical expenditure and the associated price index from 1970 to 2000 for some OECD countries. Expenditure on pharmaceutical goods has been increasing in many of the OECD countries, although in some countries the growth rate has been decreasing during the 1990s. The pharmaceutical price indexes, however, show an overall decreasing growth trend. For instance, the

Table 4.2 Growth on total expenditure pharmaceutical and other medical non-durables (million US$, PPP)

Country	1970–75	1975–80	1985–90	1990–95	1995–00
Australia	41.1	27.6	55.9	75.9	75.2
Canada	38.9	64.3	75.6	50.3	47.1
Finland	81.1	49.8	45.1	54.1	34.4
France	66.8	45.0	50.4	41.1	42.1
Germany	83.0	63.8	34.4	48.7	25.8
Ireland	57.1	59.5	46.6	34.4	59.5
Sweden	107.2	48.3	46.9	73.0	47.6
United Kingdom	49.5	73.1	35.2	60.3	
United States	47.4	68.1	66.2	37.9	74.5

Source: OECD Health Data.

Note: growth in price for Australia correspond to 1971–1975.

Table 4.3 Growth on total expenditure on pharmaceutical goods (price index, 2000 = 100)

Country	1970–75	1975–80	1985–90	1990–95	1995–00
Australia	68.7	55.4	37.0	10.8	4.1
Canada	11.3	39.4	43.3	11.7	7.0
Finland	75.0	39.8	40.3	43.7	13.0
France	13.7	34.5	1.4	3.0	0.2
Germany	24.2	17.3	16.4	27.1	12.9
Ireland	40.2	105.8	20.0	15.7	13.3
Sweden	51.7	51.8	10.5	22.1	4.0
United Kingdom	53.4	105.2	42.6	37.9	16.4
United States	14.9	41.5	42.2	25.0	16.4

Source: OECD Health Data.
Note: growth in price for Australia correspond to 1971–1975.

UK shows a drug expenditure growth of 60.3 per cent over the period 1990–1995 compared with a growth in the price index of 37.9 per cent. Differences in pharmaceutical spending growth thus cannot be solely explained by increases in prices. In fact, these differences will also be capturing increases in quantities, mainly through the combination of the expansion and substitution effect derived from the use of new technologies in the first instance. Note that this does not rule out the impact of other factors, such as increased demand derived from higher income or due to the ageing of the population. It simply recalls the minor effect on the increased quantity of non-technological factors.

It seems striking that, despite the importance of the pharmaceutical market within the heath care market, there is limited research on the diffusion of new drugs, both in theory and empirical analysis. The pharmaceutical market is typically characterized by fast technological change in which pharmaceutical companies compete in patent races to obtain a positive return on their investment in R&D, and this is indicated by the rapid rate at which new drugs are introduced. Figure 4.1 shows that the percentage of market share acquired by new medicines launched between 1997 and 2002 in several OECD countries. New drugs are shown to have an effect on the health care market, both in terms of improving health outcomes and reducing other medical expenditures. The increase in the relative importance of the pharmaceutical sector in the health care market alongside the increasing number of new medicines introduced into the market, poses the question of what are the determinants driving the diffusion pattern of new pharmaceuticals?

In this chapter we aim to review the theoretical and empirical literature on the diffusion of new pharmaceuticals and draw some lessons derived from the evidence, as well as to draw attention to potential areas of research. The following section, 'Background', depicts the diffusion process in general and as applied to the pharmaceutical sector in particular, noting the peculiarities of the health care market. 'Approaches to the modelling of demand for new drugs' (p. 60) reviews theoretical

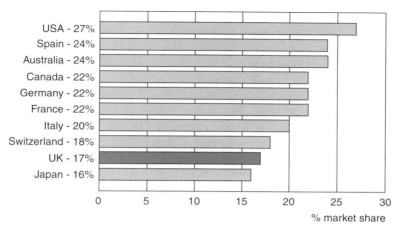

Fig. 4.1 Demand of new products over total demand. Products launched between 1997 and 2002 on primary and hospital markets. Source: IMS World Review.

models of new drug diffusion, while 'What is the empirical evidence telling us?' (p. 63) reviews the empirical evidence as it relates to the theory of diffusion. In the conclusions section (p.68) the main lessons are derived.

Background

Diffusion of new technologies has been extensively studied in neoclassic economics. It is defined as the spread of the use of technology across the relevant market in which prospective users (firms) operate. As pointed by Stoneman (2002):

> diffusion concerns issues that are among the more difficult to analyse adequately. Time is involved. Uncertainty is inherent. Change is the main topic. Imperfect markets abound. All such characteristics mean that the analysis of diffusion stands apart from much of the economic textbooks where perfect competition, full information, static models tend to hold sway.

By definition, diffusion is inherently dynamic not only in terms of the time path, but also in terms of likely regular modifications to the technology and structural changes occurring in the market/industry. In order to understand the nature of the process, it is also relevant to differentiate the different types of technology as they will represent different patterns and mechanisms of diffusion. As such, technologies are classified as process and product innovations, depending on whether they introduce a change in the production process or they are a new product themselves, respectively. At the same time diffusion can be distinguished at two levels, the first being inter-firm diffusion, which relates to the number of firms adopting the technology in a given market. On the other hand, intra-firm diffusion refers to the rates at which different firms produce goods using the new technology.[1]

---

[1] Whereas most of the work on diffusion relates to inter-firm diffusion of process innovations, there is a limited amount of evidence on intra-firm diffusion.

Empirical observations of diffusion patterns in several industries have shown that diffusion is generally characterized by an S-shaped up-take with respect to time, with an initial time span where diffusion happens at a slow rate and only a reduced number of early adopters use the technology. The next stage is characterized by quick general adoption with the number of adopters increasing gradually and a final levelling phase. The seminal work by Griliches (1957) on the diffusion of hybrid corn in the US and the research by Mansfield (1961 1968) on the diffusion of several industrial technologies first noted the S-shaped diffusion pattern. Since the publication of these works, there have been numerous empirical studies analysing the pace of different technologies over time. These works highlight the importance of 'economic incentives and profitability in the adoption of new technology', but over time other factors, such as the role of marketing, and barriers, including regulatory constraints, have been incorporated.

New pharmaceuticals represent an example of product innovation and their diffusion path in the health care market is presumed to follow the same S-shaped pattern, with a slow uptake rate in early stages and the uptake stepping up towards a point at which diffusion moves towards a convergence point. Despite these similarities, there are differences between the pharmaceutical market and other industries that reflect the particular characteristics of demand and supply in this sector – in the first place the decision unit, secondly, how the demand curve is specified, and finally the characteristics of the health care market in general and the pharmaceutical sector in particular. As for the decision unit, in contrast with other markets where firms or agents may be motivated uniquely by economic incentives in the decision to adopt, the case of physicians represents an example of an agent whose decision choice may not be driven by purely economic motives (Scott 2000). The time elapsed between the introduction and common use of the technology shows that, even in cases of new products presenting obvious competitive advantage, the adoption and diffusion are not instantaneous. After the technology has been introduced, there might be a lack of robust evidence (and uncertainty) on the product that generates a slow up-take process at early stages. As soon as the diffusion takes off there will be mechanisms that bring more evidence to the fore and decision-makers will have better information regarding the medical treatment. The profit-maximising assumption embedded in economic diffusion models may not apply to the physician case and would not be a good predictor of drug diffusion. Furthermore, the presence of third-party reimbursement systems defines a different role of prices in this market, because of the lack of price awareness or because the particularities of the health care market, to some extent, factors as altruism or ethics involved in the production function.

Demand in the health care sector does not lie within the standard definition of demand for goods and services, whereby the demand curve represents a relationship between prices and quantities. Demand for medical services reflects the decision of doctors, not the demand by the final consumer, the patient. Because of the asymmetry of information in the doctor–patient relationship the patients seeks the doctor's advise on medical treatment, and this will cover issues of safety and tolerability, as well as treatment issues relating to efficacy. Issues of product quality are therefore affected by this asymmetry of information. Hence, the medical services demanded by the patient are a reflection of the doctor's decision and will not reflect the standard quantity–price relationship. Moreover, it is usually the case that patients do not bear all the cost of the medicine, instead there are third-party payers who do so, and this may induce some degree of moral hazard from the supplier and demander of medical services.

On the supply-side, the pharmaceutical industry has some defining features that distinguishes it from other industries. New medicines emerge from the R&D efforts of manufacturers and once in the market they are protected by patents that ensure a minimum return on the R&D investment. The market for pharmaceuticals is based on a strong patent system and characterized by restrictive regulatory policies regarding pre-marketing approval and reimbursement systems (Grabowsky 1991). The vast majority of countries have regulatory bodies in charge of pharmaceutical pricing policies either directly through price controls or indirectly through profit controls. Moreover, new ethical drugs are required to go through a process to prove safety and efficacy before their approval and in many countries there is an increasing tendency to create independent bodies that set cost-effectiveness recommendations (i.e. NICE in the UK). It is only after this process is completed, and the drug is placed in the market and made available to physicians, that the diffusion process takes off and brings welfare gains derived from the superiority of the new technology.

In the health care context and, in particular, within the pharmaceutical market context diffusion (as opposed to adoption) of drugs is related to the rate at which doctors prescribe the new drugs across patients. In a general economic context the terms adoption and diffusion are used interchangeably, but in the health care context, the difference between them is clearly drawn. Adoption is accepted to be the first contact of the physician with the innovation; however, this could be a one-time contact over a period of time and does not imply that the technology would be immediately included into the doctor's routine practice. Hence, for diffusion, it is here understood the rate at which the new drug will be spread over time or, alternatively, a replacement process of the new technology, as opposed to the use of the existing technology.[2]

The seminal work by Arrow (1963) highlighted the key role of uncertainty within the medical sector. Uncertainty is present not only in terms of the unexpected nature of occurrence, but also on the effectiveness of treatment due to the heterogeneity of patients. In the particular case of diffusion, uncertainty is the main attribute of the process due to the unknown performance of the new technology. Although uncertainty has been linked to early stages of diffusion, it is still present over the whole diffusion path. Improvements and refinements in the technology are likely to arise as the technology is integrated in common practice. In the pharmaceutical sector, there are numerous examples of medicines that suffer changes in the indications the drug is approved for or after acquiring experience through use that leads to the emergence of contraindications not previously shown.

---

[2] This is opposed to the concept of diffusion as number of firms in the industry that use the new technology over time. Diffusion in the pharmaceutical context refers not only to the number of individuals but also to how disseminated the use of the innovation is.

In the presence of uncertainty, information is a key aspect. The process of information acquisition involves time and simultaneously acts as a barrier for a fast diffusion. Since uncertainty involves risk, differences in the attitudes and preferences of individual doctors will define the demand for information through different mechanisms. Self-experience is one of these mechanisms. Drugs lie within the category of experience goods: the 'quality' of pharmaceutical goods is not known *ex ante*. Experience goods were first defined by Nelson (1970) as those goods for which only repeated demand for the product provides information to consumers regarding the attributes. Thus, repeated use is related to information, with greater experience leading to more information acquisition and lowering the degree of uncertainty. Additional information channels co-exist with experience and all of them have in common the fact that information gathering is not free; there is a cost in the time and effort spent in collecting evidence on the drug's functioning. Nevertheless, on the information provider side there will be different costs and incentives to supply the correct information. For instance, there might be economic incentives to the producer of new pharmaceuticals to promote the product and disseminate the exact information (Leffler 1981). In the context of rapid technological change, the process described for a single technology interacts with the simultaneous introduction of other technologies within the health care market originating that the relationship between uncertainty and information will not be a process unique to drugs, but also a process happening with other innovations.

In all models of physician agency or doctor behaviour the technology is a non-labour input that is assumed to be constant. How would the behaviour of doctors change when these inputs change? How are they going to benefit from technological change? Which incentives arise as to use medical innovations? Why is time a main factor in the diffusion of medical technologies even when the technologies are proven to be superior to the existing ones? How is the health care market fostering or dampening the diffusion process? In general, it is assumed that new technologies have superior properties providing them with competitive advantage over existing ones. In the particular case of pharmaceuticals this superiority is expressed in terms of higher efficacy combined with lower contraindications or lower side effects, rather than advantage in terms of price. Under the assumption that new drugs are superior to incumbent products and present potential welfare gains to patients, it is important to ascertain the elements leading the diffusion path in order to understand any delays in demand.

Approaches to the modelling of demand for new drugs

Despite the relevance of the diffusion of pharmaceuticals as part of the rapid technological change in the health care sector, and their impact on expenditure and health outcomes, there are a limited number of studies that formally model the diffusion process. In general, the developments in economics in the analysis of the diffusion process have not been extended to the health care context extensively. The peculiarities of this market and the recent interest in diffusion in health care may well explain the lack of theoretical modelling in this field. In addition, it is a complex exercise to try to synthesise the elements and various agents involved in the diffusion of new drugs in a model that closely reflects the up-take process.

The analysis of the diffusion of new pharmaceuticals has been analysed from two levels of aggregation: at the market/industry level or from the individual decision-maker perspective.[3] At the individual level, the focus is on the understanding of the decision-maker's behaviour in drug choice, as driven by the physician's characteristics and organisational-related factors influencing his behaviour. At the aggregated level, modelling of the diffusion process focuses on the macro-economic variables driving the diffusion process. Differences in the analysis lie in a number of factors that may influence the individual decision, but may not be relevant at the market level because of different underlying dynamics at each level. Moreover, according to the characteristics of the health care market, there will be forces that are not relevant at the market level that may become significant at the individual level. A good example to illustrate the difference is the role of price: in countries with a national health care system in place the price of the drug is likely no to be a relevant variable taken into account by physicians in the prescription decision process as there is a third party purchaser responsible for pricing decisions and reimbursement.[4] However, the overall market demand will be affected by prices that are the product of negotiations between the manufacturer and the regulator. Thus, price may be a relevant variable at the aggregate market level, but not at the individual decision making level.[5]

Despite the numerous factors that have been listed as impacting on diffusion, the superiority of the drug appears to be the key determinant on the up-take process. It is the evidence on the medical advantages of the new drug that will shape their use. In other words, the dissemination of information regarding the drug attributes plays a key role in the diffusion process with different mechanisms available to disseminate information. Thus, how the market or the individuals become aware of this superiority hinges upon several sources of information. The importance of information dissemination does not belie the presence of other factors in the diffusion process: other factors, such as the type of incentives structure provided by the system to the prescription decision-makers are of great importance. However, the limitations provided by the system are likely to influence choice between new and existing drugs, but in order

---

[3] One might think that the distinction between the aggregated and individual approach within the diffusion process is equivalent to the analytical distinctions between inter- and intra-firm diffusion. However, this is not exactly the case for pharmaceutical products. At the market level drugs diffusion refers to the evolution of a single product over time (typically sales are used to measure diffusion) without accounting for the number of individuals that start using the technology. Opposed to that, the inter-firm diffusion measures the number of firms using the technology. At the individual (intra-firm) level, diffusion refers to the increasing proportion of output produced using the innovation and in the pharmaceutical case this reflects an increasing use of the new drug to treat a specific condition.

[4] The lack of prices awareness will give raise to the well-known problem of moral hazard, both from the supplier and the consumer side. However, it has been argued elsewhere (Ellison et al, 1997) that doctors are becoming increasingly aware of the cost of the services they provide.

[5] As noted in section 2, the price will have an effect in the health expenditure through the price elasticity of demand for health care services.

to take a well informed decision, agents require a certain degree of knowledge regarding the technology.

As an example of the information role in diffusion, Berndt *et al.* (2003) model diffusion at the market level as the increase in sales towards a saturation level that is defined as the equilibrium market share of a drug. They give an interesting perspective to the analysis of diffusion using the concept of consumption externalities as a mechanism to spread information on the drugs' attributes. They test their model using equations for four drugs within the same therapeutic class. Diffusion is thus mainly driven by consumption externalities through the usage of the drugs in the market, but also product characteristics and advertising help to drive the process. All these factors help explaining demand at the macro-level addressing the issue of how current drug consumption conveys information for future prescription. Conversely, there are additional mechanisms that complement with each other and that are not jointly examined leading to possible biased estimation results.

A growing body of literature has approached the problem of demand for new drugs as a consumer learning processes. The sources of information available to physicians vary in the degree of experimentation required to obtain information on the product quality. As such, advertising efforts or clinical evidence in scientific journals provide indirect and rather notional information, whereas the actual prescription of the drug will provide direct evidence on the products attributes. Based on drugs being experience goods, these models focus on the information obtained directly through experimentation. Uncertainty and learning are at the core of these models focusing mainly on how uncertainty is reduced through the learning process. Diffusion is generally specified as a Bayesian learning process in which doctors get feedback from the prescription of the new drug through the signals observed from the patient's drug consumption (Coscelli and Shum 2004; Crawford and Shum 2005). The definition of diffusion as a dynamic process is inherent in these models because the process runs in a time line across which the increase in experimentation reduces the degree of uncertainty.

Coscelli and Shum (2004) examine the case where doctors obtain utility from prescription, being the utility of the new drug different from that obtained with the prescription of the existing drug. The probability of prescribing the new medicine is thus a function of the update of beliefs on the unknown quality of the new drug. Note that, in these models, the learning process concerns the new product, whereas the characteristics of existing medicines are assumed to be known by doctors with certainty. In the case that uncertainty refers to all existing drugs (new and old), different implications arise as suggested in Crawford and Shum (2005). In their approach they model diffusion as a matching process between the patient and the drug. The information retrieved from the prescription allows for informational spillovers across patients of current consumption in future drugs choices. This is important because of the heterogeneity of patients, and highlights the fact that diffusion does not take place in a homogeneous context in which existing drug characteristics are completely known. Instead, it allows for some degree of uncertainty regarding the performance of both the new and the old drug, and highlights the fact they might both go through a process in which drugs undergo improvements or changes in indications and effectiveness.

An additional factor that has been analysed is the influence of the professional network in which doctors operate. In an attempt to explain variation in medical practice in a diffusion context, Bikhchandani *et al.* (2001) use a Bayesian approach to introduce imitation among physicians as a means to acquire information regarding the treatment choice. In this way, information derived from colleagues' choices will decide the path of diffusion. A major breakthrough in their contribution is the distinction between discrete versus continuous treatment choice. As such when the choice is discrete, for instance, whether or not to perform a diagnostic test, treatment, or procedure, individuals will calibrate alternatives that are dual: the choice here is a yes/no answer to whether undertake it or not. In this case, the information derived from colleagues under the assumption that physicians weight their colleagues' decision as valid as their own decisions. However their model allows for a wrong pattern of adoption through an informational cascade if the aggregated knowledge displayed by early adopters is based on erroneous initial choice. On the other hand, convergence towards a common standard is easily reached when the choice is over a continuous treatment. Doctors learn about colleagues' choice among dosage decisions that can be weighted to converge to a routine practice through the constant learning by physicians. Hence, Bikhchandani *et al.* (2001) show an alternative way to propagate diffusion of technologies based on colleagues information derived from self-experimentation.

Experimentation and learning are the main elements under scrutiny in the models described. In these models the diffusion process is driven essentially by the doctor's self-experience, keeping other informational sources grouped together under an unobserved effect. A distinctive attribute of the diffusion process is the combination of multiple forces acting together mainly at the information level, but also in terms of organisational and institutional factors of the health care market in which diffusion takes place. Whereas the demand for pharmaceuticals has been well documented, the demand for new pharmaceuticals remains unexplored mainly because of the mix of forces and interests that interact in the market when a new drug comes into force. As argued above, differences between the macro- and micro-economic approaches to the demand for new pharmaceuticals lie on the aggregation of preferences in drug choices. Despite the theoretical evidence on the physician learning process, the question of which arguments entering into the physician's utility function that will enhance the use of new drugs remain unresolved. Different models of physician behaviour have been largely discussed in the literature under the assumption that technological change was fixed. How is this behaviour modified when technological change comes into the scene? How is the process of technological change absorbed by the physician? Why some physicians immediately have a widespread use of the new drug, whereas other are followers in new drug demand? These are questions that remain unresolved on theoretical grounds and leave scope for further examination.

What is the empirical evidence telling us?

The work published in the sociological literature in 1966 by Coleman *et al.* on medical innovation diffusion was the culmination of an extensive and earlier research on the diffusion path followed by a new antibiotic. The authors examined the drug acceptance in four Mid-western cities and, despite a high rate of adoption, after a year there were still differences in the rate of adoption that raised the question of the factors that determined that differences. The degree of integration of the doctor in the social community had an important impact on adoption and informal networks were effective in speeding up the adoption. Numerous studies have been undertaken within the sociological literature and they have mainly focused on the location of consumers within the social network and, although diffusion has been analysed in other disciplines, such as marketing and economics, the approaches taken have been mainly focused on particular aspects and generally lacking a global perspective of all the forces interacting in the diffusion.

In contrast to the sociological view, Griliches (1957) argued that economic incentives and profitability were the drivers of the diffusion of hybrid corn across states in the USA. With two different fields dealing with the same problem from different perspectives, the first issue to arise is whether similar patterns of adoption prevail independent of the type of technology in place. Taking this as starting point, Skinner and Staiger (2005a,b) examined whether the adoption patterns observed by Griliches prevailed for other innovations and studied if those states that were faster adopters of hybrid corn presented the same conduct decades later and for a group of four rather different technologies – hybrid corn, tractors, computers, and beta-blockers, with an emphasis on the use of beta-blockers for the treatment of heart attack. They observed a high state-dependency on the use of new technologies given that states that were early adopters of hybrid corn in the 1930s and 1940s were also leaders in the adoption of beta-blockers. Skinner and Staiger (2005b) further studied whether this state dependency translated into convergence in the productivity of medical care from heart attack in the USA. However, their findings revealed non-convergence across states regarding mortality, costs, or quality-adjusted price. This revealed not only that there might be prevalence in trends across agents in the adoption and diffusion, but also the presence of variation in the individual performance in the demand for new technologies.

The supply of technologies has formed the basis for the analysis of the introduction of new medicines in the health care sector. On the other hand, the analysis of demand for pharmaceuticals has been studied from the perspective of drugs that are usually established in the market and in relation to competitive market issues arising after patent expiration. However, there is an intermediate step in which new medicines enter the market and are seen as an exogenous influence, a process that bridges the analysis of the initial supply and the demand of the drug in the market, which has received less attention in the literature. Typically, in the analysis of demand the innovativeness of the drug is assumed to be fixed and the focus is on the pattern of the demand of established drugs without accounting for a settling process following disturbance.

Generally, the demand side of the pharmaceutical industry has been of interest in that it is characterized as a competitive market, in which branded and generic products compete for the drug choice by the doctor. As discussed in the previous sections, in this market the individual taking the decision on drug treatment is not normally the final consumer and the consumer is not typically bearing the full cost of the drug purchase.[6] The dynamics that characterize the drug choice have been under scrutiny largely because of the importance of this market in any health care system. The prescription choice can be modelled as a two-stage process, in which, first, the doctor makes a decision over an array of drugs that are therapeutically similar for a given condition and, secondly, makes a choice between the branded drug and the generic equivalent (Ellison *et al.* 1997). The literature has been largely devoted to the competition between branded and generic drugs mainly due the observed low generic penetration in the pharmaceutical market. As Ellison *et al.* show at the aggregated level, pricing differences between branded and generic products seem to determine the prescription choice, but not the decision regarding the drug among therapeutically equivalent products. However, when the branded generic prescription choice analysis is taken to the physician level, differences in generic prescription rates seem to be remain unexplained, at least with reference to physician and patient characteristics. Information asymmetries and agency relationship issues arising in the prescription decision appear to consolidate the trend to over-prescribe branded drugs and habit persistence in demand (Hellerstein 1998).

It is worth noting before going any further in the discussion that a distinctive feature of the pharmaceutical market is the co-existence of different products within a therapeutic group that are similar in composition and close substitutes. Each therapeutic group will include different molecules that present similar characteristics, but will be different in side effects and drug interactions. The first molecule to be introduced hence defines the therapeutic group and will be the only *product* until the second molecule enters the market. Note that the incumbent and succeeding molecules will all be monopolists in that they hold patent protection until the patent expires, and only then competition between branded and generic products will start. The small differences in composition generate the right to manufacturers to benefit from patent protection. It is thus important to distinguish between diffusion at the therapeutic level, in which all the molecules are grouped together, and diffusion at the molecule level, in which molecules capture different market shares within the therapeutic market.

In light of the distinction between expansion and substitution effect by Cutler and Huckman (2003), the growth of the pharmaceutical market has been a matter of concern in the literature in that new drugs offer new characteristics that make them superior and are likely not only to displace the existing ones, but also to open treatment possibilities to other patients that were not eligible for treatment had the technology not been introduced. For diffusion of a new drug to take place, the product should offer a set of attributes that assure the higher quality and permanence in the market. Usually, the superiority of new drugs take the form of fewer side effects, fewer interactions or an advantage in the approved indication. It is expected that the size of the market will hence be determined by product quality attributes as has been the case in several markets, such as the antidepressants and anti-ulcer drug market in the US (Berndt *et al.* 1997, 2002).

---

[6] This demand setting is in contrast with the standard consumer theory of utility maximization.

The definition of pharmaceuticals as experience goods means that the product quality will be revealed after purchase characterizing the learning process involved within the diffusion process. This is only part of the dissemination of information, but marketing has been usually used as the main driver of information and determinant of increases in the market share of the new drug (Berndt *et al.* 1995). Marketing promotion has been identified as the mechanism to advertise the availability of the new drug and also, over time, to give any information of any improvement. Overall, marketing has been shown to have a positive impact on diffusion, but the main discussion has been focused on the final goal of promotion, dividing the opinion in two groups. On the one hand, some see the advertising activity as a purely informational dissemination process. On the one hand, advertising is said to be used as strategic tool to generate persistent habit prescription. Empirical evidence is not unambiguous and shows results on both directions (Leffler 1981; Hurwitz and Caves 1988).

Pharmaceutical companies spend large amounts in advertising their products. Advertising effort is of special importance when launching new products as it is used as a non-price competitive mechanism that may have amplifying effects over the monopolistic period. In the pharmaceutical sector producers may have the incentives to provide the right information regarding the drug with the expectation of future marketing returns when competitors enter the market (Leffler 1981; Klein and Leffler 1981). There are different types of promotion such as advertising in scientific journals or direct-to-consumer advertising, but detailing minutes by sales representatives is the marketing activity with the higher influence (Berndt *et al.* 1995). As the number of drugs in the therapeutic group becomes large the role of marketing as expanding the overall industry demand will have decreasing returns, and the marketing activity will become more aggressive and focused on the advertising of the differential attributes of the molecules (Berndt *et al.* 1995; Berndt *et al.* 1997).

Despite the fact that advertising has engaged the most interest in the literature there are other sources of information available that could influence the diffusion process. As such, the dissemination of information using the evidence extracted from clinical trials is also a channel available to doctors. This information is made available even before the drug starts being marketed and it has been shown to be an extra information mechanism that complements the promotion efforts (Azoulay 2002). Both the information acquired through experience and the information gained through marketing and clinical evidence are channels targeting the individual decision-maker as a user of this information. As discussed in Berndt *et al.* (2003), consumption externalities act as a market signal regarding drug acceptance that can be also used to alter the quality perception of the drug and to justify malpractice cases. Berndt *et al.* (2003) empirically show the existence of consumption externalities at the brand level, arguing that they could lead to important competitive advantage of a drug among close substitutes.

Product quality, prices, and advertising efforts are overall good predictors of the diffusion of new products, and the distribution of market shares by the different products within new therapeutic groups. However, for a better understanding of the demand for pharmaceuticals in general and for new products in particular, it is important to identify motivation behind doctors' behaviour over the drug choice. In particular, the elements influencing the choice between established brands may be different to those factors affecting the choice between drugs within a new therapeutic class and drugs in existing groups. For instance, the degree of uncertainty plays a key role in the new drug decision that is likely to shape the pattern of new drug demand. The degree of uncertainty is lower when looking at the demand of established drugs, especially when demand is related to generic products that are the bio-equivalent to an existing drug and do not require any effort in the information-seeking process. Attitude to risk and preferences at the individual level define the prescription pattern observed in doctors, such as the low generic prescription rates when branded products go off-patent (Hellerstein 1998). It is still unclear if this habit persistence is a phenomenon that also arises in the prescription of new drugs.[7]

It is reasonable to assume that the doctor being the key decision-maker in the drug choice, his socio-economic characteristics, together with the organisational restrictions imposed by the health care context in which he operates are likely to determine the demand for new pharmaceuticals. Empirical evidence suggests that variables such as gender or years of experience are not good predictors of the attitudes with respect to new products (Coscelli 1998). Instead, preferences and habit persistence formed through past prescription seems to be a strong indicator of the demand of pharmaceuticals (Hellerstein 1998; Coscelli 2000; Lundin 2000). Consistent with these results Johannesson and Lundin (2001) show also the existence of barriers to entry due to habit generation in the uptake of new drugs, thus suggesting that, in general, products in the pharmaceutical market are faced with barriers imposed due to a prescription habit formed regarding the demand for existing or competing drugs. Furthermore, this is not a feature uniquely observed from the supplier side, as the patient has also been observed to have usage dependence (Coscelli 2000). If it is the case, then habit persistence showed by the principal and the agent, in combination with the uncertainty that accompanies the introduction of new drugs, may well act as established barriers to diffusion, and therefore explain the slow uptake path showed in the pharmaceutical markets. In addition to prescription habit, uncertainty and attitudes to risk may act as a barrier to diffusion. In an empirical exercise to test their theoretical framework Coscelli and Shum (2004) consider a learning model and conclude that uncertainty regarding the new drug in conjunction with doctor's risk aversion makes those doctors reluctant to demand new products and only after first-hand experience there is an increase in the new drug prescription share. This is of special importance because their results are derived from the introduction of the molecule omeprazole, the first product to be introduced into the PPIs therapeutic market, and it represents a true learning process of a drug for which there is no close substitute among the existing drugs and no other competing molecules within the same therapeutic market.

There are two side effects of the diffusion process that refer to the cost implications of the demand for new products and the effect that the use of new drugs has on health outcomes. As for the cost implications, there are no precise quantitative estimates of

---

[7] Note that it is assumed throughout the chapter that new drugs bring higher quality attributes as compared with the existing ones. Despite their superiority there may be loyalty to existing products that deter the diffusion of new innovative drugs.

the relationship between diffusion of new pharmaceuticals and increase in the drug expenditure. However, the overall cost impact of new drugs' demand is eventually influenced by the weight given by the doctor to the burden that this cost represents to the patient and the insurer. It has been mostly claimed the doctors' lack of awareness regarding the cost of the drugs they prescribe, but recently there is some evidence of the increasing knowledge regarding prices. The evidence on the link between prescription and prices is inconclusive, with some authors having analysed the branded versus generic competition supporting the presence of no moral hazard (Hellerstein 1998; Dranove 1989) and others suggesting that the price has no influence on the doctor's behaviour (Lundin 2000). In new drug diffusion, price could be relevant to see the importance of price differences between the existing and the new (and also likely to have a higher cost) drug, but there is some evidence that shows price has no influence in the prescription choice of new drugs (Johannesson and Lundin 2001).

In terms of health outcomes generally, the diffusion process has embedded the underlying assumption of product higher superiority that will bring welfare gains to the patient. Hence, the diffusion process is expected to be intrinsically accompanied by improvements in the long-term health outcomes within the population. General measures of health outcomes, such as reduced in-patient hospitalization or declining mortality rates have been shown to be negatively related to the consumption of newer drugs (Lichtenberg 1996, 2003). In addition, health improvements brought from the use of new technologies will have spillover effects on the demand of disease-related services and will tend to decrease the total cost of treatment, which includes not only the treatment, but also days out of work (Lichtenberg 2001).

Finally, it is reasonable to assume that the higher cost of new drugs would be counterbalanced by reduced demand for other related health services through health improvements. There is some empirical evidence that has analysed specific drug treatments, but has shown opposed results in this front. The use of new drugs, and their relationship with health care expenditure and health outcomes, are mixed. There is some evidence showing clear improvements in health outcomes alongside increases in drug spending; however, the overall effect is cost-effective (Duggan and Evans 2005). In contrast, there is some evidence that demand for new drugs is showing ambiguous health improvements and pushing expenditure up (Duggan 2005). However, note first that the spending includes only health costs and does not take into account other non-health-related costs; secondly, these ambiguous relationships are disease-specific, indicating that the effect on expenditure may also depend on the condition that the technology is targeting.

Conclusions

Despite the important pharmaceutical share in total health expenditure and the fast technological change happening in this market, there is rather limited evidence to ascertain the mechanisms that shape the drugs diffusion process, both at the theoretical and empirical level, with applied studies limited to specific drugs and countries. The particular characteristics of this market make standard economics inapplicable to diffusion in this sector, as the agents taking the decisions are not the final consumers and prices do not have the same role as in classic demand theory. Also, the lack of data availability constrains empirical contribution. The underlying dynamics in the diffusion process require a long time-series in the prescription of new drugs to capture any shocks happening between introduction and establishment of the drug. Utilisation of new drugs at the market level is likely to be easily tracked down, but prescription data is not as readily available, given the need to follow consumers over a long period of time in order to have consistent data for the analysis of diffusion.

Theoretical contributions have provided insightful understanding of diffusion as a learning process. At the market level, consumption externalities have been shown to be an effective driver of the diffusion process. There is evidence on demand of established drugs, but it is not clear whether the same effects shape the demand for new pharmaceuticals. Consequently, there is scope for research on the diffusion of new drugs not only at the individual level, but also at the market level. It would appear important to look at informational sources as driving the diffusion process, as well as at the incentives and restrictions provided by the regulators of the health care system in which diffusion is taking place. The influence of physician's socio-economic characteristics may shape the diffusion process and establish the proportion of each of these factors as they affect diffusion.

Finally, even though overall drug expenditure is increasing, these costs are not without benefit; the effect of new drugs has been shown to bring health improvements. Although it is true that at the drug-specific level there is mixed evidence that new drugs bring inexorably better outcomes despite the increase in spending. To what extent the increase in expenditure originated from the introduction of new drugs is based on changes in quantities and/or changes in prices is not clear, and has not been quantified empirically. Still, the introduction and diffusion of medical innovations in general and pharmaceuticals in particular, and their link with the increasing expenditure observed over the last decades is attracting the interest of scholars and policy-makers.

References

Aaron HJ (1991). *Serious and unstable condition: financing America's health care.* Washington, DC, Brookings Institution.

Arrow KJ (1963). Uncertainty and the Welfare Economics of Medical Care. *American Economic Review*, **53**, 941–73.

Azoulay P (2002). Do pharmaceutical sales respond to scientific evidence? *Journal of Economics & Management Strategy*, **11**, 551–94.

Berndt ER, Bhattacharjya A, Mishol DN, Arcelus A and Lasky T (2002). An analysis of the diffusion of new antidepressants: variety, quality, and marketing efforts. *Journal of Mental Health Policy and Economics*, **5**, 3–19.

Berndt ER, Bui LT, Lucking-Reiley DH and Urban GL (1997). The roles of marketing, product quality, and price competition in the growth and composition of the U.S. antiulcer drug industry. In: TF Bresnahan and RJ Gordon, eds. *The economics of new goods*. Chicago, University of Chicago Press.

Berndt ER, Bui L, Reiley DR and Urban GL (1995). Information, marketing, and pricing in the U.S. antiulcer drug market. *American Economic Review*, **85**, 100–5.

Berndt ER, Pindyck RS and Azoulay P (2003). Consumption externalities and diffusion in pharmaceutical markets: antiulcer drugs. *Journal of Industrial Economics*, **51**, 243.

Berwick DM (2003). Disseminating innovations in health care. *Journal of the American Medical Association*, **289**, 1969–75.

Bikhchandani S, Chandra A, Goldman D and Welch I (2001). *The economics of iatroepidemics and quakeries: Physician learning, informational cascades and geographic variation in medical practice*. Paper prepared for the 2001 NBER Summer Institute.

Coleman JS, Katz E and Menzel H (1966). *Medical innovation: a diffusion study*. Indianapolis, Bobbs-Merrill Co.

Coscelli A (1998). *Entry of new drugs and doctors' prescriptions*, Discussion Papers in Economics 98/13. Royal Holloway, University of London.

Coscelli A (2000). The importance of doctors' and patients' preferences in the prescription decision. *Journal of Industrial Economics*, **48**, 349–69.

Coscelli A and Shum M (2004). An empirical model of learning and patient spillovers in new drug entry. *Journal of Econometrics*, **122**, 213–46.

Crawford GS and Shum M (2005). Uncertainty and learning in pharmaceutical demand. *Econometrica*, **73**, 1137–73.

Cutler DM and Huckman RS (2003). Technological development and medical productivity: The diffusion of angioplasty in New York state. *Journal of Health Economics*, **22**, 187–217.

Dranove D (1989). Medicaid drug formulary restrictions. *Journal of Law and Economics*, **32**, 143–62.

Duggan M (2005). Do new prescription drugs pay for themselves? The case of second-generation antipsychotics. *Journal of Health Economics*, **24**, 1–31.

Duggan MG and Evans WN (2005). Estimating the impact of medical innovation: the case of HIV antiretroviral treatments. *NBER* WP11109.

Ellison SF, Cockburn I, Griliches Z and Hausman J (1997). Characteristics of demand for pharmaceutical products: an examination of four cephalosporins. *Rand Journal of Economics*, **28**, 426–46.

Fuchs VR (1996). Economics, values, and health care reform. *American Economic Review*, **86**, 1–24.

Grabowsky H (1991). The changing economics of pharmaceutical research and development. In: A Gelijns and E Halm, eds. *The changing economics of medical technology*. Washington, DC, National Academy Press.

Griliches Z (1957). Hybrid corn: an exploration in the economics of technological change. *Econometrica*, **25**, 501–22.

Hellerstein JK (1998). The importance of the physician in the generic versus trade name prescription decision. *Rand Journal of Economics*, **29**, 108–36.

Hurwitz MA and Caves RE (1988). Persuasion or information? Promotion and the shares of brand name and generic pharmaceuticals. *Journal of Law and Economics*, **31**, 299–320.

Jacobzone S (2000). *Pharmaceutical policies in OECD countries: reconciling social and industrial goals*, OECD Labour Market and Social Policy Occasional Papers No. 40. OECD Publishing.

Johannesson M and Lundin D (2001). *The impact of physician preferences and patient habits on the diffusion of new drugs*, Stockholm School of Economics Working Paper Series in Economics and Finance No.2001.

Klein B and Leffler KB (1981). The role of market forces in assuring contractual performance. *Journal of Political Economy*, **89**, 615–41.

Leffler KB (1981). Persuasion or information? The economics of prescription drug advertising. *Journal of Law and Economics*, **24**, 45–74.

Lichtenberg, F. R. (1996). Do (more and better) drugs keep people out of hospitals? *American Economic Review*, **86**, 384–8.

Lichtenberg FR (2001). Are the benefits of newer drugs worth their cost? Evidence from the 1996 MEPS. *Health Affairs*, **20**, 241–51.

Lichtenberg FR (2003). Pharmaceutical innovation, mortality reduction, and economic growth. In: KM Murphy and RH Topel, eds. *Measuring the gains from medical research: an economic approach*. Chicago, University of Chicago Press.

Lundin D (2000). Moral hazard in physician prescription behavior. *Journal of Health Economics*, **19**, 639–62.

Mansfield E (1961). Technical change and the rate of imitation. *Econometrica: Journal of the Econometric Society*, **29**, 741–66.

Mansfield E (1968). *Industrial research and technological innovation: An econometric analysis*. New York: Norton.

Nelson P (1970). Information and consumer behavior. *Journal of Political Economy*, **78**, 311–29.

Newhouse JP (1992). Medical care costs: how much welfare loss? *Journal of Economic Perspectives*, **6**, 3–21.

Newhouse JP (1993). An iconoclastic view of health cost containment. *Health Affairs*, **12**(Supplement), 152–71.

Scott A (2000). Economics of general practice. In: AJ Culyer and JP Newhouse, eds. *Handbook of health economics*, Vol. 1B. Amsterdam, Elsevier Science B.V.

Skinner J and Staiger D (2005a). *The diffusion of health care technology*, Mimeo. Dartmouth, Dartmouth College.

Skinner J and Staiger D (2005b). Technology adoption from hybrid corn to beta blockers. *NBER* WP11251.

Stoneman P (2002). *The economics of technological diffusion*. Oxford, Blackwell Publishers.

Weisbrod BA (1991). The health care quadrilemma: an essay on technological change, insurance, quality of care, and cost containment. *Journal of Economic Literature*, **29**, 523–52.

Part 3

Technological change and health insurance

Chapter 5

Insurance and new technology

Mark V. Pauly and Adam Isen

Introduction

In all developed countries real medical care spending has been growing over time. The bulk of this growth cannot be attributed to demographic changes, or to increases in prices (and profits or net income) of physicians, hospitals, or drug and device firms. Instead, analysts usually impute the bulk of spending growth to changes in 'technology,' broadly defined to include all changes in the way medical inputs are combined to produce outputs. One unanswered question about this conclusion is how to get beyond its essentially tautological nature and identify specific changes in technology, their precise health effects (relative to health outcomes in the absence of technological change), and judge whether the health benefits from new technology are worth their higher costs. This question has been answered affirmatively for cardiovascular disease and some other diseases in the United States (Cutler and McClellan 2001; Cutler 2004). However, an equally important positive question with normative implications is that of the reasons or the causes of the changes in technology. At one extreme of possible explanations is the so-called 'technological imperative:' discoveries and implementation of beneficial, but costly new medical technologies are said to occur because of exogenous positive advances in science. Once the science behind a product or service has been discovered, medical care providers and payers have no alternative, but to bring that discovery to the market, prescribe the use of it, and pay the price charged. Prices are potentially affected by the temporary market power conferred on technologies embodied in products by the patent or intellectual property system. At the other extreme is the view that technological change (and higher quality or improved outcomes) in health care is a normal or even a luxury good whose demand ebbs and flows as real income changes. Technological change in the aggregate is therefore largely driven by rising household incomes (and other demand influences) in all developed countries; on average, scientific breakthroughs can be produced with confidence by the application of enough investment in research and development.

Neither of the extreme views is persuasive on face value and neither of them gives a role to insurance. We know that investments in research and development are largely made by for-profit or at least profit-motivated firms, and we generally hypothesize that there is some connection (although by no means a precise one) between the size of investment in research and development and the flow of new discoveries. We know that fortuitous discoveries can lead to substantial increases in outputs and spending. We know that there is a correlation between growing real income and growing medical spending, but we do not know what process might link the one with the other.

In this chapter we explore whether and how the linking mechanism is affected by health insurance. We strongly suspect that the design of health insurance can facilitate and even distort the pattern of technology adoption. We hypothesize that changes in health insurance in individual countries and variations in health insurance across countries might be expected to influence the pace, shape, and cost of technological change. In particular, we derive some economic models of the relationship between insurance, and the demand for and supply of new technology in a market-based setting with a private supply of both medical care and insurance. An innovation in modelling in this essay is to take specific account of the key role that physician advice, judgment, and action must play in both interesting patients in new technology and supporting higher demands for it. That is, rather than just assume that what happens is a result of richer consumers somehow going out and buying new technology, we try to model the intervening effects of insurance, physician recommendations, and patient adherence under insurance, and possible feedback effects from insurance effects on new technology to public and private insurance design and functioning. In particular, virtually all new technology a patient might use requires physician recommendation in the form of a prescription or medical order of some type, but generally the patient must consent and often must take some action (like going to a pharmacy) as well. We want to explore how this filtering process might work. Because of the importance of government in financing and managing insurance in all countries (including the United States), we also discuss how such activities might modify the results of a market based model with physician prescribing.

Some basic premises and some avoidable distractions

Medical insurance policies, public or private, affect the introduction and subsequent use of new technologies in three basic ways:

- *Payment matters.* Insurance payment or reimbursement policies determine the expected profitability of technologies, and consequently the flow of new discoveries. That is, we assume that firms invest in research and development of new technologies with a view to the expected profits that might be collected should discovery and development of a product occur. Expected profit, in turn, depends in part on the demand for the new product, and that demand depends on the extent and form of insurance. In addition, the relationship between payment to the seller of a medical service or product that embodies new technology and the marginal cost of that technology determines the effort sellers of new technology will make to achieve high rates of use of the technology. Because of the uncertainty, and the long time lag between initiation of costly research and introduction of a new product, investors must form expectations of the future insurance market (and the time at which the new technology is introduced); changes in the insurance market will influence decisions to accelerate or slow the process; Finkelstein 2004).

- *Physicians matter.* Virtually all new technology in all developed countries is consumed jointly with physician-provided information (and usually with physician services). Thus, a key element regarding the prospective introduction of a new discovery and its diffusion is how physicians (either in private practice or as employees) view the desirability of recommending the new technology to their patients. Insurance coverage and payment both for the technology, and for physician services can affect this decision-making process.

♦ *Patients matter.* There is strong evidence that patients do not always do what physicians advise (namely, that 'compliance' with or 'adherence' to physician recommendations is far from perfect). Differences in patient adherence between new and old technologies may affect both what physicians recommend and what patients end up consuming.

There has been considerable controversy in the health economics literature over the extent to which physicians 'induce' patient demands, primarily for physician-supplied services, but also for goods and services provided by others (McGuire and Pauly 1991). In our discussion in this chapter we do not take a prior position on this question, but instead try to derive what physicians say or recommend to patients from the incentives and constraints they face in the model. Moreover, while we assume that patients seek physician advice largely because the patients wish to modify their demands for medical services and products, we do not assume that physician advice wholly determines realized patient demand. Instead, we allow both patients' prior beliefs and the level of any insurance benefits (and resulting patient cost sharing) as having an influence on the patient's final consumption decision, given a physician recommendation and prescription. That is, in our model, use of medical goods or services requires both that a physician advises (and prescribes) and that patients consent. Use will not occur if a physician prescribes, but a patient does not adhere, or if a patient desires, but a physician will not prescribe.

The fundamentals of a positive model that incorporates physician orders, patient behaviour, and new technology

The ultimate behaviour which prospectively influences what new technologies will be made available at what prices is patient use; patients must use and pay for a technology to make any difference in annual medical care spending and use. Therefore, specification of the patient's combined willingness and ability to generate payment for technology used is important.

For virtually all the costly technologies we might consider and, for that matter, for virtually all medical care use other than initial patient visits and over-the-counter remedies, patient use requires not only that the patient have the desire and the means to pay for the care, but that a physician recommend, and prescribe or order it. It might seem then that the only economically relevant demand would be that by a physician (although on behalf of a patient), and not the demand of the patient himself. However, while a physician order may be necessary for a patient to receive some amount of a medical care or product, it is not sufficient; patients sometimes (and in some cases often) do not comply with physician recommendations. One might suppose that insurance would affect compliance, and that is surely the case for a given pattern of prescribing, but because physician prescribing behaviour may also be affected by insurance, the effect of insurance on the compliance rate is ambiguous.

Patient non-compliance with physician recommendations occurs frequently and sometime to a surprisingly great extent. Here, we consider the question of whether (other things equal) the novelty of a technology influences use by influencing compliance. Since both industry investments in research and development (R&D), and prices set when a new product is ready to be introduced depend on the shape of the demand function for that product, and since non-compliance (by definition) affects demand compared with perfect compliance, consideration of non-compliance may have a profound effect on what is offered and at what price.

To have non-compliance occur, a physician must first prescribe or recommend a product to a patient. Tautologically, the more persuasive the physician's recommendation (assertion that this product will improve patient health with small side effects), the lower the predicted extent of non-compliance. Do we know anything about the nature of physician recommendations and/or about patient–physician communication about newer products as opposed to older ones? Superficially, we can think of conflicting influences: physicians being less familiar with new products may not be able to recommend them as strongly as older ones, but the novelty of the new medicine (which patients may have heard about) may lead to stronger recommendations and more compliance. Even more fundamentally, if the new technology yields more net health benefit than its older comparators, patients who are aware of this improvement will be more likely to use it.

What effect does research have on this interaction? There is evidence that compliance or adherence is greater for new technologies than for older ones. For example, multiple studies have looked at the relationship between compliance and anti-hypertension medicine, a field of drugs for which there has been significant innovation. Although we cannot rule out non-random selection into the prescribing of different classes of drugs in terms of underlying proclivity to comply, patients prescribed newer blood pressure agents are more likely to adhere to their medication. Monane et al. (1997) found that compliance was highest with angiotensin converting enzyme (ACE's) and calcium channel blockers (CCbs) versus older drugs, such as beta blockers and diuretics at the time when they were the newest agents. Wannemacher et al. (2002) found that the latest class of drug on the market, angiotensin II receptor blockers (ARBs), compared favourably in levels of compliance while Bloom (1998), Degli Esposti et al. (2002), and others found that compliance was highest with ARB's than all other anti-hypertension medications. On the other hand, there is no systematic evidence on compliance with or effects of new technology on markets for expensive treatments (e.g. positron emission tomography [PET] scans, expensive cancer drugs). It seems unlikely that compliance should be a problem in these cases, however.

How might we explain the apparent effect of the newness of technology on compliance? As noted above, the most obvious explanation is that, at least for the patients for whom it is prescribed, the new technology provides greater net health benefits than the older ones available for that condition, and so the patient is less likely to allow forgetfulness or inattention to deter use. If the patient must pay a higher out of pocket price for the better technology, higher gross health benefit alone may not be enough, but we can assume for the present that insurance covers the bulk of any incremental price over older technologies with less adherence. The other potential influence is newness per se. On the one hand, the patient may have heard about the new product (and indeed such external information, even in the form of direct to consumer advertising, does often trigger a patient visit), or the information that the treatment is not only good but new may cause the patient to believe that its gross benefits are higher than if it had been around for years. Another difference is that the information from friends or from the patient's previous experience with a new product is much less than would be the case for an older product. The patient might eventually decide that the new product doesn't work well enough or has side effects, but it will take longer to come to that conclusion than if the product is old and familiar to the patient or his friends. Finally, the new technology may be better known to or more appreciated by the physician, who responds by prescribing it and accompanying the prescription with strong advice to the patient that the new product is worth taking, even if the patient does not see immediate benefits, experiences side effects, or has to pay something (but on the other hand doctors are almost always going to be more familiar with older treatments).

The other issue is the effect of insurance on prescribing: will insurance affect the rate of prescribing of new products? The existence of moral hazard in health insurance has been well documented; at a minimum, the use of both new and older technologies will be higher with insurance than without. However, is there any differential effect by vintage of technology? To answer this question, we first need to model physician choice of recommendation. One possible, but unfortunately implausible assumption would be that physicians would only recommend care whose benefits are greater than its full cost; physicians inhibit moral hazard. A more plausible assumption is that they recommend technology to patients as long as the marginal benefit from that technology exceeds the cost sharing they experience. With this assumption, moral hazard would have neutral effects on old versus new technology. However, as we shall see below, the coverage a consumer would want to have may be different between new and old technology.

The fundamental normative model

Here, we briefly describe the characteristics of the normative model that we will be using; we will offer a more formal presentation of the model later in the chapter. We assume that the inventor of new technology is able to obtain patent protection for the intellectual property represented by that technology. While most patented products have some substitutes available, we assume that perfect substitution is impossible so that the firm with the patent faces a monopoly demand curve. The socially optimal rate of use of the new product will be at that quantity at which the consumer's marginal benefit equals marginal cost, but assuming constant marginal costs of production, a price equal to marginal cost will not generate enough profit to cover the sunk costs of research and development. Rather, the first best optimal arrangement would be one in which the monopolist produces the optimal quantity and earns profits equal to the full consumers' surplus at that quantity. With such an arrangement, the flow of new products will be optimal given the trade-off between their value to consumers, and the expected cost of research and development.

A simple monopoly price, made possible by patent protection, will generally yield positive profit, but that profit will always be less than the excess of full consumers' surplus over the cost of production. Thus, even an award of a permanent patent will fail to lead to the optimal supply of new products. A system of perfectly price discriminating monopolists would choose the optimal supply of new products. Without such discrimination possibilities, the supply of new products will be suboptimal and the rate of use of offered products will be suboptimal as well.

Because market insurance shifts out the demand curve, it potentially might offset the inefficiencies just discussed, depending on both the form of patient cost sharing and the level of cost sharing that consumers will choose. Gaynor *et al.* (2000) show that, in equilibrium with competitive insurance markets, the demand can never increase so much as to make monopoly more efficient than under competitive product pricing; monopoly-generated price increases set in place higher levels of cost sharing than would have prevailed under competitive pricing. Pauly (2003) argues that, when insurers have the power to refuse to cover a new product, no new product will be introduced that makes consumers worse off—so the rate of introduction can never be excessive on this score.

In between the two extremes of full coverage and no coverage, there must be a level of co-insurance that, taking monopoly pricing into account, maximizes the expected utility of insurance purchasers. One question is whether we should assume that the insurers take possible price effects into account when they change co-insurance and so change the demand curve for the new technology, or whether they adjust in a Cournot-Nash way to each possible price. The issue here is complex. If insurers do adjust atomistically, taking any monopoly price level as given, then choosing the best co-insurance rate that sums health benefit and financial risk protection, the demand curve facing the monopolist will not be the no insurance demand curve multiplied by any particular co-insurance rate. Setting aside possible anomalies, in equilibrium, consumers must be better off than without the new technology, but the profit signals to innovators may be somewhat distorted.

That is, the normative question is whether, at such an interior equilibrium, the signals for investment in new technology are correct. Can the profit level from a new product that makes insured patients better off (given its price) over-state the true consumers' and producers' surplus from that product?

The basics of a model incorporating prescription and compliance

Now we add to the insurance new product model the necessity that physicians prescribe and patients comply for use of a product to occur. To construct a complete model based on the literature on prescribing and compliance, we need a theory of physician prescribing and information transfer, given that the patient has made an initial visit and given expectations about patient compliance. We also need a theory of patient behaviour, conditional on what physicians are expected to do, which explains both the initial contact with the physician, and the decision to comply or not comply with the physician's advice conditional on a contact and a prescription.

The literature offers some guidance on how to model physician prescribing behaviour and patient compliance. Armantier and Namoro (2006) assumed that the physician's maximand depends on choosing to prescribe the medical service or product that maximizes the health-related utility of the average patient in some class of patients with similar diagnoses, minus a disutility cost (to the physician) of non-compliance. Ellickson *et al.* (1999) assumed that the physician maximizes a utility function that takes account of both the positive benefits to patient health, and the negative costs of side effects, out of pocket payments, and psychic 'bother' associated with the frequency of dosage; these are the same arguments as those in the patient consumer's utility function, but the physician may attach different weights to them, relative even to the average patient's valuation, and patients may differ especially on the values they attach to the explicit and implicit costs of compliance. In both cases, a patient decides not to comply if the costs of compliance relative to the benefits from compliance as perceived by the patient yield a lower level of utility than would be achieved in the no-care state.

Patient judgments about their utility are taken as valid measures of eventual patient welfare; this is a 'rational non-compliance' story. The last step in such a backwards induction model is to insert expectations of patient behaviour back into the doctor's maximand. A model like this is plausible for interventions whose good and bad effects are immediate and immediately perceived by patients, such as prescription analgesics. However, it is substantially less plausible for costly and uncomfortable prevention measures for asymptomatic patients that are supposed to yield health benefits at a later point in time.

In both models, equilibrium occurs as physicians choose recommendations based on the benefits they expect the average patient to receive and the costs, signalled by non-compliance, experienced by patients with above-average side effects, out of pocket payment, or administration burden. Equilibrium occurs when actual patient non-compliance rates, given some physician prescribing pattern, equal the non-compliance rates that prescribing physicians expect. In both models insurance coverage is either assumed away or taken as given; Ellickson *et al.* (1999) offered the reassurance that 'insurance can easily be incorporated' into their model, but did not do so. These models assumed that the rate of physician contact that patients will choose is given, although they permit physician selection of patients for whom prescriptions are written; physicians may choose not to prescribe for patients who would be expected to be non-compliant.

Beginning at the beginning

We need to model how physicians and patients make the choices that result in the patient making contact with a physician in a setting where a recommendation or a prescription might occur. McGuire (2000) offered a benchmark model in which physicians care only about their real net income (gross revenue minus practice expenses and minus the opportunity cost of physician time and effort), but compete with other physicians in the market. The market is monopolistically competitive, so physician practices potentially have some market power (whether or not they earn economic rents). Critically, McGuire (2000) assumed that physicians do not offer each potential buyer the option of buying varying amounts of services at a given price, but rather they confront each buyer with an all-or-nothing treatment option, which specifies the amounts of the physician's own services, the effort the physician makes to choose their own and outside services to match the patient's condition, and the average amount and cost of those outside services, and a price for the package. Competitive physicians would take actions that increase patients' expected utility if they can obtain additional profit from doing so, by permitting them to charge higher prices for own services or furnish larger quantities of profitable own services.

How would insurance affect this model? The general effect of insurance is to lower user prices given some gross pricing structure. In some cases those gross prices can be set by physicians; in other cases the level of such prices are administratively set by a large insurer. If insurance reduces the firm-level price elasticity of the all-or-nothing demand curve, greater insurance should lead to higher prices even if long-term marginal costs are constant.

What about the impact of new technology? We assume that any new technology that makes it through the regulatory process and into the market will have been determined to offer positive net health benefits (gross benefits minus adverse health side effects) to at least some sub-segment of the patient population. Should we also assume that the value of these health benefits to the patient is always greater than the cost of making the new technology available, or are there situations in which new technology generates costs that exceed benefits? The standard application of the welfare cost of moral hazard suggests that there might be inefficient supply (Goddeeris 1984; Baumgardner 1988); conventional insurance lowers the user price below the market price and potentially below resource cost. Moreover, some countries have regulatory bodies that compare benefits of some new technologies (principally those embodied in new drugs) with their cost to the national insurance system before permitting the technology to be offered or insured; other countries do not have such a requirement, but will approve for potential sale products and services with positive net health benefits, and will leave it up to competing (public or private) insurers to make choices (potentially differing across different insurance plans) about whether they will cover these innovations and, if so, to what extent. We therefore need a model of insurance coverage determination.

A key issue for insurance is whether the insurer can precisely determine the patient's medical condition and limit coverage for a new technology only to those patients whose conditions are ones where there is positive net economic benefit (i.e. with a cost-benefit ratio greater than one). If so, ideal insurance will cover completely new technologies when and where they are efficient; the patient cost share will be zero and all informed patients will comply with prescriptions. Insurance will provide no coverage for technologies in settings when they are not efficient; cost sharing then will be 100 per cent of the price, but fully informed patients will never demand these services at that level of cost sharing. In this case, the relationship between new technology and insurance is obvious: all new technologies that would have met the market test in a no insurance world will be covered, and it is efficient for all such new technologies to be introduced and used at the levels insurance permits. It is possible that some new technologies with very high costs or which reduce risk might be covered by insurance even though they would not meet the no-insurance market test. However, generally, this simple model says that the introduction of insurance should have minimal effects on the rate of introduction of new technology, and there should be little or no non-compliance.

If the insurer is imperfectly informed about the patient's medical condition or illness severity, relative to information possessed by the patient or the physician, moral hazard will occur. It will also be impossible to have a fully effective pay for performance reimbursement system for physicians. This case of imperfect information on patient health state is the more interesting one to analyse.

One possibility is that both patient and physician have the same knowledge of the patient's health state, but the insurer does not. Then there may be moral hazard. A technology may generate more benefits than costs for severely ill patients, but benefits (although positive) that fall short of costs for mildly ill patients. With full insurance coverage, physicians and patients will pretend that the mildly ill patients have high severity, and expenses that are inefficient will be incurred. Cost-sharing just exceeding the gross health benefits in the mildly ill state will potentially reduce the welfare cost of moral hazard and be efficient as long as the increased exposure to risk is not too costly. In this second-best model, informed patients with a mild illness furnished with a prescription will all decide, in the face of cost sharing, not to fill the prescription. If physicians anticipate this problem as the models in the literature imply, however, they will not write the prescription, but if there is heterogeneity among consumers in risk aversion there may be heterogeneity in levels of cost sharing that physicians do not take into account; there will then be non-compliance no matter what, but the non-compliance (among those facing higher than average cost sharing) will be efficient.

Insurance at any given level of co-insurance should, in a market where patients are fully informed (by their physician or in other ways) about marginal benefit from care, lead to the introduction of more efficient new products in absolute numbers than in the absence of insurance, although its effect on the percentage rate of increase is ambiguous. If co-insurance can be chosen in the market, one question is whether it must be uniform for all products covered or whether it can be varied. (Our assumption that insurance can refuse to cover a product implies that the option of 100 per cent co-insurance is always available).

Figure 5.1 illustrates the issues. Suppose the actual demand and marginal benefit curve is $D(A)$, and the marginal cost is constant at MC. Without insurance the price will be $P(W)$ and the quantity $Q(W)$, yielding the (expected) profit of the lightly shaded area. Now suppose insurance is offered with a 50 per cent co-insurance rate. The demand curve pivots out to $D(I)$, the price rises substantially to $P(I)$, and the quantity increases modestly to $Q(I)$. (Had the marginal cost been zero, the quantity would have been left unchanged.) Profits increase by the darkly shaded area. The question is the relationship of this addition to profit compared with the excess of the true consumers' surplus over the uninsured monopoly situation—that is, the two cross-hatched triangles. The other question is whether 50 per cent (or any other particular amount) would be chosen as the ideal level of co-insurance. That depends to some extent on whether insurance coverage is chosen under the assumption that a particular pricing level is given or whether the insurance market takes into account possible changes in monopoly prices as the extent of coverage is varied.

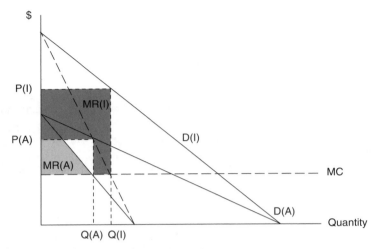

Fig. 5.1 Monopoly Price Determination with Insurance

Finally, we need to admit the fundamental ambiguity about whether the equilibrium co-insurance rate chosen by atomistic insurers and atomistic buyers will be the optimal one (in the sense of delivering the maximum consumers' surplus, given the existence of the product). It would seem that insurance should reduce the chances that a product with positive net benefit will fail to be introduced, compared with a world with no insurance and non-discriminating monopoly, since the only additional introductions generated by insurance coverage will be efficient (or they would not be covered). More needs to be known about this case.

The other possibility is that patients are not fully informed or fully rational. They have different estimates of how sick they are (and, therefore, how much good the technology would do) than what physicians have. Viewed from the point of ex post 'truth,' non-compliance by these patients will reduce their realized welfare, but patients will not know that when they are deciding what to do or not do. Patients might have different opinions about the health benefit of an intervention, again leading to irrational and ex post welfare reducing non-compliance.

New technology will have a different impact on compliance (and hence on welfare) depending on the initial cause of non-compliance and the reason for improvements in compliance associated with the new technology. Let us assume for the moment that both the new and old technologies are offered at prices, which equal a constant marginal cost; the supply of products fits the perfectly competitive paradigm. If the causes of non-compliance are 'rational' physician-unobserved differences in patient side effects, it is obvious that a new technology that increased compliance because it reduced side effects would, other things equal, be efficiency improving. Insurance coverage for the new technology would be chosen according to the usual analysis of moral hazard, with higher cost sharing the more responsive (inefficient) demand is to cost sharing. A second possibility is that compliance improves because the new technology generates improved health outcomes compared with the old. While this increases net benefits as well, in the usual models both physician and patient previously knew net benefits, so the main reasons for increased compliance is that higher gross benefits cause net benefit to be positive in cases of side effects or cost sharing. Here again, however, we would expect market based insurance to be efficient.

The more interesting case is the one in which patients had different beliefs about gross benefits than do physicians, because physicians were unable to convince patients of the true value of the benefit from the new technology. That is, adequate demand inducement was somehow not accomplished. We will explore possible reasons for physician failure to communicate shortly, but for the present we note that if the new technology, in addition to providing higher than average net benefit, also somehow convinces patients of the magnitude of those net benefits (perhaps because of the publicity surrounding the new technology or because of advertising of the new technology to patients), compliance will increase at any level of cost sharing. Somewhat surprisingly, the impact of this kind of change on the optimal level of cost sharing may be to increase the level of cost sharing (and reduce the risk protection benefits from insurance) because better information may lead to stronger moral hazard (Pauly and Blavin 2007).

A more complicated analysis arises if new technology products or services are protected by patent, and a result of spending on research and development. Then the prospective supplier of new technology will have long run increasing returns to scale (because of the high initial R&D cost), and will have some market power once the product becomes available (depending on the terms of patent protection and the presence or absence of close substitutes). The first best optimum here is easy to describe. Think of the quantity of the new product that would have been demanded by informed patients at a user price equal to its marginal cost (for some drugs, this cost could be less than 10 per cent of the simple monopoly market price). Calculate the present discounted value of consumers' surplus at this rate of use over the lifetime of the product, and see if it exceeds the present discounted value of research and development costs. Any potential product that has a positive expected surplus should then be brought to market and any product that does not have a positive surplus should not be offered at all. The problem, of course, is that even if the seller has a legal monopoly through a patent, it may not be able to behave as a perfectly discriminating monopolist who would achieve the first best solution.

Economists have worried about this problem. Lakdawalla and Sood (2004) assumed that a single insurer can arrange all-or-nothing contracts with potential suppliers of new products, and thus achieve a first best outcome. Pauly (2007) and Garber *et al.* (2006) worry that, with insurance and moral hazard, setting user price equal to marginal cost of production, while allowing gross price per unit to be set at the simple monopoly level (given the insurance-affected demand curve) might lead to excess investment in R&D, although whether it would do so or not would depend on the amount of consumers' surplus that would be lost by an inability to perfectly price discriminate. None of these models deal with physician prescriptions and patient compliance. What happens if we add these elements?

Non-compliance will be welfare improving in the first best model, so adding these elements does not alter the main conclusion. It does require that physicians somehow be able to persuade patients who ought to use the drug to use it all the time, and somehow winnow out patients whose net health benefit is positive, but less than the marginal cost.

In the second-best world, but with no non-compliance, the level of insurance coverage (and, hence, the level of cost sharing) will be chosen in competitive insurance markets so that the gross market price times the level of co-insurance always exceeds the marginal cost (Gaynor *et al.* 2000); there will still be under-use relative to the optimum.

Patient cost sharing and compliance are an uncomfortable match. If physician prescribing behaviour is independent of insurance coverage, the only purpose of having patient cost sharing is to cause non-compliance. If, instead, physicians take patient cost sharing into account, even if imperfectly, then cost sharing may reduce moral hazard even if patients comply perfectly. If insurance makes demand (the responsiveness of non-compliance to price) less price responsive, it will allow a higher unit price to be accompanied by welfare improving increases in use. Up to a point, this higher price can help to bring forth new products with positive, but unevenly distributed true health benefits. Into this setting, the addition of new technology with more persuasive or more transparent health benefits may paradoxically require reducing insurance protection, and reducing the incentive to innovate by cutting prices.

The main conclusion of analysis of insurance design that incorporates physician prescribing and patient compliance into the model is that ideal insurance ought to set cost sharing to take both moral hazard and non-compliance arising from patient ignorance of the true marginal benefit schedule into account (Pauly and Blavin 2007). How does this phenomenon interact with the potential availability of new technology?

The new technology, as already noted, may itself have an independent effect on the rate of compliance. For treatments whose benefits were previously under-estimated, the availability of a new technology that patients appreciate means, paradoxically, that the potential for moral hazard increases, and so cost sharing must increase despite its effect of exposing the household to more financial risk. On balance, these negative insurance effects are surely offset by higher levels of real benefit from more appropriate use of the treatments, but the effect on coverage is still noteworthy.

What about the case where patients over-estimate the benefit of treatment? If they can obtain additional care to satisfy their perceived demand, optimal insurance will have to have a higher level of cost sharing. However, there is a constraint; physicians may be unwilling to prescribe treatment that they think will have little benefit. If so, cost sharing can remain low. New technology which patients better understand can relieve the physician of the burden of explaining why he or she is not willing to prescribe something the patient incorrectly believes to be highly effective.

Insurance, physician prescribing, patient compliance, and technological progress

The first best outcome would be to bring to market every technologies whose expected discounted consumer surplus above the marginal cost of production at the optimal quantity exceeds the present discounted value of its research and development cost. For patented new technologies, the price that would prevail in a market setting with no additional government intervention would be the undifferentiated monopoly price, given the insurance-affected demand curve. How will the quantity in this setting compare with that in the uninsured setting? There are offsetting effects: at any given gross price the lower insurance-affected user price will increase the quantity demanded, but if insurance makes the market demand curve less elastic, the gross price will be higher. However, whatever the outcome, the quantity is not certain to be at the first best level, nor will the supplier's profit equal the total consumers' surplus above variable cost. The profit cannot be greater than the consumers' surplus because then the insurer would refuse to cover the service, since making it available would make consumers worse off than if they did not use the product at all.

This is the argument made earlier Pauly (2003). How is it modified by consideration of physician prescribing and patient compliance? Compliance is only an issue if patient demand differs from better informed physician demand. If patient demand does fall short of better informed demand, that would lead to potential under-use of treatment. If product novelty improves compliance in the case of under-use, that would definitely lead to more efficient use of a given treatment. If patient demand exceeds informed demand, the key issue is whether physicians will acquiesce and provide prescriptions for care of low or no benefit. If physicians would prescribe, the higher patient demand would lead to higher profits on these types of care, which might offset the lowered profits for under-demanded care. If firms investing in R&D do not know whether the product that might result from their investment will be over-demanded or under-demanded, there might be no net effect of consideration of prescribing and compliance, depending on the distribution of errors. However, if investors can anticipate future prescribing and compliance, product by product, there will be more investment in R&D for products that are likely to be over-used relative to others. To the extent that new technologies have benefits that are less likely to be biased by patient misinformation, investment will follow a more efficient pattern. It would seem then that any compliance increasing properties of new products (relative to older competitors) will be captured by the innovating firm. Compared with a model in which compliance was the same with new treatments as with old ones, this additional effect will make more new products profitable and those new products will be ones that improve efficiency.

Other models of price setting and cost sharing

In most countries, and even in the United States, holders of patents are often not able to set their prices at the monopoly price level. Instead, large insurers, public and private, negotiate both prices and quantities. For the patent-protected product, the only economic leverage a large insurer has is a threat to refuse to let the product be used by its insurees, or to curtail their use through either cost sharing or managerial limits. The 'triple tier' cost sharing structures that have become dominant in the United States are a good example of insurer counter-pressure.

Of course, if the public insurer sets a low level of cost sharing for political or institutional reasons, then as Zweifel (2003) noted, the form of technological change is likely to be distorted. If consumers benefit little from choosing a lower priced new product, the incentive to invent such products will be blunted. Conversely, if consumers are insulated from prices, they and their physicians may select new technologies that are slightly better in terms of quality, but much higher in terms of price. The solution to this problem, we have noted, is a system of competitive insurers who are free to set their own cost sharing levels (including 100 per cent) for new products. A single public insurer or a set of regulated insurance plans could make the same choices in principle, but whether they will do so or not will depend on politics and not economics.

What effects are such public or private imposed procedures likely to have on the supply of new technology? The most obvious point is that the short-term attractiveness of low prices means that profits may be forced too low to provide efficient incentives for R&D. However, short-term political advantage may be offset by longer-term losses of beneficial new products. However, 'may' is not the same thing as 'will'; it is probably impossible for even a public insurer or regulator to know how to get the balance right. Perhaps the observation that, even without regulation, the rate of flow of new products is likely to be suboptimal suggests attention be directed at too restrictive, rather than too permissive regulatory strategies.

Research may help; it should be possible to determine what the marginal cost of production is for various health care goods and services. If one can also determine the marginal benefit schedule (a more complex task than estimating the single measure of effectiveness as is done in cost effectiveness analysis), one might be able to determine the user price that will lead to the optimal quantity and to the total payment that would cover R&D costs for products that are efficient to introduce. However, for public or private insurers to develop payment policies for the present that yield the right incentives for R&D on products that will appear years if not decades into the future is an enormous task, perhaps exceeded only by the need to develop a reputation of rewarding useful R&D on a sensible basis. That is, the insurer must be thought by investors as willing to set prices and quantities in ways which cover the cost of R&D when it should be covered; we crucially assume that the insurer can refuse to pay for products that are not worth what they cost. This kind of dynamic cost-plus pricing is challenging indeed.

Other issues in the efficiency of technological change and insurance

There are other reasons why the supply of new technology may differ from the optimum that insurance might potentially affect.

◆ *Research as a public good.* The discovery of new knowledge can be very costly in both money and effort, but the diffusion of this knowledge into practical and beneficial applications usually has a very low or zero cost. In this sense, innovative discoveries are public goods and, going back to Schumpeter, economists have been willing to accept the monopoly power implied by patents as a second-best trade-off to encourage the supply and use of new information. However, medical technology is often sold not in a traditional market; in many cases, its price is covered by public or private insurers. In such cases, insurers with large or complete market shares need not accept even a monopoly price as given, but can instead bargain with suppliers of patented medical products over the price in a setting in which the usual threats of withdrawing business can be accompanied by political pressures.

Government insurers around the world generally view it as desirable to negotiate, cajole, or extract lower prices. While such behaviour may benefit current consumers, by reducing expected profits it also reduces the incentive for innovation. If we assume that the terms of patent protection are set to bring for the optimal supply of new technologies in ordinary markets with many buyers, these downward pressures in health technology markets must lead to a suboptimal supply of new technology. If there was a single welfare maximizing world health insurer, that insurer might be expected to take lost innovation into account in negotiating prices for new medical technologies. In fact, many different countries have separate public systems, and so there is a strong tendency—stronger the smaller the country—to engage in free rider behaviour by negotiating lower than globally optimal prices. Even in the United States (with about 50 per cent of global pharmacy revenues), public payers often negotiate low prices, then bemoan the scarcity of new products. This has been most obvious in the market for paediatric vaccines, where the national government is a major buyer in the USA and where, until recently, innovation was low and even seller efforts to assure consistent supply were deficient.

- *Medical arms race.* As already suggested in connection with Zweifel's comment, insurance that is not properly structured can lead to markets that reward technologies of low net value. Even when public policy or private conspiracy forces insurers to offer policies with cost sharing so low that consumers pay little attention to cost, this should still not lead to inefficiently high technical change as long as insurers are able and willing to refuse to cover new technology. In the example of a technology arms race that prevailed in the United States before the advent of managed care, one reason for this phenomenon was that the dominant and government-favoured insurers (the so-called 'Blue' plans) were created by and managed in the interests of hospitals and doctors, who would have had little interest in discouraging technologies that they might be able to profit from. There was (and still is) another impediment to efficient insurance design, however: frequently political regulation and political interests force insurers to cover new technologies while they are still experimental and unproven. Why does this happen? One obvious answer notes that the set of patients and their providers who have the disease for which the new technology might help, even if only a little, are an intense minority and are able to exert political pressure often without opposition. The other impediment to efficient decision-making is a belief on the part of many citizens and politicians that a regulation mandating coverage will impose costs on others—either insurers and their stockholders, or (in the case of self-insured employer provided coverage) on firm owners, rather than on workers. Full transparency that would display the connection between higher insurance benefit payments and larger reductions in consumer incomes from high premiums often does not exist.

- *Imperfect information about medical benefits.* If consumer-patients have systematically incorrect views of the net benefits of new technologies, the rate of introduction will obviously be non-optimal. Upward-biased estimates of benefits lead to too much technology, while downward biased estimates cause there to be too little innovation. Examples of both phenomena can be cited, and it is not possible to judge what the overall effect is. There is evidence that patients are more willing to comply with physician advice when it involves a technology that is new, so there may be a partial offset here (with previous under-compliance, another takeaway might be with systematic under-use, the incentives to overinvest due to moral hazard are not as large). Insurers are now being urged to use the level of cost sharing to foster use of those technologies where benefits are under-estimated and discourage the use of technologies where benefits are over-estimated, but it will take a long while for such changes to actually make a difference to the flow. Information imperfection can lead to another kind of influence: sellers of new technologies may find that direct to consumer (DTC) advertising can increase demand and possibly reduce its price elasticity, allowing more technologies to be profitable. There is, however, an offsetting effect: insurers may seek to hide the benefits of costly new technology (at least in the short term) in order to avoid paying out more as benefits rise. DTC advertising has grown in the United States; we know that one reason was a change in the law that made such advertising permissible. Regulation and law both forbid false advertising, but do not prevent correct, but selective presentation of information. To some extent, there is reason to believe DTC advertising represents an attempt to counter incentives and policies used by managed care insurers to limit their payment for costly new services. It is surely likely that consumers have become sceptical consumers of both advertising by sellers of products that selectively emphasize their benefits, and advertising by insurance plans that boast of their trustworthiness and interest in quality of care.

♦ *Heterogeneity of preferences.* It is highly likely that households differ on the values they attach to new technologies, and on the kind of evidence they would require before wanting to have access to an experimental treatment or process. Probably, the value of technology increases with income, but there are almost surely additional differences in taste that are large enough to matter. Finally, the extent of variation in values probably varies across countries, which surely differ in the extent to which incomes vary and perhaps differ, as well on the size of variation in tastes for novelty and risk-benefit trade-offs.

In principle, markets could deal better with such variation in preferences than could public programmes, precisely because, as long as economies of scale are not large, markets can efficiently offer a wide variety of options, whereas collective provision and collective choice almost always leads to greater uniformity. However, although the US market would appear to permit such product differentiation in insurance, at present there are generally not competing plans that offer different innovation adoption strategies at different prices. The insurance plan that will pay for any new technology patients and physicians desire would have to carry a high premium and potentially exhibit high rates of premiums growth, while more limited and limiting plans (potentially basing their technology choice on the kind of cost effectiveness measures not favoured by many public systems) could offer coverage with premiums that are lower and grow more slowly (Pauly 2005). Perhaps the absence of such variety is due to the difficulty of marketing plans that are explicitly constraining; the backlash against managed care plans has surely made insurers apprehensive about promising cost containment if it has to be accompanied by some imposed limitations on the use of resources. However, since the current growth patterns in premiums for private US insurance plans are unsustainable, those plans will either need to discover a so far overlooked model to greatly improve their efficiency or will eventually offer plans that cost less and do less.

Conclusion

New technology is probably the single most important defining characteristic of modern medical care systems and the insurances that pay for them, but the efficiency of the patterns of technology adoption that are exhibited by both public and market plans may be questioned. One reason for potential inefficiency and certain confusion is that we have no well-developed and tested models of medical choices when physician prescribe and patients comply; in this chapter we have offered some thoughts about how to model such an interaction, and we have linked it to the empirical observation that patient compliance tends to be greater for newer technologies than for older ones.

The other theme in this paper as that, as long as market insurers are permitted to choose *not* to cover new technologies, the rate of introduction of new technology that would prevail in such settings can never be too high. In contrast, there is a large number of reasons why the rate of addition of beneficial, but costly new technology can be too low in systems with competitive insurance plans or with public plans. Against this theoretical proposition we must set the visceral political feeling in most countries that spending growth must be reined in, no matter what. We outline a possible market arrangement to achieve that goal, but we anticipate a greater deal of anxiety and turmoil before any effective solutions to the problem of structuring insurance coverage of new technologies is achieved.

References

Armantier O, Namoro S (2006). Prescription drug advertising and patient compliance: a physician agency approach. *Advances in Economic Analysis & Policy*, **6**(1). Available at: http://www.bepress.com/bejeap/advances/vol6/iss1/art5 (accessed 3 March 2008).

Baumgardner JR (1988). Physicians' services and the division of labor across local markets. *Journal of Political Economy*, **96**, 948–82.

Bloom B (1998). Continuation of initial antihypertensive medication after one year of therapy. *Clinical Therapeutics*, **20**, 671–81.

Cutler DM (2004). *Your money or your life: strong medicine for America's health care system*. New York, Oxford University Press.

Cutler DM and McClellan M (2001). Is technological change in medicine worth it? *Health Affairs*, **20**(5), 11–29.

Degli Esposti E, Sturani A, Di Martino M, *et al.* (2002). Long-term persistence with antihypertensive drugs in new patients. *Journal of Human Hypertension*, **16**(6), 439–44.

Ellickson P, Stern S and Trajtenberg M (1999). *Patient welfare and patient compliance: an empirical framework for measuring the benefits from pharmaceutical innovation*, NBER Working Paper No. 6890. Available at: http://papers.nber.org/papers/w6890 (accessed 3 March 2008).

Finkelstein A (2004). Static and dynamic effects of health policy: evidence from the vaccine industry. *Quarterly Journal of Economics*, **119**, 527–64.

Garber A, Jones C and Romer P (2006). Insurance and incentives for medical innovation – Biomedical research and the economy, Article 4. *Forum for Health Economics & Policy*, **9**(2). Available at: http://www.bepress.com/fhep/biomedical_research/4/ (accessed 3 March 2008).

Gaynor M, Haas-Wilson D and Vogt WB (2000). Are invisible hands good hands? Moral hazard, competition, and the second-best in health care markets. *Journal of Political Economy*, **108**, 992–1005.

Goddeeris JH (1984). Medical insurance, technological change, and welfare. *Economic Inquiry*, **22**, 56–67.

Lakdawalla D, Sood N (2004). Social insurance and the design of innovation incentives. *Economics Letters*, **85**, 57–61.

McGuire TG (2000). Physician agency. In: AJ Culyer and JP Newhouse, eds. *Handbook of health economics*, Vol. 1A. Amsterdam, North-Holland/Elsevier Science.

McGuire TG and Pauly MV (1991). Physician response to fee changes with multiple payers. *Journal of Health Economics*, **10**, 385–410.

Monane M, Bohn RL, Gurwitz JH, Glynn RJ, Levin R and Avorn J (1997). The effects of initial drug choice and comorbidity on antihypertensive therapy compliance: results from a population-based study in the elderly. *American Journal of Hypertension*, **10**, 697–704.

Pauly MV (2003). Market insurance, public insurance, and the rate of technological change in medical care. *Geneva Papers on Risk & Insurance - Issues & Practice*, **28**, 180–93.

Pauly, MV (2005). Competition and new technology. *Health Affairs*, **24**, 1523–35.

Pauly MV (2007). Measures of costs and benefits for drugs in cost effectiveness analysis. In: FA Sloan and CR Hsieh, eds. *Pharmaceutical innovation: incentives, competition, and cost-benefit analysis in international perspective*, pp. 199–214. New York, Cambridge University Press.

Pauly MV and Blavin FE (2007). Value based cost sharing meets the theory of moral hazard: medical effectiveness in insurance benefits design, NBER Working Paper No. 13044. Available at: http://www.nber.org/papers/w13044 (accessed 3 March 2008).

Wannemacher AJ, Schepers GP and Townsend KA (2002). Antihypertensive medication compliance in a veterans affairs healthcare system. *Annals of Pharmacotherapy*, **36**, 986–91.

Zweifel P (2003). Medical innovation: a challenge to society and insurance. *Geneva Papers on Risk & Insurance - Issues & Practice*, **28**, 194–202.

Chapter 6

Technological change and health insurance*

Peter Zweifel

Introduction and motivation

This chapter argues that there is a dual causal link between technological change and insurance. On the one hand, technological change often presents new opportunities, but also challenges to insurers. However, what has been rarely recognized up to now is that insurance also may induce technological change, in the guise of both product innovation and process innovation. Therefore, the aim of this chapter is as follows. In the first part, the impact of innovation on insurance in general will be discussed with emphasis then changing to innovation in medicine and its impact on health insurance. The second half of the chapter is devoted to the reverse causal relationship, again starting with the feedback from insurance to innovation, in general, and ending with the feedback from health insurance to technological change in medicine. Figure 6.1 illustrates the structure of the chapter.

General technological change and its impact on insurance in general

The impact of product and process innovation (the latter often called technological change) on insurance has been the subject of *The limits to certainty* (Giarini and Stahel 1993), emphasizing the vulnerability of a society that relies on an ever-increasing degree of division of labour. Indeed, the division of labour with its new ways of organizing production is very much driven by process innovation, which means that the same goods or service are to be produced at a lower cost. Vulnerability is the consequence of an increasing number of agents being involved in the process of value creation. If one of them fails, the process is stalled, calling for risk management and potentially creating a demand for insurance coverage. Since the objective is to produce at lower cost, i.e. faster as a rule, process interruptions become more costly, motivating additional risk management. The challenge to insurers is to find ways to deal with this type of risk, rather than routinely excluding it as *force majeure*. Turning to product innovation, a consumer product is bestowed with changed or new attributes. However, some of these new features may be unfamiliar to consumers, possibly causing damage

* Excellent research assistance was provided by Patrick Eugster (University of Zurich).

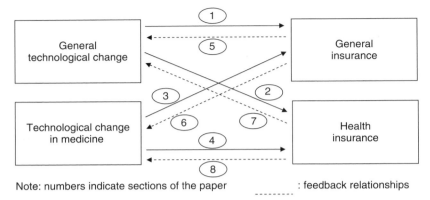

Note: numbers indicate sections of the paper   - - - - - - - : feedback relationships

Fig. 6.1 Relationships between innovation and insurance.

or injury. They thus give rise to the risk of product liability, which in turn may be met by pertinent insurance coverage.

Conclusion 1

Both types of innovation—process and product—may trigger the demand for several types of insurance.

The impact of general technological change on health insurance

Both product and process innovation have effects specifically on health insurance. Historically, process innovation changed the nature of the workplace. Many of the illnesses at the time were caused by work-related health risks. The original aim of health insurance was to secure an income to workers who fell ill and were not able to work. Process innovation has been modifying (in the main reducing) these risks. In addition, product innovation resulting in new consumer products may pose health risks. On the one hand, these changes serve to increase the demand for health insurance coverage. On the other hand, they challenge insurers because they cause the probability of illness to increase, possibly calling for costly medical treatment.

Apart from this direct effect, innovation has an indirect effect on health insurance. The argument is due to old-age longevity and mortality-contingent claims (Philipson and Becker 1998). It establishes a spillover from the provision for old-age (which itself depends on innovation) to health insurance (see Fig. 6.2).

If capital is paid out when a life insurance matures, the beneficiaries have to weigh two things against each other. On the one hand, an increase in remaining life duration implies a decreasing per-period consumption, as shown by the transformation curve $K'K$. If an annuity or a pension benefit is paid (as is typical of today's collective systems), this trade-off is much less pronounced. By surviving for one more year, beneficiaries obtain an additional year's pension (resulting in the transformation curve $R'R$). Now consider the reference point Q^*, which can be reached under both variants.

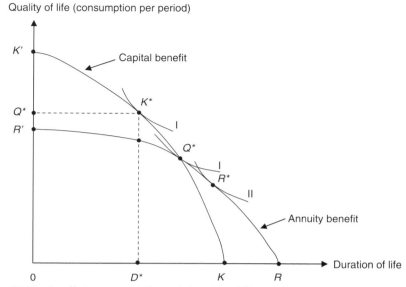

Fig. 6.2 Trade-offs between quality and duration of life.

Let there be two types of individuals (depicted by two indifference curve systems). Type I would prefer K^* and would want to opt for the capital benefit. However, in the context of today's social security, this alternative usually is not available. Therefore, individuals of type I are constrained to be at Q^*. Now consider type II, who is more interested in long life. Given the availability of collective old-age provision, type II individuals move away from Q^* to point R^*, trying to achieve a longer duration of life. However, in order to spend their additional life years in good health, these individuals will rely heavily on medical services and, hence, have a high demand for health insurance. In this way, innovation outside the health care sector has both direct and indirect effects, notably on health insurance.

Conclusion 2

General innovation both of the product and the process type has both a direct and an indirect effect on health insurance. The direct one is due to possible health effects of innovation, while the indirect one works through a heightened interest in long life and, hence, medical care induced by collective provision for old-age.

Technological change in medicine and its impact on insurance in general

To see that innovation in medicine may have effects that impact on insurance quite generally, consider an innovation that adds to the longevity of people. This means that individuals might work longer, exerting additional demand for insurance against workplace accidents. However, they also will be active longer as consumers (with implications for a product liability, travel, and homeowner's insurance). A major problem facing insurers in this context is selection. Those workers and consumers carrying on are not representative of the general population. Indeed, the mere fact that they are more active than average may make them more likely to cause damage. Another influence comes from the 'medicalization' of the 'production of health' that probably goes along with innovation in medicine. The concomitant growth of the health care sector puts particular pressure on public budgets (Zweifel *et al.* 2006). This means that, for example, investment in infrastructure is pushed back, with clear implications for building insurance.

Conclusion 3

Innovation in medicine has effects on insurance in general, which typically are of the indirect type.

Technological change in medicine and its impact on health insurance

Innovation in medicine is usually of the product type (for reasons that will become clear in the section leading up to Conclusion 8). As such, it induces more demand for (typically more costly) treatment and also health insurance. The challenge to health insurers is that with each additional product comes an ex post moral hazard effect. This effect can be illustrated as follows (see Fig. 6.3).

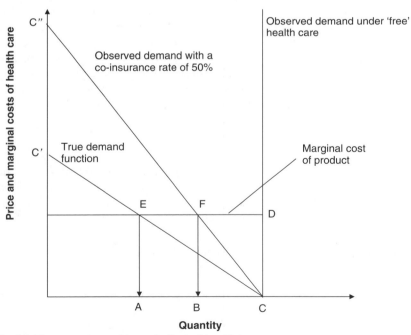

Fig. 6.3 The ex post moral hazard effect of health insurance.

Assuming that consumers' willingness to pay out-of-pocket for a medical service or product is approximately given by the linear demand function $C'C$ shown in Fig. 6.3, in the case of health insurance with a 50 per cent co-insurance rate, maximum willingness to pay is doubled, from C' to C''. More generally, the demand function is rotated outward to become the effective demand function CC''. The lower the rate of co-insurance, the more pronounced this rotation. With no co-payment at all (as is often the case with tax-funded schemes), the curve runs fully vertical from C.

Therefore, the market equilibrium shifts from point E to F, with a higher quantity of the service or product transacted. The benefits to be paid increase, resulting in an ex post moral hazard effect. In the long-term, this causes the premium to increase, creating a negative income effect (shifting the demand curve inward) that is neglected for simplicity.

The moral hazard effect is of relevance to the choice of benefit package because it comes to bear with each additional item in the package. The more complete the package, the larger the loading component in the gross premium and, hence, the larger the net cost of insurance. Therefore, moral hazard considerations should lead an insurer to exercise caution in expanding the package. Specifically, it would want to add services characterized by low price elasticity of demand because the moral hazard effect is more limited in this case. In Fig. 6.1, lower price elasticity means that, for a given maximum willingness to pay such as C', the demand function runs steeper, causing point C to shift towards the origin. This serves to reduce the difference between the true and the observed demand curve, and hence the size of the ex post moral hazard effect. Indeed, modelling health insurance as a two-part pricing scheme that levies a price on access to medical innovation, while subsidizing its use (Ladawalla and Sood 2005) find that, in a social optimum, insurance coverage cannot be complete.

Conclusion 4

Innovation in medicine being mainly of the product innovation type, causes the demand for health insurance to increase, but also aggravates ex post moral hazard.

If the innovator yields a monopoly, however, ex post moral hazard can be beneficial because insurance coverage corrects the monopolist's tendency towards undersupply (Crew 1969). Extending this argument to dynamic efficiency (i.e. the likelihood that innovation in fact occurs), Garber et al. (2006) show that depending on the price elasticity of demand, there is an upper limit to the monopoly price beyond which the innovation ceases to convey a net benefit to society. To derive this result, they need to posit a distribution function of benefits. The model to be presented in Section 5 is distribution free; on the other hand, it only permits prediction of the behaviour of a firm that has to weigh product against process innovation.

The impact of general insurance on technological change in general

This section deals with the feedback effects displayed in Fig. 6.1. The impact of general insurance on innovation in general is a topic that has been little researched. In the pertinent literature, the emphasis has been very much on moral hazard effects of insurance coverage. However, insurance also is a facilitator of innovation in general. Indeed, one may argue that without insurance, many innovations would not be performed because of their risk. An early example, given by Zweifel (1987), has been adapted to the present context.

In Fig. 6.4, a decision situation is depicted, relating to a management that thinks of launching a new product, but considers the risk of being sued for product liability. The decision tree is as follows. The main decision is whether or not to invest $480 m in medical innovation, rather than in securities. At present $ 480 m can be considered a fair estimate of the cost of developing a new drug (relying on estimates for a new pharmaceutical product; see Grabowski *et al.* 2002; DiMasi *et al.* 2003). Let the planning horizon be 20 years, a realistic value for the pharmaceutical industry. The present value of a $480 m investment in securities at 6 per cent real interest and discounted at 3 per cent is $852 m. In case of unfavourable economic development, let the real rate

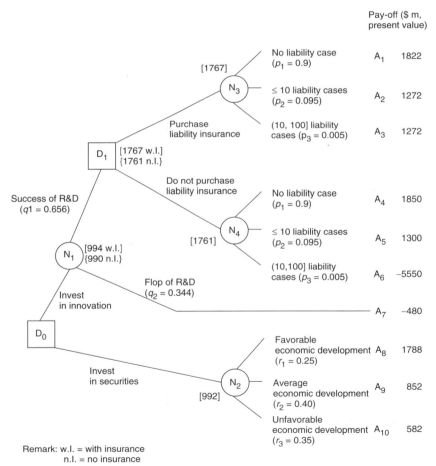

Fig. 6.4 Economic viability of an innovation through product liability insurance.

of return drop to 4 per cent. Together with a 3 per cent discount rate, the present value becomes $582 m. Given a favourable development (10 per cent real, discounted at 3 per cent), it even attains $1788 m. With assumed probabilities (0.35, 0.40, 0.25), the expected value of this investment is $992 m (see N_2).

In the case of an investment in the new product, a flop would cause the whole investment to be lost (see A_7). However, assuming that a breakthrough occurs in the market, very high returns can be achieved, always provided there are no cases of liability (nodes A_1 and A_4, respectively). Let the innovator estimate the probability of this favourable outcome $p_1 = 0.9$; the achievable present value of returns is $1850 m ($A_4$). This is an estimate for the top two percentiles taken from Grabowski *et al.* (2002). Also, let there be a 9.5 per cent probability associated with the maximum of 10 liability cases (uniformly distributed) that cause returns to be reduced by $100 m per case to an expected $1300 m (see A_5). However, there is a remaining risk of 0.5 per cent that the company is successfully sued, making the innovation a bad investment (pay-off equal to –$5550 m at node A_6 in Fig. 6.4.

However, the innovator can purchase liability insurance for insurable claims, which is assumed to be of the stop loss type. Let this mean that the first 10 claims (at $100 m each by assumption) must be borne by the innovator itself; beyond this limit, claims will be settled by the insurer. The fair premium for this coverage, given a uniform probability density, amounts to $27.75 m [= (100 + 11)/2 · 100 m · 0.005], which have been deducted from pay-offs A_4 to A_6 to yield pay-offs A_1 to A_3.

Considering the decision tree of Fig. 6.4 and using the criterion of maximum expected present value (appropriate for a risk-neutral investor), the innovator will first compare the chance nodes N_3 and N_4. On average, it pays to have liability insurance because the expected pay-off is $1767 m, compared with $ 1,761 m without insurance. After having made this conditional decision, the innovator will work back to the decision note D_1, to see that expected profit due to the innovation is $1767 m in present value. However, this node will be reached only with probability $q_1 = 0.656$ [= $1 - 0.344 = 1 - (6/7)^7$], because for one successful innovation in the pharmaceutical industry, there traditionally have been seven failures (Hansen 1979; for a more recent and somewhat more favourable estimate, see DiMasi *et al.* 2003). This causes the present value of the profit in the case of investment to shrink to $994 m, which just about suffices to have an edge on investment in security that amounts to $992 m.

However, if there had not been the possibility of buying liability insurance for product liability, then the expected pay-off at N_1 would only be 990 m, which is below the value at the other node N_2 ($992 m) in case of an investment in securities. Therefore, insurance achieves a stabilization of the income stream from an innovation whereas without insurance, innovation would lose out against an investment in (e.g. business interruption) securities. Clearly, other types of insurance (e.g. business interruption) have a similar effect, encouraging innovation.

More generally, the decision-making situation of an innovator weighing a product against a process innovation can be described as follows:

$$\max_{i,e} E\Pi = \pi\{Y(i) - C(e)\} + (1 - \pi)\{\overline{Y} + I(i) - C(e)\} - P(\lambda, i, e) - i - e$$

with EΠ as expected profit. In the probability of success in the sense of having no liability, Y revenue if successful, depending positively on product innovation effort (= expenditure) i, C production cost depending negatively on process innovation effort (expenditure) e, l insurance benefit, P premium, and λ loading on premiums. Comparative static analysis (see Appendix) yields the predictions:

$$\frac{di}{d\lambda} < 0 \text{ in general};$$

$$= 0 \text{ if } \lambda \to \infty \text{ and } Y(i) \to \infty.$$

Therefore, the existence of insurance or its availability at lower cost ($d\lambda < 0$) encourages product innovation almost certainly. With regard to process innovation, one obtains

$$\frac{de}{d\lambda} < 0 \text{ in general};$$

$$= 0 \text{ if } Y(i) \to \infty$$

$$> 0 \text{ if } \pi \to 1 \text{ or } I \to 0.$$

Therefore, the availability of less costly insurance ($d\lambda < 0$) does not encourage process innovation under all circumstances. In particular, it may even hamper it if the probability of success is high anyway or if insurance coverage is very limited initially.

Conclusion 5

Insurance coverage may encourage both product and process innovation, but usually favours product innovation, possibly to the detriment of process innovation.

The impact of general insurance on technological change in medicine

Innovation in medicine is especially risky if it is of the breakthrough type. The reason is that authorities deciding on admission do not usually reflect trade-offs in preference to patients with regard to product attributes. Rather, the innovation must dominate incumbent products on all counts; this holds true of pharmaceutical and biomedical innovation in particular (Zweifel *et al.* 2008, chapter 12). The claim that patients trade-off between attributes can be substantiated using the (admittedly very mundane) example of hip protectors. Some 520 elderly Swiss participated in a market experiment of the discrete choice type in 1996 (Telser and Zweifel 2007). From their repeated stated choices between the status quo and a hip protector with varying attributes, among them an out-of-pocket price, the willingness to pay values shown in Table 6.1 could be inferred. Now a typical authority can be expected to exclusively value the protective effect of a hip protector. Consumers also value this attribute highly in that they are willing to pay $3.35 for a one percentage point reduction in the probability of breaking their femur. Therefore, an existing product reducing this probability by 50 per cent triggers a willingness to pay of US$168, *ceteris paribus*. However, other attributes, such as ease of handling and wearing comfort, are of

Table 6.1 Marginal willingness to pay (WTP) for hip protectors, in US$

Product attribute	Marginal WTP	SD
Protective effect (PROT)	3.35	0.71
Ease of handling (HAND)	56.96	15.25
Wearing comfort (COMF)	122.93	23.59
Status quo bias	−685.84	68.54

importance to consumers as well. Specifically, consider the producer of a hip protector who can promise only a 25 per cent risk reduction, but an improvement of wearing comfort by 1 point on a 1–4 scale. Overall, its innovation has the higher willingness to pay than the incumbent product since the negative effect of reduced protection ($-84 = 25 \cdot 3.35$) is more than neutralized by the advantage of better wearing comfort ($123 = 1 \cdot 123$). Nevertheless, a typical authority would reject the innovation on the grounds that it fails to increase medical effectiveness.

While general insurance cannot mitigate this crucial risk facing innovators, it may at least relieve them from other risks. For example, many production processes in the pharmaceutical industry can have detrimental effects on the environment due to toxic smoke and effluents. Environmental impairment liability insurance may play a similar role as product liability insurance. Thus, the example depicted in Fig. 6.4 can be used again to show that insurance coverage not related to health (environmental impairment liability coverage in this instance) may make investment in a medical innovation worthwhile. Since insurance coverage causes this decision to be made differently, one has a moral hazard effect here. However, the change being advantageous for society in this instance, one could speak of a 'benign moral hazard effect', to paraphrase a term coined by Pauly and Held (1990).

Conclusion 6

General insurance probably has an encouraging impact on technological change in medicine.

The impact of health insurance on technological change in general

Although this relationship has hardly ever been addressed by research, it is likely for health insurance to have an influence on innovation in general. It suffices to consider the fact that many inventions are marketed by a small or medium enterprise. If inventors, acting as independent workers, were not covered by health insurance, they would be less likely to engage in their highly risky activity because their economic survival would be very quickly threatened by a spell of illness. Figure 6.4 can be used to illustrate after the pertinent modifications. Its lower part need not be changed, except for pay-offs, in the tens of thousand, rather than millions. In its upper part, the issue is now to purchase supplementary health, rather than liability insurance, noting that outside the United States, the purchase of basic health insurance is mandatory. Supplementary coverage then could be for days in a clinic that has no contract with social health insurance. Accordingly, let there be a 0.9 probability of no hospital stay during the coming year (node A_4). The probability of up to 10 days in one of these (expensive) clinics is 0.095 costing \$55,000 [= (1850 − 1300), the unit of account now being \$100 in Fig. 6.4] without insurance. However, with a probability of 0.005, a costly treatment lasting up to 100 days may be necessary, amounting to \$740,000 [= {= [1850 − (−5550)]}, see node A_6] without insurance. Given supplementary insurance coverage, however, co-payment is limited to \$10,000 (= 1822 − 1727). Therefore, with (supplementary) health insurance, the expected value of engaging in innovation is \$99,400 (see node N_1). Without insurance coverage, the \$99,000 would not have been sufficient to motivate the individual to become an innovator. Therefore, health insurance tips the balance in favour of innovation in this example.

However, it should be noted that the effect of health insurance may even be larger than indicated by the difference in expected pay-offs (\$99,400 −99,000). Contrary to the owners of an established company in the previous liability insurance example, here the decision maker considered has his or her assets invested in that one R&D project. Due to this lack of risk diversification, risk aversion plays a role, but for a risk-averse decision maker, pay-offs ranging between \$185,000 (node A_4 of Figure 4) and \$555,000 (node A_6) in the case of innovation without health insurance quite likely would compare unfavourably with securities, where pay-offs range between \$178,000 (node A_8) and \$58,200 (node A_{10}), whereas pay-offs between \$182,200 (node A_1) and \$127,200 (node A_3), associated with health insurance, are quite acceptable. Therefore, the beneficial effect of health insurance can be considerably stronger than indicated by the mere difference in expected financial pay-offs when it comes to individual innovators.

Conclusion 7

Health insurance may well have an accelerating effect on innovation in general, although the magnitude of its effect is unknown.

The impact of health insurance on technological change in medicine

The very existence of health insurance imparts a bias in favour of product innovation to the health care sector, with cost-saving process innovation getting short thrift. To illustrate this statement as well as the model underlying Fig. 6.3, let health insurance be of the conventional type, with (small) co-payment. Its effect can be seen from the following example (Table 6.2). Initially, let the maximum willingness to pay of a patient be \$20 for an innovation, e.g. a new drug. With a rate of co-payment of 10 per cent, the price of the drug may be as high \$200 because in that case, the out-pocket-cost to the patient is precisely \$20. Moreover, assume that the actual purchase and administration of the drug uses 1 h worth of patient time, valued at \$30. Therefore, initially the effective cost of the therapy is \$50 to the insured patient.

Table 6.2 Medical innovation and effective cost to the insured

Product	US$
Existing	
Willingness to pay of insured (assumed)	20
Maximum price of product on the market (assumed rate of co-insurance 10 per cent	200
Time cost to patient (assumed 1 h at US$30)	30
Total effective cost to patient	50
Innovation	
Maximum willingness to pay of insured (assumed)	25
Maximum price of product on the market (assumed rate of co-insurance of 10 per cent)	250
Time cost to patient (assumed 0.5 h at US$30)	15
Total effective cost to patient	40

Now let there be a product innovation, with two effects. First, patients' maximum willingness to pay increases to $25, for example, in view of improved quality attributes. Accordingly, the market price of the drug may rise to a maximum of $250. For simplicity, assume that the innovator actually charges that price. Secondly, another improved feature of the drug may well be its less frequent administration, saving patients one-half of their time by assumption. Accordingly, taking the new drug entails a time cost of $15 rather than $30 initially.

In this example, the drug's total effective cost to the patient decreases from $50 to 40. Therefore, more patients are likely to demand the product innovation. At the same time, its money price (which must be reimbursed by health insurance) has increased, from $180 (90 per cent of $200) to $225 (90 per cent of $250). This simple example may explain why health insurers are so nervous about medical innovation (Zweifel 2003).

Conclusion 8

Health insurance has a clear feedback effect on technological change in medicine, impacting a bias in favour of product, rather than cost-saving process innovation.

Concluding remarks

The basic argument of this contribution is that both product and process innovation are not exogenous to insurance, contradicting the widespread notion innovation just happens regardless of insurance coverage. For instance, many of today's innovations would not occur or be delayed if product liability insurance were not available. In turn, it is, of course, true that new products may create risks that trigger a demand for liability insurance or health insurance by their users. The most prominent example of this interrelationship is health insurance. Even today, most health insurers conceive of technological change in medicine (and especially biomedical innovation these days) as a threat to the financial viability of their business because it almost always causes health care expenditure to increase. They tend to overlook the fact that patients who are protected by health insurance coverage are much more likely to opt for the new, more costly treatment alternative. The new alternative is more costly because physicians, hospitals, pharmaceutical companies, and medical innovators are aware of patients' choices, causing them to compete with product innovation rather than price. Therefore, when launching a new, more comprehensive policy, health insurers may be well advised to take this dynamic moral hazard effect into account. However, they should also heed the latent (true) willingness to pay for innovation of their clients, which may be substantial. As a piece of indirect evidence, Zweifel *et al.* (2006) found, using discrete choice experiments, that Swiss consumers would have to be compensated to the tune of 30 per cent of the average contribution to social health insurance for accepting a delay of just 3 years in their access to medical innovation.

References

Crew M (1969). Coinsurance and the welfare economics of medical care. *American Economic Review*, 59, 906–8.

DiMasi J, *et al.* (2003). The price of innovation: news estimates of drug development costs. *Journal of Health Economics*, **22**, 150–85.

Garber AM, Jones RI and Romer P (2006). Insurance and incentives for medical innovation. *Forum for Health Economics and Policy*, 9(2).

Giarini O and Stahel W (1993). *The limits to certainty*, 2nd edn. Dordrecht, Kluwer.

Grabowski HG, Vernon J and DiMasi JA (2002). Returns on research and development for 1990s new drug introductions. *PharmacoEconomics* 20(Supplement 3), 11–29.

Hansen RW (1979). The pharmaceutical development process: estimate of current development costs and times and the effects of regulatory change. In: RI Chien, eds. *Issues in pharmaceutical economics*, pp. 151–87. Lexington, Lexington Books.

Ladawalla D and Sood N (2005). *Insurance and innovation in health care markets*, NBER Working Paper 11602. Cambridge, MA, National Bureau of Economic Research.

Pauly MV and Held (1990). Benign moral hazard and the cost-effectiveness analysis of insurance coverage. *Journal of Health Economics*, 9, 447–61.

Philipson TJ and Becker GS (1998). Old-age longevity and mortality-contingent claims. *Journal of Political Economy*, **106**, 551–73.

Telser H and Zweifel P (2007). Validity of Discrete choice experiments: evidence for health risk reduction. *Applied Economics*, **39**, 69–78.

Zweifel P (1987). Was ist Versicherung? – Funktionelle und institutionelle Aspekte (What is insurance? functional and institutional aspects). In: Gesamtverband der Deutschen Versicherungswirtschaft, ed. *Was ist Versicherung?* pp. 38–61. Köln.

Zweifel P (2003). Medical innovation: a challenge to society and insurance. *Geneva Papers on Risk and Insurance, Issues and Practice*, **28**, 194–202.

Zweifel P, Breyer F and Kifmann M (2008). *Health economics*, 2nd edn. Boston, Springer.

Zweifel P, Telser H and Vaterlaus S (2006). Consumer resistance against regulation: the case of health care. *Journal of Regulatory Economics*, 29, 329–32.

Appendix: formal model of innovating firm

$$\max_{i,e} E\Pi = \pi\{Y(i) - C(e)\} + (1-\pi)\{\overline{Y} + I(i) - C(e)\} - P(\lambda,i,e) - i - e.$$

[A.1]

Where $E\Pi$ is expected profit, π is probability of success/no liability, i is innovative effort (at the price of 1), $Y(i)$ is the revenue if success/no liability, C production cost, $\overline{Y}$ is the revenue if innovation triggers liability, e is the cost-reducing effort, I is the insurance benefit, P is insurance premium, and λ is the loading contained in premium.

The first order condition (FOC) w. r. t. innovative effort reads

$$\frac{\partial E\Pi}{\partial i} = \pi\frac{\partial Y}{\partial i} + (1-\pi)\frac{\partial I}{\partial i} - \frac{\partial P}{\partial i}(\lambda,i,e) - 1 = 0.$$

[A.2]

The first order condition w. r. t. cost-reducing effort is given by

$$\frac{\partial E\Pi}{\partial e} = -\pi\frac{\partial C}{\partial e} - (1-\pi)\frac{\partial C}{\partial e} - \frac{\partial P}{\partial e}(\lambda,i,e) - 1 = 0.$$

[A.3]

The two conditions can be rewritten in terms of elasticities,

$$\pi\left(\frac{\partial Y}{\partial i}\frac{i}{Y}\right) + (1-\pi)\left(\frac{\partial I}{\partial i}\frac{i}{I}\right)\frac{I(i)}{Y(i)} - \left(\frac{\partial P}{\partial i}\frac{i}{P}\right)\frac{P(\lambda,i,e)}{Y(i)} - \frac{i}{Y(i)} = 0$$

[A.4]

$$-\left(\frac{\partial C}{\partial e}\frac{e}{C}\right)\frac{C(e)}{e} - \left(\frac{\partial P}{\partial e}\frac{e}{P}\right)\frac{P(\lambda,i,e)}{e} - 1 = 0.$$

[A.5]

In the following, the elasticities

$$\varepsilon(Y,i) := \left(\frac{\partial Y}{\partial i}\right)\left(\frac{i}{Y}\right), \quad \varepsilon(I,i) := \left(\frac{\partial I}{\partial i}\right)\left(\frac{i}{I}\right), \quad \varepsilon(P,i) = \left(\frac{\partial P}{\partial i}\right)\left(\frac{i}{P}\right),$$

$$\varepsilon(C,e) := \left(\frac{\partial C}{\partial e}\right)\left(\frac{e}{C}\right) \text{ and } \varepsilon(P,e) := \left(\frac{\partial P}{\partial e}\right)\left(\frac{e}{P}\right)$$

are treated as constant.

Now let the FOCs [A.4] and [A.5] be disturbed by a shock $d\lambda > 1050$ (insurance coverage becoming more expensive). This yields

$$
\begin{bmatrix}
(1-\pi)\cdot\varepsilon(I,i)\cdot\dfrac{\dfrac{\partial I}{\partial i}Y-I\dfrac{\partial Y}{\partial i}}{Y^2} & \varepsilon(P,i)\cdot\dfrac{\dfrac{\partial P}{\partial e}}{Y} \\[2em]
-\varepsilon(P,i)\cdot\dfrac{\dfrac{\partial P}{\partial i}Y-P\dfrac{\partial Y}{\partial i}}{Y^2}-\dfrac{Y-\dfrac{\partial Y}{\partial i}\cdot i}{Y^2} & \\[2em]
-\varepsilon(P,e)\cdot\dfrac{\dfrac{\partial P}{\partial i}}{e} & -\varepsilon(C,e)\cdot\dfrac{\dfrac{\partial C}{\partial e}e-C}{e^2} \\[2em]
& \varepsilon(P,e)\cdot\dfrac{\left[\dfrac{\partial P}{\partial e}\cdot e-P\right]}{e^2}
\end{bmatrix}
\begin{bmatrix} di \\[3em] de \end{bmatrix}
=
\begin{bmatrix} \varepsilon(P,i)\cdot\dfrac{\partial P}{\partial\lambda}\cdot\dfrac{1}{Y} \\[3em] \varepsilon(P,e)\cdot\dfrac{\partial P}{\partial\lambda}\cdot\dfrac{1}{e} \end{bmatrix}
d\lambda
$$

[A.6]

Using elasticity notation once more, one obtains

$$
\begin{bmatrix}
(1-\pi)\cdot\varepsilon(I,i)\cdot\dfrac{\varepsilon(I,i)I-\varepsilon(Y,i)\cdot I}{Y\cdot i} & -\varepsilon(P,i)\cdot\varepsilon(P,e)\cdot\dfrac{P}{e\cdot Y} \\[2em]
-\varepsilon(P,i)\cdot\dfrac{\varepsilon(P,e)P-\varepsilon(Y,i)P}{Y\cdot i}-\dfrac{1-\varepsilon(Y,i)}{Y} & \\[2em]
-\dfrac{\varepsilon(P,e)\cdot\varepsilon(P,i)C\cdot P}{e\cdot i} & -\varepsilon(C,e)\cdot\dfrac{\varepsilon(C,e)C-C}{e^2} \\[2em]
& -\dfrac{\left[\varepsilon(P,e)\right]^2 P-\varepsilon(P,e)\cdot P}{e^2}
\end{bmatrix}
\begin{bmatrix} di \\[3em] de \end{bmatrix}
=
\begin{bmatrix} \varepsilon(P,i)\cdot\varepsilon(P,\lambda)\cdot\dfrac{P}{\lambda\cdot Y} \\[3em] \varepsilon(P,e)\cdot\varepsilon(P,\lambda)\cdot\dfrac{P}{e\cdot\lambda} \end{bmatrix}
d\lambda
$$

[A.7]

Using Cramer's rule, one can solve this equation system for $\dfrac{di}{d\lambda}$, with $|H|<0$ denoting the value of the determinant of the Hessian,

$$
\frac{di}{d\lambda}=\frac{1}{|H|}
\begin{vmatrix}
\overset{(+)}{\varepsilon(P,i)}\cdot\overset{(+)}{\varepsilon(P,\lambda)}\cdot\dfrac{P}{\lambda\cdot Y} & -\overset{(-)}{\varepsilon(P,i)}\cdot\overset{(-)}{\varepsilon(P,e)}\cdot\dfrac{P}{e\cdot Y} \\[3em]
\overset{(-)}{\varepsilon(P,e)}\cdot\overset{(+)}{\varepsilon(P,\lambda)}\cdot\dfrac{P}{e\cdot\lambda} & -\overset{(+)}{\varepsilon(C,e)}\cdot\dfrac{\left[\overset{(-)}{\varepsilon(C,e)}-1\right]C}{e^2} \\[3em]
& -\dfrac{\left[\overset{(-)}{\varepsilon(P,e)}\right]^2\varepsilon(P,e)P}{e^2}
\end{vmatrix}
$$

[A.8]

The signs entered reflect the assumptions that $|\varepsilon(P,e)|<1$ and that premium P is large in comparison to elasticities. Then, one obtains

$$\frac{di}{d\lambda} < 0 \text{ in general;}$$

$$= 0 \text{ if } \lambda \to \infty \text{ and } Y(i) \to \infty. \qquad [A.9]$$

In full analogy, one can solve for $\dfrac{de}{d\lambda}$, assuming $\varepsilon(I, i) < \varepsilon(Y, i)$,

$$\frac{de}{d\lambda} = \frac{1}{\underset{(-)}{|H|}} \begin{vmatrix} (1-\pi)\cdot\overset{(+)}{\varepsilon(I,i)}\cdot\dfrac{\overset{(-)}{\varepsilon(I,i)I}-\varepsilon(Y,i)\cdot I}{Y\cdot i} & \overset{(+)}{\varepsilon(P,i)}\cdot\overset{(+)}{\varepsilon(P,\lambda)}\cdot\dfrac{P}{\lambda\cdot Y} \\[2em] -\varepsilon(P,i)\cdot\dfrac{\overset{(-)}{\varepsilon(P,e)}P-\overset{(+)}{\varepsilon(Y,i)}P}{Y\cdot i}-\dfrac{1-\overset{(+)}{\varepsilon(Y,i)}}{Y} & \\[2em] -\dfrac{\overset{(-)}{\varepsilon(P,e)}\cdot\overset{(+)}{\varepsilon(P,i)}\cdot P}{e\cdot i} & \overset{(-)}{\varepsilon(P,e)}\cdot\overset{(+)}{\varepsilon(P,\lambda)}\cdot\dfrac{P}{e\cdot\lambda} \end{vmatrix}$$

$$[A.10]$$

From [A.10], one obtains

$$\frac{de}{d\lambda} < 0 \text{ in general;}$$

$$= 0 \text{ if } Y(i) \to \infty$$

$$> 0 \text{ if } I \to \infty \text{ or } i \to \infty \qquad [A.11]$$

Chapter 7

Health insurance and the uptake of new drugs in the United States

Marin Gemmill, Victoria Serra-Sastre, and Joan Costa-Font

Introduction

Other chapters in this book have addressed the mechanisms underlying the process of invention, innovation, and diffusion, and indicated that technological change is an important area of research, particularly given the importance of technology as the main driver of health expenditure growth. In relation to the theories and ideas put forward in other chapters, there is scope to develop additional conceptual and empirical models that extend the analysis of diffusion to areas in which research is still scarce. As pointed out in the chapter by Serra-Sastre and McGuire (p. 59), technological change has mainly been analysed as the process through which new goods are brought to the market, and hospitals and physicians uptake these new innovations. There is extensive literature on the incentives given to firms to develop new products, but there are few papers that explore how these products are diffused into the market.[1] For instance, what factors shape a physician's prescribing of new medical technologies? What characteristics determine the demand for new technologies at the individual level?

Understanding the entry of new technologies into the market provides insights into the diffusion of technologies that have high development costs and low marginal transportation costs, and that are susceptible to rapid replacement by subsequent innovators. However, diffusion is normally characterized by a slow process in which time elapses between the introduction of the technology and its spread. It has been empirically observed not only in the health care sector, but also in other markets that the diffusion of new technologies follows an S-shaped curve, with low demand during the initial period and demand rising more steeply at later stages of diffusion. Despite the fact that innovations typically have a competitive advantage, diffusion is initially a slow process.

---

[1] Of course, assuming that new technologies are more expensive, these innovations must have embedded characteristics which make them superior to existing products to generate the expected welfare gains.

Pharmaceuticals are a natural focal point for research into technological change because of the growing share of the health care bill that drugs comprise. Researchers have primarily concentrated on incentives to develop new drugs, while analyses of adoption and diffusion have been limited, mainly because the characteristics of the market are such that the principles of standard economic theory are not conducive to explaining the behaviour of individuals. Moreover, the existing evidence on adoption primarily considers how the market and doctors disseminate new pharmaceuticals, but there is little evidence related to adoption at the consumer level.

While consumers should benefit from innovative technologies via improvements in health, these improvements may not be distributed evenly across the population. In fact, researchers such as Goldman and Smith (2005) argue that the introduction of new technologies is partially responsible for a socio-economic gradient in health. That is, the adoption of better health technologies is correlated with education and socio-economic status, which exacerbates existing disparities in health. Although evidence highlighting this effect is still lacking, an alternative explanation for health disparities might be that insurance coverage is a more important determinant of the adoption of new pharmaceuticals. Numerous other studies have found that insurance coverage is an important determinant of general prescription drug use (Lexchin and Grootendorst 2004) and, by extension, the same may be true for the use of new pharmaceutical technologies.

Despite the possibility of insurance being an important predictor of adoption, as mentioned earlier, this is still a relatively unexplored idea within the pharmaceutical arena where individuals share the risks with third-party payers. Yet, insurance schemes are continually expanding the financial burden of prescription drugs that individuals bear, especially for new and relatively more expensive drugs. New drugs are usually priced higher than the older medications, but they may offer benefits in terms of better health outcomes (Lichtenberg 2001).

To account for this gap in the literature and shed more light on the determinants of pharmaceutical adoption, this chapter investigates the effect of health insurance coverage on the use of relatively new prescription drugs. We focus the analysis on statins, a class of lipid-lowering drugs[2] that were considered a major breakthrough after a number of important clinical trials were published (Scandinavian Simvastatin Survival Study Group 4S Group 1994; Shepherd *et al.* 1995). To examine various aspects of adoption, we explore two dependent variables: the probability of statin uptake and the number of statins consumed adjusted by the defined daily dose. The United States (US) is an ideal setting for the research question as insurance is fragmented between public and private insurers, and the spread of new medications can potentially begin upon market approval.

The organization of this chapter is as follows: Section 2 is devoted to a brief review of the literature on technology diffusion and the relationship between insurance and consumption, and also covers the institutional setting in the United States. Section 3

---

[2] We include the following drugs in the lipid-lowering drug class: statins, fibrates, anion exchange resins, nicotinic acids, fish oils, and ezetimibe.

offers a model of pharmaceutical adoption, while Section 4 provides the results of the analysis. Section 5 concludes the chapter with a discussion of the results and the policy implications.

Literature review and background on insurance coverage

Literature review of technology diffusion and demand-side cost sharing

Technology diffusion within health care has been under scrutiny because of its recent role in increasing health care expenditure. Indeed, Glied (2003) and Newhouse (1992) argue that, across the developed world, medical innovation accounts for a substantial proportion of the increase in medical expenditure. Teitelbaum *et al.* (2002) also found that in 1999, 40.8 per cent of total pharmaceutical expenditures in the US were for drugs introduced since 1992. The literature has approached the diffusion of new pharmaceuticals from the supply side, mainly looking at how new drugs capture a percentage of the market, controlling for other macro-level determinants like marketing, prices, and product quality (Berndt *et al.* 2003).

From the demand side, namely doctors and patients, the evidence has been more restricted. For existing and well-established drugs in the market, studies have researched the presence of supply-side moral hazard and habit persistence in prescribing from the physician's perspective (Hellerstein 1998). Results on the presence of supply-side moral hazard are mixed and all studies have examined providers' attitudes towards the existence of third-party payers. Yet, there is little evidence on the factors determining the actual purchase of the medicine from the perspective of the consumer. For instance, the imperfect agency relationship between the patient and physician may be an important determinant of consumption. Other factors, such as socio-economic characteristics, may directly affect the patient. As an example, education has been shown to limit the access to new drugs (Lleras-Muney and Lichtenberg 2002). Because patients are sometimes covered by health insurance, the type of insurance coverage may be an important determinant of new drug use. The extent to which health insurance enhances or limits the use of medical innovations has been discussed by Weisbrod (1991), but the relationship between health insurance and the demand for new drugs remains unexplored.

Although the literature on the relationship between insurance and the uptake of new technologies is scant, there is a significant body of literature that investigates the existence of moral hazard in prescription drug markets; these studies examine the relationship between health insurance and the use of prescription drugs. Perhaps the most seminal dataset is from the RAND health insurance study, where a group of non-elderly residents was randomly assigned to different co-insurance regimes and their consumption was tracked over time. All of the studies that used RAND data found that more generous insurance coverage increased consumption of prescription drugs (Newhouse 1993). It has been more than 25 years since the RAND study, but recent evidence still points to a positive relationship between the generosity of insurance coverage and consumption. Literature reviews from Gemmill *et al.* (2008), and Lexchin and Grootendorst (2004) also find that more generous insurance coverage increases prescription drug consumption, in particular, supplementary prescription drug coverage is an important determinant of consumption.

Research has also focused on the effects of different reimbursement systems on the adoption and diffusion of new medical technologies. Under the theory of dynamic, ex post, moral hazard, health insurance is likely to exaggerate the consumption effect of moral hazard (Zweifel and Manning 2000). The empirical evidence is mainly based on the effect of several insurance contracts between the provider and the insurer on the adoption of physical capital among hospitals. As such, there is evidence that prospective reimbursement systems dampen the speed of diffusion by increasing hospital concern about the economic burden that capital-embodied technologies generally place on hospital finances (Romeo et al. 1984; Lee and Waldman 1985). Motivated by the increasing presence of HMOs in the US health care market, the effect of managed care has also been examined. Baker and Phibbs (2000) shows that the greater the presence of managed care, the lower the speed of adoption and the lower the availability of technological innovations. It is important to note that these are 'big-ticket' technologies, i.e. capital-intensive technologies, for which hospital management is a crucial determinant in the adoption process. The link between the restrictions imposed by different forms of insurance contracts and hospital adoption of medical innovations leaves scope for the analysis of how insurance coverage may also influence the demand for innovations at a different level, that is, the relationship between the insurance coverage and demand for new drugs from the patient perspective.

Thus, the implication of this literature review is that, despite the potential gains from the introduction of new technologies (Lichtenberg 1996), there may be financial and other barriers to the consumption of these new medicines. Typically, the provider has been blamed for delays in the uptake of new drugs, and the patient and third-party payer sides have been largely ignored. Yet, the type of insurance coverage that the patient has may be an important predictor of demand for new technologies, particularly because insurance is an important predictor of demand for prescription drugs in general. The literature review highlights that it is also important to distinguish between insurance coverage that includes prescription drugs and insurance coverage that does not. As a result, we provide an explanation of the insurance coverage variable in the next section.

Background on insurance coverage in the US

The health insurance system in the US is fragmented between public and private insurers, with around 16 per cent of the population having no coverage (US Census Bureau 2007). Medicaid and Medicare are the main public insurance programmes offering health coverage to low-income beneficiaries and individuals over 65, respectively. Insured individuals not included in these groups mostly receive coverage from private sources. With the exception of some public insurance programmes, third-party payers rely heavily on cost sharing to limit moral hazard and constrain health care expenditure, particularly cost sharing for pharmaceuticals. In fact, the generosity of prescription drug benefits under private insurance has been declining due to increased deductibles and cost sharing across all medication tiers [Kaiser Family

Foundation and Health Research and Educational Trust (KFF/HRET) 2006]. Although pharmaceutical expenditure comprised about 10 per cent of total national health spending in 2004, prescription drugs contributed 14.7 per cent of total health care spending growth from 1994 to 2005 (Kaiser Family Foundation 2006).

There are many different pharmaceutical cost sharing regimes that individuals face. All Medicaid programmes cover prescription drugs, and although the co-payments are generally not more than $3, many states impose limitations on the number of medications that beneficiaries can obtain in a given period. Within Medicare many of the elderly did not have prescription drug coverage until 2006, as Medicare did not offer outpatient prescription drug benefits before that year. Thus, Medicare recipients had to purchase supplementary private insurance coverage or be covered by Medicaid to receive prescription drug benefits.

The implication of this background explanation is that insurance coverage can be partially distinguished according to public/private/none and whether the coverage includes prescription drugs in the package. Specifically, non-Medicare public coverage generally includes prescription drugs, and these programmes can be grouped together to form public insurance coverage. Private insurance also covers prescription drugs in most cases and this type of coverage can be set as a second group. We set a third group as those with both public and private insurance coverage, as this is likely to encompass individuals with Medicare who purchase supplementary insurance coverage. Respondents with Medicare as their sole source of coverage comprise a fourth group, as Medicare did not cover outpatient prescription drugs during the study time period. Finally, we classify individuals with no insurance coverage as a stand-alone group.

Conceptualizing technology adoption

As mentioned above, technology adoption is typically investigated from the supply side, but the actual uptake of an innovative medicine is an interaction between the supply and demand sides of the market. In essence, this is a reduced form of the agency relationship. The process begins with the physician who acts as an agent for the patient. When determining the optimal treatment for the patient's condition, the physician can choose between the innovative technology, which is assumed to be more effective, and older substitutes. We assume that the doctor acts on the patient's behalf as a perfect agent; that is, the doctor maximizes the patient's utility given the available information, and there is no supplier-induced demand.

For the purpose of the analysis, we take this stage as exogenous and, instead, consider the next stage in the process where the patient makes the decision regarding consumption. Specifically, the patient compares the marginal benefit and marginal cost of drug consumption to determine whether the prescription purchase yields a positive net benefit. The generosity of insurance coverage lends itself to the marginal cost calculation, while the factors that influence the marginal benefit calculation are discussed below.

From the patient's side, factors such as information, need, and access to care play an important role in the marginal benefit calculation, and there are a number of variables that directly measure or proxy these factors. Age and income may proxy information. That is, because of declining cognitive ability and potential separation from newer technologies (such as the Internet), where information is widely available, groups such as the elderly may have access to less information. Income[3] is a proxy for the information held by the patient because higher income generally reflects greater training and education, and thus a greater ability to learn. However, there is evidence that better educated individuals might not make the most beneficial decisions as a result of greater reliance on their own knowledge (Lleras-Muney 2005).

The racial/ethnic background of the patient may also be a proxy for information. For instance, language may be a barrier to information for certain groups. Finally, the existence of cardiovascular disease or a risk factor for cardiovascular disease (measurable conditions from MEPS include coronary heart disease, acute myocardial infarction, stroke, diabetes, hypertension, and hypercholesterolemia) could proxy information as these individuals have likely been informed of their risk and available treatments by their physicians.

In terms of need factors, the existence of cardiovascular disease or a cardiovascular risk factor are clear indicators of need for lipid-lowering drugs. However, there are other factors not listed in the MEPS database (for instance, waist circumference) that are important considerations, and a general health variable may capture some of these other possibilities. Gender and age are also related to need, as males are typically at greater risk of cardiovascular disease and the risk of cardiovascular disease increases with age up until a point.

Barriers to access to new prescription drugs are also important factors influencing adoption, and some of the variables discussed above as proxies for information are proxies for access. Income influences uptake as it implies a greater ability to afford new medications. Racial and ethnic background may also influence access as racial and ethnic groups are sometimes concentrated in certain areas, and the supply of physicians and pharmacists could differ in these areas. Whether the individual lives in an urban or rural area may also proxy access to physicians, hospitals, and pharmacies.

The final result of this interaction between the patient and the physician suggests that uptake arises from a trade-off between need and the income loss resulting from the out-of-pocket price. The level of information on the side of the patient along with other barriers that the patient may face could be important determinants of the purchase decision.

To provide insight into different aspects of the diffusion process, we investigate two main dependent variables. The first variable is the probability of positive statin consumption, which is meant to capture trends in initial purchases of statins. Another variable employed is the annual number of statins purchased, based on the defined daily dose (DDD), which is meant to provide a standardized measure of annual consumption.

---

[3] While there is an education variable in the MEPS, there are a number of measurement problems with this variable, and we chose not to include it in the analysis.

Data and results

Data

The dataset used for the empirical strategy is the Medical Expenditure Panel Survey (MEPS), which is available from 1996 to 2005 (Agency for Healthcare Research and Quality (AHRQ) 2007). The dataset is a nationally representative sample of the US civilian, non-institutionalized population, and there is over-sampling of Hispanics and blacks. Data is collected from a new sample of households annually, which creates overlapping panels of survey data. We excluded respondents below the age of 18 as children generally do not make health insurance coverage or consumption decisions; these decisions are usually taken by parents and guardians. The raw data consisted of 306,238 observations and after removing individuals under the age of 18 (93,662 observations) and excluding observations with missing data (1767 observations), our final sample consisted of 210,809 observations.

The MEPS dataset contains information regarding the type of insurance coverage that the individual holds. We are able to identify if the respondent has public insurance coverage (through Medicaid, the Veterans Administration, the military health care system, or some other public form of assistance). Individuals with Medicare as a sole source of coverage are not defined as having public insurance coverage. Instead, we categorize individuals with Medicare only as a separate group. We are also able to identify if the individual has private insurance, both private and public insurance, or no health insurance coverage.

Descriptive statistics

Figure 7.1 depicts the progression of statin and other lipid-lowering drug use over time. While the probability of statin use increased over time, the probability of consumption of other lipid-lowering drugs remained relatively constant. Although major

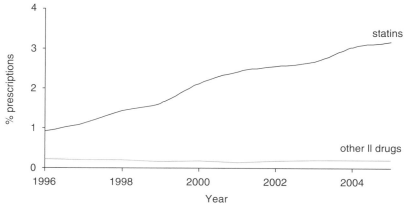

Fig. 7.1 Percentage of total prescriptions that statins and other lipid-lowering drugs comprise, 1996–2005.

clinical trials providing evidence of the benefits of statin use were published as early as 1994 (4S Group 1994), the largest increases in statin use did not occur until after 1999.

Table 7.1 provides information and basic descriptive statistics on the independent variables. Over 53 per cent of the sample had private health insurance only, while 12.3 per cent of the sample had public insurance only (excluding individuals with Medicare only), 11.1 per cent had both public and private insurance, and 5.3 per cent of the

Table 7.1 Means and standard errors of variables included in the analysis

Explanatory variable	Definition	Mean	SE
Public insurance only	Respondent had public health insurance only (Medicaid, Veterans Administration coverage, TRICARE, and other state and federal sources) - respondents with Medicare as a sole source of coverage were not included here	0.123	0.001
Private insurance only	Respondent had private health insurance coverage only	0.538	0.001
Public and private insurance	Respondent had both public and private health insurance coverage	0.111	0.001
Medicare only	Respondent had Medicare as a sole source of health insurance coverage	0.053	0.000
No insurance	Respondent had no health insurance coverage	0.174	0.001
Age	Age of the respondent	44.62	0.038
Male	Respondent was male	0.462	0.001
Female	Respondent was female	0.538	0.001
White	Individual was white	0.595	0.001
Black	Individual was black	0.139	0.001
Hispanic	Individual was Hispanic	0.220	0.001
Other race/ethnicity	Individual was of another race or ethnicity than white, black, or Hispanic	0.047	0.000
Income	Amount of income remaining after total out-of-pocket prescription drug costs are subtracted out	22,252	50.34
Urban area	Individual lived in an urban area	0.790	0.001
Non-urban area	Individual lived in non-urban area	0.210	0.001
Excellent health	Individual reported being in excellent health	0.245	0.001
Very good health	Individual reported being in very good health	0.318	0.001

Table 7.1 (continued) Means and standard errors of variables included in the analysis

Explanatory variable	Definition	Mean	SE
Good health	Individual reported being in good health	0.290	0.001
Fair health	Individual reported being in fair health	0.108	0.001
Poor health	Individual reported being in poor health	0.040	0.000
Coronary heart disease	Individual has been diagnosed with coronary heart disease	0.017	0.000
No coronary heart disease	Individual has not been diagnosed with coronary heart disease	0.983	0.000
Acute myocardial infarction	Individual has experienced an acute myocardial infarction	0.007	0.000
No acute myocardial infarction	Individual has not experienced an acute myocardial infarction	0.993	0.000
Stroke	Individual has suffered a stroke	0.003	0.000
No stroke	Individual has not suffered a stroke	0.997	0.000
Diabetes	Individual has been diagnosed with diabetes	0.069	0.001
No diabetes	Individual has not been diagnosed with diabetes	0.931	0.001
Hypertension	Individual has been diagnosed with hypertension	0.174	0.001
No hypertension	Individual has not been diagnosed with hypertension	0.826	0.001
Hypercholesterolemia	Individual has been diagnosed with hypercholesterolemia	0.081	0.001
No hypercholesterolemia	Individual has not been diagnosed with hypercholesterolemia	0.919	0.001

sample used Medicare as a sole source of coverage. The average age was 44.62 years, and 46.2 per cent of the sample was male. Whites accounted for nearly 60 per cent of the sample followed by Hispanics, blacks, and individuals of another race or ethnicity. The average annual income was about $22,252 (in 1996 dollars), and most respondents lived in an urban area. Most reported being in excellent health (31.8 per cent) or very good health (29.0 per cent), and only 4.0 per cent claimed to be in poor health. The proportions of the sample with coronary heart disease, acute myocardial infarction, stroke, diabetes, hypertension, and hypercholesterolemia ranged from 0.3 per cent to 17.4 per cent.

Table 7.2 offers descriptive evidence of the relationship between the independent variables, and prescription drug and statin consumption. Uninsured individuals had the lowest probability of positive drug consumption followed by those with private insurance only. The likelihood of drug consumption was highest among those with

Table 7.2 Descriptive results

Explanatory variable	Probability of positive prescription drug use	Probability of positive statin use[a]	Number of statins (in DDD)[a]
Public insurance only	75.98	14.04	50.8
Private insurance only	64.51	8.82	27.3
Public and private insurance	87.20	24.70	77.9
Medicare only	86.43	24.56	76.9
No insurance	36.92	4.67	12.2
Age <=45	53.42	2.37	6.5
Age, 46 – 65	74.11	18.14	59.0
Age > 65	89.84	27.03	86.4
Male	54.87	15.85	50.6
Female	73.34	10.60	33.6
White	72.00	14.03	45.5
Black	61.43	10.41	34.0
Hispanic	49.45	8.90	25.0
Other race/ethnicity	55.58	13.10	39.0
Income < $6,843	62.56	11.15	37.2
Income, $6,843–$16,201	64.38	14.18	45.4
Income, $16,201–$30,610	64.31	12.21	38.0
Income > $30,610	68.04	13.04	40.4
Urban area	63.53	12.56	39.4
Non-urban area	69.63	12.97	43.2
Excellent health	50.26	6.69	20.3
Very good health	61.85	11.10	33.7
Good health	69.06	13.82	43.2
Fair health	84.69	18.11	61.0
Poor health	93.12	20.94	74.3
Has coronary heart disease	97.74	51.95	189.4
Does not have coronary heart disease	64.25	11.64	36.4
Has acute myocardial infarction	96.31	50.00	173.8
Does not have acute myocardial infarction	64.60	12.29	39.0
Has stroke	97.25	45.42	146.4
Does not have stroke	64.72	12.51	39.8

Table 7.2 (continued) Descriptive results

Explanatory variable	Probability of positive prescription drug use	Probability of positive statin use[a]	Number of statins (in DDD)[a]
Has diabetes	97.53	32.18	111.1
Does not have diabetes	62.40	10.41	32.1
Has hypertension	97.26	26.49	89.4
Does not have hypertension	57.98	7.77	22.9
Has hypercholesterolemia	96.66	75.47	246.7
Does not have hypercholesterolemia	62.00	4.00	11.8
Year is 1996	66.61	4.58	10.9
Year is 1997	63.94	6.26	14.1
Year is 1998	64.81	7.92	17.6
Year is 1999	64.70	8.85	22.7
Year is 2000	64.84	11.34	31.3
Year is 2001	66.50	13.06	39.9
Year is 2002	65.23	14.38	44.4
Year is 2003	64.61	15.82	61.8
Year is 2004	63.76	18.69	64.1
Year is 2005	63.63	20.11	72.7

[a] Calculated on the sample with at least one prescription drug (N=136,632)

any type of public insurance. The insurance trends were similar for the likelihood of positive statin use. Interestingly, individuals with public and private insurance or Medicare only purchased the most number of statins adjusted by the defined daily dose (conditional upon positive drug use), while consumption was lowest for uninsured respondents.

The probabilities of positive prescription drug and statin consumption increased with age. Females were more likely to obtain at least one prescription drug, but males were more likely to obtain at least one statin and consumed more statins. Whites were the most likely to receive at least one prescription drug, followed by blacks, those of another race or ethnicity, and Hispanics. A similar pattern held for the probability of positive statin consumption and the number of statins purchased.

While the likelihood of prescription consumption increased with income, the probability of statin consumption and the number of statins consumed was highest for those with incomes between $6843 and $16,201 (in 1996 dollars). The differences in prescription drug and statin consumption were relatively small for urban and non-urban respondents. In addition, health status was negatively correlated with prescription drug use, statin use, and the number of statins purchased. Those with at least one of the risk factors for cardiovascular disease experienced higher probabilities of positive drug and statin use, and consumed more statins (adjusted by DDD).

Table 7.3 Influence of health insurance coverage on statin adoption

Health insurance variables	Probability of positive statin use[a,b]	Log number of statins (in DDD)[c,d]
Public insurance only	0.037[§]	0.132[§]
	(0.005)	(0.015)
Private insurance only	0.019[§]	0.060[§]
	(0.003)	(0.011)
Public and private insurance	0.034[§]	0.108[§]
	(0.005)	(0.021)
Medicare only	0.031[§]	0.065[§]
	(0.006)	(0.029)

[§]Significant at the 5 per cent level, *significant at the 10 per cent level.
[a]Calculated on the sample with at least one prescription drug (n = 136,632); [b]marginal effects reported with standard errors in parentheses; [c]calculated on the sample with at least one statin (n = 17,054); [d]coefficients reported with standard errors in parentheses.

Regression results

In addition to the descriptive statistics, we ran regressions for both of the dependent variables. For the probability of positive statin use, we used a simple probit, conditioned upon positive prescription drug use. For the number of statins purchased adjusted by the defined daily dose, we ran a simple two-step model where the first step was a probit on the probability of positive drug use and the second step was an ordinary least squares of the number of statins purchased. To account for the skewed nature of the number of statins purchased, this variable was transformed into logs. Because MEPS is a rotating sample, in both regression models clustering was used to account for individuals that were observed more than once in the sample. The independent variables in the regressions were all of the variables listed in Table 7.2. Table 7.3 reports only the insurance coefficients from the models,[4] and the omitted category is respondents with no health insurance.

According to the results, those with public insurance only had a probability of statin consumption that was 3.7 per cent higher than those with no health insurance coverage. Individuals with both public and private health insurance coverage had a 3.4 greater chance of positive statin consumption than those with no coverage, while those with Medicare had a 3.1 greater probability of positive statin consumption. The probability of positive statin consumption was the second lowest for respondents with private insurance only as they were 1.9 per cent more likely than individuals with no health insurance to obtain at least one statin.

Once an individual received a statin, the number of statins consumed adjusted by the DDD was also the highest for individuals with public insurance coverage. A respondent with public insurance coverage only purchased 14.1 per cent more statins (adjusted by

---

4 For interpretation we report the marginal effects instead of the coefficients from the probability of positive consumption regression.

the DDD) than a respondent with no health insurance coverage. The increases in statin use experienced by individuals with private insurance only, individuals with public and private insurance, and individuals with Medicare only were similar. Specifically, the increase in statin use ranged from 6.1 per cent (adjusted by DDD) for those with private insurance only to 11.4 per cent (adjusted by DDD) for those with public and private insurance, where the baseline comparator is individuals with no health insurance coverage. An interesting finding was that there was a significant difference in consumption between those with no insurance and those with Medicare only.

Discussion

This chapter has empirically examined the relationship between cost sharing for prescription drugs and the uptake of new technologies. The focus has been on statins, an innovative technology that provided a means of treating a condition where few pharmaceutical treatments previously existed. To examine statin adoption from various angles, we employed two dependent variables, including the probability of positive statin use and the number of statins consumed (adjusted by the defined daily dose).

Our findings suggest that insurance is an important determinant of positive statin use and the number of statins purchased. Interestingly, statin use is highest among those with public insurance coverage only and those with both public and private insurance coverage, even after adjusting for other important determinants like health status. Those with Medicare only also experienced greater use of statins than those with no health insurance, even after adjusting for age and health status. Not surprisingly, statin adoption was also higher among those with private insurance only in comparison with the uninsured. The implication is that insurance coverage is an important stimulant of the uptake of new drugs, with access being better for those with public insurance or a combination of public and private insurance. Overall, this could be interpreted as private insurance being more restrictive than public insurance in limiting the use of newer and generally more expensive innovative drugs.

The findings are also in line with Chapter 6 of this book, where Zweifel argues that health insurance leads to a bias in product over cost-saving process innovation. Given that many new drug technologies are more expensive than their older substitutes, it is not surprising that we find a positive effect of health insurance on new drug consumption.

In terms of other variables from the descriptive statistics, statin adoption appeared to depend on information, need, and access. That is, those with greater information, such as individuals with higher incomes, whites, and respondents with cardiovascular disease or at risk for cardiovascular disease experienced greater use of statins. Age as a proxy for information did not appear to be a significant deterrent to statin use, although the oldest age band did not consume any more prescriptions than individuals between the ages of 46 and 65. The results of the need variables (age, gender, cardiovascular risk, general health indicators) indicated that need was an important predictor of statin uptake. Finally, access appeared to be an important determinant of statin adoption. Those with higher incomes experienced higher probabilities of statin consumption, while access was generally worse for Hispanics, blacks, and individuals of another race or ethnicity as compared with whites.

The implication is that, although diffusion partially depends on the need for new medical technologies, there does still appear to be a socio-economic gradient that is not overcome by public insurance coverage. That is, individuals with lower incomes and individuals in certain racial/ethnic groups experience lower probabilities of statin consumption and consume fewer statins adjusted by DDDs. This is in line with the results reported in Lleras-Muney and Lichtenberg (2002) and suggests that there may indeed be a socio-economic gradient in the uptake of statins.

There are a few policy implications that can be drawn from these results. Regarding insurance coverage, there is a clear difference in consumption between those with any insurance coverage and those with no insurance coverage, even after adjusting for other socio-economic, demographic, and need characteristics. Extending insurance coverage to everyone, even if the insurance coverage is not for prescription drugs, could help alleviate some of these access issues. Yet, even within individuals that had insurance coverage, access to statins differed according to the type of coverage. Interestingly, access appeared to be highest for those with public insurance only; this group is mostly made up of individuals with Medicaid coverage. Thus, Medicaid appears to be achieving access to prescription drugs relatively well. In fact, it seems that private insurance coverage is restricting access to statins more than the public programmes.

As with any study, it is important to keep the potential limitations in mind. One limitation is our inability to measure compliance with the MEPS dataset. While the purchase of the prescription drug is an important step in the adoption process, arguably, another important step is the actual consumption of the medication. Again, socio-economic and demographic characteristics, and the nature of the illness may be important predictors of compliance. Another limitation is our inability to use education as a predictor of statin uptake as education may be a proxy for the information level of the patient. Although an education variable exists in the MEPS database, there are a number of inconsistencies with this variable, particularly over time. However, income is typically related to education and should partially measure the information level of the patient.

References

Agency for Healthcare Research and Quality (AHRQ) (2007). *MEPS HC-097: 2005 Full Year Consolidated Data File*. Rockville, Agency for Healthcare Research and Quality.

Baker LC and Phibbs CS (2000). *Managed care, technology adoption, and health care: the adoption of neonatal intensive care*. Cambridge, MA, National Bureau of Economic Research, WP 7883.

Berndt ER, Pindyck RS and Azoulay P (2003). Consumption externalities and diffusion in pharmaceutical markets: antiulcer drugs. *Journal of Industrial Economics*, **51**, 243–70.

Gemmill M, Thomson S and Mossialos E (2008). What impact do prescription drug charges have on efficiency and equity? Evidence from high-income countries. *International Journal for Equity in Health*, 7, doi:10.1186/1475-9276-7-12.

Glied S. (2003). Health care costs: on the rise again. *Journal of Economic Perspectives*, **17**, 125–48.

Goldman D and Smith JP (2005). *Socioeconomic differences in the adoption of new medical technologies*. Cambridge, National Bureau of Economic Research. Available at: http://papers.nber.org/papers/w11218 (accessed 22 January 2008).

Hellerstein JK (1998). The importance of the physician in the generic versus trade-name prescription decision. *Rand Journal of Economics*, **29**, 108–36.

Kaiser Family Foundation (KFF) (2006). *Trends and indicators in the changing health care marketplace*. Washington DC, Henry J. Kaiser Family Foundation. Available at: http://www.kff.org/insurance/7031/print-sec1.cfm (accessed 16 August 2007).

Kaiser Family Foundation and Health Research and Educational Trust (KFF/HRET) (2006). *Employer health benefits: 2006 annual survey*. Washington DC, Henry J. Kaiser Family Foundation. Available at: http://www.kff.org/insurance/7527/upload/7527.pdf (accessed 16 August 2007).

Lee RH and Waldman DM (1985). The diffusion of innovations in hospitals: some econometric considerations. *Journal of Health Economics*, **4**, 373–80.

Lexchin J and Grootendorst P (2004). Effects of prescription drug user fees on drug and health services use and on health status in vulnerable populations: a systematic review of the evidence. *International Journal of Health Services*, **34**, 101–22.

Lichtenberg FR (1996). Do (more and better) drugs keep people out of hospitals? *American Economic Review*, **86**, 384–8.

Lichtenberg FR (2001). Are the benefits of newer drugs worth their cost? Evidence from the 1996 MEPS. *Health Affairs*, **20**(5), 241–51.

Lleras-Muney A (2005). The relationship between education and adult mortality in the United States. *Review of Economic Studies* **72**, 189–221.

Lleras-Muney A and Lichtenberg FR (2002). *The effect of education on medical technology adoption. are more educated more likely to use new drugs?* Cambridge, National Bureau of Economic Research. Available at: http://papers.nber.org/papers/w11218 (accessed 22 January 2008).

Newhouse J (1992). Medical care costs: how much welfare loss? *Journal of Economic Perspectives* **6**(3), 3–21.

Newhouse J (1993). *Free for All? Lessons from the RAND Health Insurance Experiment*. Cambridge, Harvard University Press.

Romeo AA, Wagner JL and Lee RH (1984). Prospective reimbursement and the diffusion of new technologies in hospitals. *Journal of Health Economics*, **3**, 1–24.

Scandinavian Simvastatin Survival Study Group (4S Group) (1994). Randomized trial of cholesterol lowering in 4444 patients with coronary heart disease: the Scandinavian Simvastatin Survival Study (4S). *Lancet*, **344**(8934), 1383–9.

Shepherd J, Cobbe SM, Ford I, Isles CG, Lorimer AR, MacFarlane PW, McKillop JH and Packard CJ (1995). Prevention of coronary heart disease with pravastatin in men with hypercholesterolemia. *New England Journal of Medicine* **333**(20), 1301–8.

Teitelbaum F, Martinez R, Parker A, Henderson R, Kolling B, Roe C and Ellis S (2002). *Express Scripts 2001 Drug Trend Report*. St Louis, Express Scripts.

US Census Bureau (2007). *People with or without health insurance coverage by selected characteristics*. Washington US Census Bureau. Available at: http://www.census.gov/hhes/www/hlthins/hlthin06/p60no233_table6.pdf (accessed 22 January 2008).

Weisbrod BA (1991). The Health Care Quadrilemma: an essay on technological change, insurance, quality of care, and cost containment. *Journal of Economic Literature*, **29**, 523–52.

Zweifel P, Manning WG (2000). *Moral hazard and consumer incentives in health care. Handbook of health economics*. New York, Elsevier, 409–59.

Chapter 8

Genetic advances and health insurance

Lilia Filipova and Michael Hoy

Introduction

The Human Genome Project (HGP), which began in 1990 and was declared completed in 2003, provided a rough road map of the human genome that is often referred to as the blueprint of life. Now work has moved onto finding the myriad of genetic variants and how this knowledge can improve the health of individuals. Reports about new gene variants (alleles) being discovered and new genetic tests becoming available appear almost daily in newspapers. One could be forgiven for thinking that we are well into the so-called 'genetic revolution' and that medicine has fundamentally changed as a result. What would such a world be like (at least in developed countries)? It would involve hundreds, if not thousands, of genetic tests being available to everyone. Pharmaceuticals that are designed for individual-specific genomes will have replaced one-size-fits-all drug treatments. New genetic therapies will have eliminated diseases such as Huntington's chorea. Prenatal therapies will have eliminated the birth of children with debilitating diseases and deformities. However, work on such advances is still in the early stages, and the pace of future developments is not easy to predict or even imagine. Considering the lack of high profile applications, like a cure for Huntington's disease (HD), one could also be excused for thinking of the HGP as a promise unfulfilled. Nonetheless, advances in genetic technologies and treatments will come, and possibly in spurts, so it is important to anticipate the benefits and challenges that such information will provide to society, and how these will be related to country-specific health insurance plans. Of particular interest here is whether such plans are primarily private or public.[1]

One can think of the progress towards the genetic revolution, as characterized above as involving three stages, although this is perhaps rather simplistic and optimistic.

----

[1] The announcement on September 3, 2007, that Craig Vetner's detailed DNA sequence (96 per cent coverage) has been made publicly available – the first such complete detailed genome to be sequenced – was perhaps less important to predicting the future impact of genetic technology than a related news item that Dr. George Church, a professor of genetics at Harvard University, is working to develop a DNA test that would identify 1 percent of an individual's DNA at a cost of $1,000 (see Gajlan 2007).

The first stage is completion of the Human Genome Project and we think of this as really just the preliminary phase. The second stage, or first phase of the actual revolution in medicine, we think of as occurring in the current, near, and medium-term future, in which many genes that are responsible for onset of diseases, in varying degrees of importance and predictability, are identified and genetic tests for such genes become increasingly available. In this first phase, the use of genetic tests will improve predictability of diseases for individuals, but be of limited use in helping to prevent or cure them. This phase, in fact, is underway with many tests such as the genetic test for the Huntington's disease gene or the test for the so-called *BRCA1/2* genes now available. There has been substantial research in economics on the implications of this sort of information and the impact of regulating this information on insurance markets. In the subsequent section we discuss what this means for health insurance and what further thinking and research would be helpful in establishing an appropriate regulatory framework in response to this phase of the revolution.

By the second phase of the genetic revolution we mean that period in which the knowledge gained from scientific research leads to the practical means of treating, and in some cases curing or preventing diseases through knowledge of their genetic components. In this chapter we try to anticipate potential benefits and challenges that the genetic revolution may create for health care provision and for insurers. We pay special attention to how the health insurance industry can and should react to the new information and technologies that we can eventually expect to arise. Health care systems and insurers are typically heavily regulated, and so we must also consider possible responses of government regulatory bodies as well. The issue of genetic privacy and discrimination have framed much of the debate concerning legislative measures. A great deal of attention has been paid to the issue of government regulation of genetic information not only for health insurers, but for life and disability insurance as well. The effects of genetic information on individual behaviour are also crucial to consider. Government regulation is driven by voter concerns and effective medical interventions based on genetic information will depend on elements of individual behaviour that may not be easy to predict. The interaction of all of these factors will determine societal effectiveness of the new information and related technologies that we can expect to be developed.

Besides regulation of the use of genetic information, governments directly determine the types of medical interventions provided to society in countries with public healthcare systems and have indirect influence through regulation in countries where private insurance companies are relevant players. A major challenge is to determine which genetic tests and subsequent medical treatments should be provided to members of society and at what cost. A woman who tests positive for one of the *BRCA1/2* genes may choose from a list of prophylactic measures including double mastectomy, a variety of drugs including tamoxifen, or no medical treatment at all. Alternatively, or in conjunction with a specific prophylactic measure, such information may well change the degree of surveillance taken (e.g. mammography). There is evidence that information about the relative risk of such diseases does affect such decisions, which in turn affect the cost and effectiveness of providing health care.[2] However, it is important to model how different types of genetic information may affect such behaviour and what are the implications. This is one of our main objectives in this paper.

Implications from phase I of the genetic revolution

Although most people do not yet hold detailed information about their genetic predispositions to a wide range of diseases, the potential to obtain such information seems to be very near.[3] For countries that rely primarily on private health insurance, most notably the USA, this creates a conundrum.[4] Restricting private insurers from basing premiums on individuals' genetic profiles creates a situation of asymmetric information and potentially serious efficiency issues for the insurance market due to adverse selection. However, allowing risk-rating based on such information is, for many, a serious equity concern that must be dealt with through legislation. Indeed, in the areas of life and disability insurance, there has been a wide range of responses, from no action to voluntary moratoria by the insurance industry to government guidelines to strict regulation. Several countries in Europe have legislation that regulates the use of genetic information by the insurance industry. In the USA, more concern has been voiced and more regulation directed at this issue in the context of the private health insurance market.[5]

To better understand how to trade-off the advantages and disadvantages of regulation, we need to understand how one would expect insurers to react. If insurance buyers are allowed to keep private from insurers any information such as that derived from genetic tests, a situation of asymmetric information will persist. The economics literature has identified two basic strategies used by insurance providers in reaction to the informational advantage of consumers when asymmetric information prevails. One strategy is to use so-called price-quantity competition to screen risk types.[6] Consumers with higher risk of making claims will value insurance coverage more. Thus, an insurer may be able to design a menu of contracts (two in the case of two risk types) such that each risk type self-selects the appropriate contract. The contract designed for the high risk types will have full coverage, but offered at a higher price than the contract designed for the low risk types, which will have lower coverage and

---

[2] In a study on the demand for three measures for early detection of breast and cervical cancer, Picone, Sloan and Taylor Picone *et al.* 2004 find that information on an increased risk of illness increases the demand for surveillance, while uncertainty about the effectiveness of treatment might decrease the demand for surveillance. Witt 2007 also finds that women who are at a higher risk of breast cancer are more likely to demand a mammography.

[3] According to the GENETESTS website www.genetests.org 2007 as of August 30, 2007 there are currently over 1,300 genetic tests available, with 1,147 of these available for clinical use and the others only for research. See also www.23andme.com 2008.

[4] This issue could also become more relevant in many other countries. As noted in (Wagstaff *et al.* 1999, p. 269), 'It is well known that during the last decade or so, there has been a shift in many OECD countries away from public sources of finance (*for health care*) to private sources.'

[5] For a discussion on various regulatory approaches see Lemmens 2003 and Kn0ppers *et al.* 2004.

[6] See the seminal papers by Rothschild and Stiglitz 1976 and Wilson 1977. See also Hoy 1982 and Crocker and Shaw 1986.

have a lower per unit price. By offering a sufficiently low coverage level on the contract designed for and chosen by lower risk types, the high risk types can be discouraged from purchasing it. Thus, lower risk types end up being under-insured, and this is the efficiency or welfare loss due to adverse selection.

The ability of insurers to screen risk types implicitly as discussed above requires that contracts can be offered exclusively; that is, each insurance buyer cannot buy coverage from more than one insurer. If the principle of exclusivity did not prevail, the high risk types would buy several policies with partial coverage that are designed for low risk types in order to obtain their desired level of coverage at 'the low price'. Thus, insurers would end up losing money on these contracts and overall high risk types would be purchasing as much (or more) insurance as low risk types. Exclusivity of contracts is the norm in health insurance and some other lines of insurance, such as automotive insurance, but not in other lines, such as life insurance.[7] For the above strategy of screening risk types to be effective, it must also be the case that the fraction of high risk types is sufficiently large. Otherwise, the low risk types would prefer that they be pooled together with the high risks and pay what would be only a small addition to the premium relative to what they would pay if they were charged according to their risk type-specific actuarially fair rate. Since insurance companies want to compete for low risk types, the separating pair of contracts would not be sustainable as a market equilibrium. In this circumstance it turns out that a Nash equilibrium would not exist. However, Wilson (1977) showed that, with a plausible assumption about firm foresight, a pooling equilibrium will exist in these circumstances.[8] This pooling equilibrium is characterized by a price set at the population weighted pooled price (i.e. actuarially fair for the entire population) with a coverage level that, given this price, is most desired by the low risk types. This latter characteristic follows naturally from the insurance companies wanting to compete for low risk clients.

The pooling outcome described above is also inefficient in that the coverage level that low risk clients will desire will be at least a little bit less than the 'full coverage' that they would choose if charged their (lower) risk-type specific price under symmetric information. However, in the pooling scenario everyone receives insurance at the same terms and so, in this sense, a ban on insurers using genetic information to risk-rate contracts leads to a more equitable outcome. Thus, there seems to be no clear and uncontroversial decision on the appropriate response to the debate about whether to ban insurers from using genetic test results to risk-rate premiums. However, if the amount of such information that is held by the public is 'not too significant', we would accept that a ban on its use is likely to be welfare enhancing. The reason is that the equity benefits are clear. Individuals with 'bad genetic luck' will not be penalized in the insurance market in the presence of such a ban. This means that income net of insurance costs would not depend on one's genetic luck and so there would be less

---

[7] See Polborn *et al.* 2006 for some possible reasons why exclusivity does not prevail in the life insurance market.

[8] Wilson's foresight Wilson 1977 assumption implies that firms would not offer contracts that lead to negative expected profits after other firms react to those contract offers.

inequality as a result.[9] The condition that the amount of information that is held by the public is 'not too significant' is important because this condition limits the size of the efficiency loss due to adverse selection. If sufficient private information is held by insurance buyers, then those at higher risk, i.e. those with 'bad' genes, can, on average, be expected to purchase more insurance than those with 'normal genes'. The result is that for the lower risk individuals the price of insurance will increase relative to what is actuarially fair for them and this induces them to reduce their purchases leaving them effectively uninsured. The loss of welfare due to this distortion created by a ban on the insurers' use of information must be compared with any gain in welfare due to the distributive advantage created by the implicit transfers of income from low risk to high risk (unlucky) types in the pooling equilibrium.

Actuarial and economic studies suggest that, given the present state of genetic information, the price effects of such a ban, as well as the efficiency costs due to adverse selection are likely insignificant.[10] Therefore, a ban on such information at this point in time seems appropriate. Even in countries where private health insurance plays a limited role, the way the information is regulated in life and related insurance markets is still somewhat important. People may be deterred from having genetic tests that could improve decisions concerning healthcare if they think the information could also be used by life insurers to restrict their potential future coverage.[11] As more genetic tests become available, and as they become more useful in terms of guiding improved heath care decisions, this will become a greater concern. However, it is also the case that, as the amount of such privately held information grows, the concern about adverse selection costs may become serious enough to revisit the argument about whether the equity benefits of a ban exceeds the welfare loss due to adverse selection. For countries that rely heavily on private health insurance, and in particular the USA, this means that strict regulation banning genetic test results being usedto risk-rate premiums may make sense now, but not necessarily in the medium-term future. One method of avoiding the adverse selection costs, created by insurers' cream-skimming behaviours involving price-quantity competition for low risks, is to impose mandated coverage in addition to a ban on genetic categorization. This naturally creates a complex problem in deciding what medical procedures to include on the list (see, for example, Barrett and Conlon 2001; Butler 2003).

Although we don't claim to be clairvoyants, we will presume that, over time, the use of genetic tests will eventually become significantly more predictive about the onset of disease for individuals, and also that substantial medical treatments and cures will be

---

[9] For formal arguments see Hoy 1984, Hoy 2006, Hoy and Polborn 2000, and Hoy and Ruse 2005.

[10] See, for example, MacDonald 2000, MacDonald 2005, Subramanian *et al.* 1999, Hoy *et al.* 2003, Hoy and Witt 2007.

[11] As Hall 2005 notes, the use of such information is sometimes used by life and health insurers in the US, for example, although the practice is not widespread. Nonetheless, 'the fear of genetic discrimination by insurers is much greater than the reality.' (Hall 2005, p.1). A ban of such information use would therefore remove an important, albeit perhaps exaggerated, deterrent.

developed as a result of genetic research, including the use of drugs based on specific genotypes. This will generate a different class of issues for insurers and society in general, and it is these to which we now turn.

Phase II of the genetic revolution: potential future uses of genetic information

Without intending to be exhaustive, we present below some of the many potential uses of genetic information and technology. The conceptual approach to use in order to anticipate the potential impact of genetic technology will vary across these cases. For some types of information uses it may be relatively easy, at least conceptually, to determine the social and private values of the information, as well as to estimate the cost implications of adopting relevant health technologies. In some cases, however, the uncertainty of expected benefits and costs might be too large to make clear-cut predictions. The relative importance for health improvements and predictability of behavioural reactions will also vary across types of information use. We will discuss these implications for several types of genetic information and technologies briefly in this section, then focus on one of the particular cases (see 'Predictive and pre-symptomatic testing', p. 131) in the following section.[12]

Prenatal genetic tests

In this use, individuals obtain genetic tests on foetuses (including embryos created through IVF techniques). For example, amniocentesis is a procedure that extracts amniotic fluid to obtain various biomedical substances besides DNA material of the foetus and has been available for more than 50 years. The first documented case of using this procedure to identify a foetus with Down syndrome, followed by an abortion, was in 1968. The decision to abort after determination of a genetic 'abnormality' is not a straightforward one and must be considered in the context of existing social norms.[13] Recent evidence [Mansfield et al., on behalf of a European concerted Action: Decision-making After the Diagnosis of a foetal Abnormality(DADA) 1999] suggests that the decision to abort a foetus carrying an abnormal gene varies across diseases, not surprisingly, and may vary across time.[14] Various reasons besides social norms, including factors such as directives to genetic counsellors, could influence individuals' decisions to use prenatal screening that is followed by a decision to abort.

The cost of prenatal screening using amniocentesis and relevant genetic tests is not difficult to determine. It is also conceptually straightforward to estimate the medical cost of abortion, although not so easy to estimate the psychological cost to

---

[12] Taborrok 1994 discusses some of the costs and benefits of genetic testing in light of altered medical treatments.

[13] See Cowan 1994 for an interesting discussion.

[14] Interestingly, Mansfield, et al. 1999 report that from a societal perspective, abortion decisions in the case of prenatal testing for Down Syndrome has not been found to vary over the 1980s and 1990s.

the individuals concerned. It is not a straightforward exercise to estimate the future cost – both personal and medical – for the treatment and accommodation of a child born with a particular genetic abnormality since that depends on future developments in medical technology.[15] Moreover, the decision to abort may well depend on the level of publicly provided benefits for the care of affected individuals and that can change over time. This makes the decision on what types of genetic diseases one should screen for and what services to offer on the basis of a positive test result, including the option of abortion, a thorny one indeed, even ignoring the sort of debates on morality that arise. A recent study concerning the genetic test for Gaucher disease (2007) highlights the controversial nature of such tests. Gaucher disease is often realized as low penetrance and effective treatments already exist. However, the disease can also be severe and essentially untreatable, and so the decision to abort is a difficult one.

Overall, however, we suspect this is not one of the more quantitatively important applications of genetic information from the cost-benefit analysis perspective. Although it is not a clear-cut case, we also suspect that, if one includes the cost of caring for individuals with genetic abnormalities in the overall (financial) cost to insurers and society, then increased use of this type of genetic information will not lead to inflated health care costs and may well lead to some cost savings.

Genetic testing of newborns

There are genetic abnormalities, such as phenylketonuria (PKU), which if treated early in life significantly improves a child's chances for normal development.[16] If not treated through appropriate choice of diet, children will develop progressive impairment of cerebral function, including conditions such as hyperactivity, seizures, and severe mental retardation. Since the cost of treatment is low, involving restricting foods high in phenylalanine, such as meat, fish, nuts, and dairy products, expanding opportunities for newborn genetic testing, such as the test for PKU, seem likely to be even more straightforward to analyse in terms of costs and benefits than prenatal screening. However, testing for some abnormal genes may present more complicated considerations. For example, if a child is born to a family with a history of HD for one of the parents or grandparents, especially while there are no feasible treatment options for this disease, it is not so easy to decide whether the child should be tested as a newborn or young child. The result of a positive test could lead to substantial psychological problems for the family (see Procter 2006, for a discussion of these issues).

Predictive and pre-symptomatic testing for adults

In one way, the primary difference distinguishing the first three uses of genetic testing that we have listed here is the timing of when the test is taken. Of course, only for

---

[15] One of the costs of testing, of course, is the risk of miscarriage that includes both personal costs as well as medical costs. Recent evidence suggests this rate to be 1 in 1600 procedures (see Eddleman *et al.* 2006).

[16] PKU has been a part of many core newborn screening programs since the late 1960s. Treatment is through choice of a diet low in phenylalanine and high in tyrosine.

prenatal testing is abortion an option. If abortion is the only relevant response to a positive test result, then it can be argued that prenatal screening should be restricted to those diseases which are sufficiently severe to justify the procedure. For newborn testing, one can start preventative treatments very early in life and, for some diseases, such as PKU, this is essential for effective intervention. However, if early treatment is not a factor, then it is probably sensible to offer genetic tests only to adults (see Procter 2006). This set of tests, it seems to us, may well become the biggest use of genetic testing in the medium term future. Moreover, it seems this set creates one of the bigger challenges for analysis in terms of predicting how such tests will affect the cost of health insurance and the future effectiveness of health care.

An interesting historical example of the use (take-up) of predictive genetic testing is that of the test for the Huntington's disease (HD) gene. In general terms, classical decision theory in the context of uncertainty predicts that provided an individual would change one's actions conditional on at least one possible outcome of the information (test) about the future, then obtaining the information would be worthwhile.[17] The intuition underlying this prediction is that if an individual would *not* respond to information in any meaningful (action-orientated) manner, then getting the information just means the uncertainty is resolved sooner in life, but that the probabilities of good and bad outcomes, from an ex ante perspective, would be neither better nor worse. On the other hand, if the individual *would* respond in one way or another, by being able to better plan his/her life on the basis of such information, then the test would hold positive value. Despite this latter condition being almost certainly relevant for a test to HD, it has been discovered, through various clinical trials, that individuals are not always interested in obtaining such information. Even when offered at zero cost the actual take-up rate of such information has been found to be quite low.[18] One reason could be the psychological implications of possibly learning that one has to live with such a disease (see Biesecker 2005). These potential psychological effects may not be adequately addressed by classical decision theory; also, there are possibly complex family and social implications of such knowledge. Once the information is known to the individual, he/she would probably find it very difficult to hide a positive test result from family members, friends, and others. This could affect, in a negative way, the manner in which people treat the tested individual.[19] Moreover, people may worry about their ability to obtain life insurance in the future as a result of predictive genetic

---

[17] By classical decision theory under uncertainty we mean the application of the expected utility hypothesis. We recognize that this approach is a narrow one even in the absence of external and psychological effects that are likely to be very important in the context of genetic information. For criticism of this standard decision making hypothesis see, for example, Machina 1987 and Rabin and Thaler 2001. Also see Cox and Mcnellin 1999.

[18] For example, in various clinical testing environments, when anonymous genetic tests were offered at zero cost, Meiser and Dunn 2000 found that the percentage at risk who requested testing varied from 9 per cent to 20 per cent in various centers in UK cities and Vancouver, Canada. For further discussion, see also Babul *et al.* 1993 and Quaid and Morris 1993.

[19] Note that for these reasons it may be best, except in the circumstances noted above, to let decisions about whether to obtain genetic information of this sort wait until later in life (again, see Procter 2006).

test results. Whatever the reasons underlying actual behaviour, it seems that predicting the demand for such information and how this demand may change over time is difficult to understand.

Although some diseases, such as Huntington's disease, as yet have no viable preventive or treatment strategies, this is not the case with many diseases that have, along with other risk factors, a genetic component; that is, multifactorial diseases, such as diabetes, cardiovascular diseases, colon cancer, or breast cancer. For these diseases, knowing one has a susceptibility gene can at least lead to improved surveillance activity. Consider the example of the so-called *BRCA1* or *BRCA2* genes.[20] A woman with one of these genes has a much higher risk of breast cancer and so one could expect that increased surveillance, such as increased frequency of mammograms would be worthwhile. Therefore, it is of interest to individuals, healthcare providers, and health insurers to understand how the use of such information may change in the future, and what this means for healthcare costs and outcomes. Given the quantitative importance that we expect from this aspect of genetic information, we spend considerable space in the next section of this chapter addressing a way to think about this application of genetic information.

An important additional issue to be addressed for this class of genetic tests is targeting. In the case of HD, for example, the probability of receiving a positive test result is effectively 50 per cent for someone with a family history of HD (i.e. existence of an affected parent) and 0 per cent for anyone else. With the strong relationship between the probability of testing positive and the family background of the disease, the target group for a test is clearly those with a family history, and only those with a family history. However, for the *BRCA1/2* genes the likelihood of testing positive depends, in a rather complicated manner, on family history.[21] Determining the target group for a test for the *BRCA1/2* genes requires, besides the family history, also the consideration of such factors as the resulting surveillance, prevention, and treatment activities, and their expected costs, as well as the accuracy (specificity and sensitivity) of the test and the cost of the test itself. Whether a woman tests negative or positive for the *BRCA1/2* gene, or whether the woman doesn't have a test at all, determines an optimal (or appropriate) surveillance and prevention strategy that, in turn, depends not only on family history, but on personal views as to the relative (personal) cost of pro-phylactic measures, such as having a double mastectomy or taking a drug such as tamoxifen should a positive test result be received. The value of offering a genetic test for *BRCA1/2* genes could also change dramatically if improved prophylactic measures are developed in the future. We address these and other issues in the following section of this chapter.

---

[20] This is also a good example of a genetic test that probably should be offered primarily for adults. The probability of getting breast cancer up to age 25 is very low (1 in 15,000) but rises to 1 in 200 by age 40 in the general population but much higher for a woman with one of the breast cancer genes (statistics due to 'Breast Cancer Care, UK, www.breastcancercare.org.uk 2008).

[21] See, for example Hoy and Witt 2007 – especially Table 1, p. 531–which demonstrates how the likelihood of having one of the BRCA1/2 genes depends in a rather complex manner on family history.

Genetic tests as diagnostic tools

Another important use of genetic testing is to provide improved diagnosis. The use of genetic tests in these cases is certainly less controversial than when testing for pre-symptomatic diseases, since the health of the patient is presumably already in a compromised state, and arguments concerning the psychological impact of knowing about having a disease that is already creating symptoms are less relevant. Thus, the decision about whether such a test is worthwhile is a simpler matter involving the relative costs of alternative diagnostic procedures and the benefit of knowing the genetic component of the disease in question in making appropriate health interventions. Thus, although an important source of the developing technology, this case does not seem to present as much difficulty in determining its appropriate use, or in assessing the economic and medical value of such uses on insurers and health providers as the other cases we have listed.

Pharmacogenetics

Advances in genetic technology to develop new drugs or to better use existing ones, is likely to be quantitatively important in terms of costs and benefits for insurers and health care providers. In fact, the use of drugs in general has expanded significantly over the past couple of decades and now represents a much larger fraction of health-care costs. For example, in Canada, between 1975 and 2004, expenditure on prescribed drugs has risen from 6.3 per cent of total health expenditure to 13.8 per cent (as noted by Zhong 2007, p. 488). This raises important distributional concerns regarding how drug costs are covered. The response in Canada has been an increase in the public subsidy on prescribed drugs for low income individuals.

Gene therapy

It is possible that gene therapies will be developed in the rather more distant future. Such therapies will allow transfer of 'healthy genes' to replace or offset the failings of 'faulty genes'. If low cost effective therapies can be developed, then the cost savings to the health care system and private insurers, where relevant, could be substantial. Such therapies, if curative, would obviate the need for expensive treatments or costly increased surveillance and/or precautionary activities. For example, if one could 'correct' the effects of a person's *BRCA1/2* gene, this would eliminate the need for increased surveillance (e.g. mammograms), and the possible use of prophylactic measures such as taking a drug like tamoxifen or having a double mastectomy. The financial and personal costs of the presence of the *BRCA1/2* gene could be drastically reduced. Despite the fact that some attempts at clinically viable genetic therapies are currently taking place, we think it is likely to be a long time before such procedures are quantitatively important in the context of overall health care. We suggest this might represent a third phase of the genetic revolution.

A more detailed consideration of predictive and pre-symptomatic testing

From the perspective of cost and health implications of advances in genetic technologies in Phase II of the genetic revolution, perhaps the most important type of use is that for predictive and pre-symptomatic testing for adults. This is also an area that is potentially quite complex to understand, both in terms of how individuals will react to this knowledge, and what implications this will have for the cost of health care delivery and the improvement to quality of health outcomes. One reason for the complexity is the unpredictability of the types of health care strategies that will be developed in relation to the genetic knowledge that accumulates. Another reason, which we focus on in this section, is that even once genetic advancements are better understood in terms of what treatment options are best applied and developed, behavioural responses of individuals to this information may be wide ranging and unpredictable. Besides privacy issues and the apparent strength of the 'desire-not-to-know preference' that is often displayed in the context of some genetic information (e.g. the test for the HD gene discussed earlier in this paper), it is difficult to judge how people will react to the options of increased surveillance and/or precautionary actions that may become available. Not only are individuals likely to display a range of different responses to the same genetic information, but population trends in behavioural responses may be significant and difficult to predict. Consider, for example, the recent trend in obesity in so many developed countries. Such a significant change in behaviour at the population level, even in the absence of the introduction of a new and qualitatively different regime in medical knowledge, suggests a major challenge awaits health researchers in understanding how populations will react to increased genetic information about susceptibility to disease. Below we propose an approach to analyse the costs and benefits—both financial and non-financial—that may arise from genetic testing in the context of susceptibility genes.

For the most part, it is both less costly and more effective in improving health outcomes to treat disease onset early, most notably in cancers. The advantage of genetic tests that indicate heightened risk to a cancer, such as breast cancer or colon cancer, is that it offers the opportunity for those who test positive to increase their level of surveillance in order to improve the chances of early rather than late detection. Similarly, those who test positive may adopt precautionary actions that could increase the chance of avoiding onset of disease altogether. Since the two types of issues are conceptually quite similar, we focus here on the surveillance decision. Later we explain how decisions about levels of precautionary actions can be considered in a similar manner.

One can expect that at least some individuals who receive a positive test result for the presence of a multifactorial or so-called susceptibility gene[22] will avail themselves

---

[22] A multifactorial gene is one that is a component in the likelihood of future disease but other components, such as other genes, environmental and personal behavioural considerations are also relevant in determining the likelihood of onset of disease. We will focus on cases where it is individual behavioural choices that affect susceptibility to disease differentially according to the individuals' genotypes as well as the impact of early versus late detection in determining the effectiveness of treatment for the disease.

of increased surveillance. This increases the overall surveillance cost to the health care system, but of course creates the advantage of increasing the rate of early, rather than late detection for the disease. In this way the overall health outcomes are improved and the overall financial cost of treating the disease may be reduced. The balance of these costs and benefits to the health care system, as well as the direct cost of the genetic tests, are important inputs into a cost-benefit consideration for the development and use of genetic information. It is important to recognize, however, that individuals can be expected to take decisions that are *personally* optimal. These decisions will depend on the financial cost of surveillance to the individual, which in turn depends on the type of health insurance plan held, as well as on non-pecuniary costs of surveillance (e.g. discomfort and possible negative side effects). As an example, consider the case of colon cancer. In the absence of genetic testing that provides individuals with differential susceptibility levels to incurring colon cancer, each individual decides on what level of surveillance to adopt based on the relevant factors, including those mentioned above. If an individual discovers he is at a relatively high risk for colon cancer due to him having a susceptibility gene, then he may well increase his surveillance level. This sort of information seems likely to improve overall social welfare (ex post) for the group who discover their increased risk status and also quite possibly reduces the financial cost to the overall health care system. However, one must trade-off these sorts of benefits with the overall cost of the genetic testing program.

It is often recommended that only those individuals with a family history suggestive of a relatively high risk of disease should take the associated genetic test(s). Given current availability and costs of genetic tests for susceptibility genes like those for breast cancer and colon cancer, this seems a rational social policy. Moreover, since most incidents of cancers within the population are not related to known susceptibility genes (e.g. only 10 per cent of breast cancers are thought to be related to known breast cancer genes), those who either do not have a test for the gene or who test negative should not presume that they have a perceptibly different risk of incurring the disease than for the pre-test population average and so should not adopt a significantly different level of surveillance compared with that chosen before the introduction of the relevant genetic tests. In what follows, we assume for the most part that these people do not switch their approach to surveillance. However, if the fraction of individuals in the population who are identified by genetic testing to be 'high risk types' for a particular disease becomes significant, as it may in the future as more susceptibility genes are discovered, then those who test negative will perceive a reduced risk to incur the disease and so may well change their surveillance behaviour. This may or may not be an individually or socially rational behavioural change. We suggest how this consideration may affect the cost-benefit analysis of the use of genetic tests, especially as population screening devices. In what follows, we make several simplifying assumptions in order to get at what we believe are the core issues that need to be considered.

From an ex ante perspective (i.e. before realization of the disease state) the individual chooses a level of surveillance in order to maximize expected utility. The expected utility depends both on his income net of total cost of medical care and the health status. The cost of medical care may be recovered through taxation, as in many countries, such as Canada, or through private health insurance premiums. In either case, the healthcare cost to the individual may or may not depend on the level of surveillance he chooses.[23] The individual holds a perceived probability of incurring the disease. If the individual does incur the disease, there is a probability of early detection that grows in the level of surveillance (e.g. frequency of mammograms or colonoscopies). The disease causes a perceived loss of health status to the individual, which is, however, smaller if the disease is detected early than if it is detected late. Engaging in surveillance in turn produces a non-financial or psychological cost, which is increasing in the level of surveillance.

For simplicity, we suppose that there are two surveillance levels available for the individual to choose in order to maximize his expected utility. We refer to these as low and high surveillance strategies. In the absence of genetic tests, all individuals hold the same probability of incurring a disease and the same probabilities of early (respectively late) detection given that the individual has incurred the disease. As long as the total cost of medical care and, hence, net income does not depend on the particular level of surveillance, the optimal decision on which level of surveillance to opt for depends only on the trade-off between the benefit one obtains from improving the probability of early versus late detection and the personal (non-financial) cost that reflects the psychological cost – and potential medical risk in some cases – of the surveillance activity. For now, we assume individuals have homogeneous preferences in that they hold similar views on the changes to health status, which depends on whether disease occurs, and whether the disease is detected early or late, and on the psychological cost of surveillance. Furthermore, assume that the relative levels of these variables are such that individuals in the scenario with no genetic testing choose the lower level of surveillance.

In contrast, the expected benefit from switching to a higher level of surveillance would exceed the additional personal (psychological) cost of increased surveillance if the probability of disease is high enough (which makes the expected benefit of early detection higher). Now, suppose a genetic test for a susceptibility gene becomes available and all individuals have the test (i.e. population screening takes place). Furthermore, suppose that the test is sufficiently informative that those who test positive have a sufficiently high probability of disease (which is higher than the initially perceived probability of disease before the test) that they switch to the higher level of surveillance. If this occurs, then the value of the test from the individual's ex ante perspective is positive. The reason for this is that, by conveying additional information on the probability of disease, the genetic test allows the individuals to adjust their demand for surveillance according to it. To summarize, the following factors enhance the private valuation of obtaining a genetic test for a susceptibility gene conditional on the presumption that those who test positive opt for a higher level of surveillance:

---

23 For example, in the US private insurers typically cover only a fraction of the cost of colonoscopies while in Canada such a cost would be covered entirely by the state health system but only provided the procedure fell under the list of covered items and it is recommended by the individual's physician.

Conditions 1

◆ A significant increase in the probability of incurring the disease due to the presence of the gene (i.e. if the probability of disease for those who test positive is substantially greater than the perceived probability of disease before the genetic test).

◆ The improvement in the probability of early detection due to the higher level of surveillance and the improvement of the health impact due to early detection are high.

◆ The additional psychic cost of a higher level of surveillance is not too great.

All of the above factors are relevant, not only from the perspective of private decision-making, but also from the social perspective in coming to a conclusion about whether the introduction of genetic testing on a population wide basis is worthwhile. However, there are other costs that individuals do not typically take into account if they do not pay directly (i.e. on a user-pays basis). If medical insurance is provided by the state, then the cost of the health care system is borne by individuals in a way that is unrelated to the health tests and treatments that the individual receives.[24] Therefore, to make a judgment on the social value of a particular genetic test, these additional costs must be taken into account.

One of these 'other costs' that is obviously relevant is the cost of the genetic test itself. From an ex ante perspective the value of a test naturally depends, in part, on the cost of the test. Moreover, the higher is the probability that the test will be positive and, hence, induce a switch in behaviour (from a low to a high level of surveillance), the higher is the ex ante value of the test. This is the reason underlying the well-known result that screening is often valuable only for individuals who, ex ante, are at high risk of having a faulty gene.[25] Although we return to the possibility of cost sharing between the health care provider (or insurer) and the individual, here we assume that the share of the financial costs of the health care system borne by an individual is independent of the particular individual's level of use. The expected financial costs (per capita) of providing for all aspects of health care (surveillance and treatment costs) are made up of the expected cost of treatment conditional on disease occurring, the financial costs of providing surveillance, and if genetic testing is offered, that cost needs to be accounted for as well. The expected cost of treatment in itself depends on the probability of disease and, presuming that the financial cost of treatment is lower if the disease is detected early, rather than late, on the probability of early detection.

In switching from the low to the high level of surveillance there is a saving in financial cost of treatment resulting from increased early detection in per capita terms.

---

[24] If individuals' coverage is through private insurance with positive coinsurance, at least some fraction of some of these other costs may be incurred by the individual.

[25] That is, population wide screening may not be socially worthwhile but screening of those at high risk, say as indicated by family background, may be. This is an especially important consideration if the genetic test is not perfect (i.e., if false positives and false negatives occur). We do not explicitly take into consideration the test accuracy in terms of specificity and sensitivity here either for the genetic test or the surveillance procedure. For such models, see Hoy 1989 and Hoy and Lambert 2000.

With a higher probability of disease the expected value of this saving is more significant. This cost saving is offset by the increased cost of a higher level of surveillance, as well as the cost of the genetic test. Thus, factors that enhance the financial value (WRT provision of health care services) due to the introduction of genetic testing for a susceptibility gene with the consequence that those who test positive opt for a higher level of surveillance are listed under 'Condition 2'.

Conditions 2

+ A significant increase in the probability of incurring the disease due to the presence of the gene (i.e. if the probability of disease for those who test positive is substantially greater than the perceived probability of disease before the genetic test).

+ The improvement in the probability of early detection due to the higher level of surveillance and the improvement in treatment costs due to early detection are high.

+ The additional financial cost of providing a higher level of surveillance is not too great.

+ The cost of the genetic test is low.

We see from the above set of conditions 1 and 2 that some factors that would lead to a genetic test reducing the financial cost imposed on the health care system due to a switch from a low to a high level of surveillance are in common with the factors that would influence private decisions in the same way. In particular, the greater is the salient information discovered from a positive test (i.e. the greater is the difference between the probability of disease for those who test positive and the initially perceived probability of disease) and the greater is the effectiveness of increased surveillance in arriving at an early diagnosis (i.e. the greater is the difference between the probabilities of early detection of the disease with the low and with the high level of surveillance), the more likely is an individual to make such a switch and the more likely such a switch will reduce the financial costs of the health care system. Consider the example of hereditary haemochromatosis, which causes the continuous accumulation of excess iron in the blood and various organs, and leads to their impairment. It has a relatively high prevalence in people with north European descent and the risk of developing the condition for individuals with the gene mutation goes up to 90 per cent. Because of the non-specific nature of the symptoms, such as fatigue and joint pain, it might remain undetected and cause cirrhosis, diabetes, or heart disease. The treatment of this condition, once it is detected by measuring the iron level in the blood, involves regular bloodletting. This is an inexpensive treatment measure that results in normal quality of life and life expectancy as long as the disease is detected early (Miller *et al.* 2002). In this particular example the individual's private valuation of a genetic test and its cost effectiveness for the healthcare system are likely to be aligned. In other cases, however, private and social evaluations may diverge, since insured individuals can be expected to ignore the financial costs of healthcare procedures whether they are covered privately or publicly.

In a public health care system, such as in Canada, the cost of an individual's medical procedures is typically not borne by the individual, but rather is shared by all those who contribute to the overall cost of the health care system through taxation or other payment systems. This is also true for those in jurisdictions where private health insurance is the usual form of coverage, such as in the USA, if the particular procedures/tests are covered by the plan. To an individual whose health care costs are covered by the community the financial consequences of his behaviour, in particular of his demand for surveillance, will be irrelevant.

Thus, even those enrolled in private health insurance plans may face incentives to 'over use' the health care system if the financial costs of health care, which the individuals do not account for, increase due to their behaviour. This is often described as a classic moral hazard effect due to insurance. In the case of private insurance, however, co-insurance payments are a more common feature and can be used to correct, to some extent, this moral hazard problem. Of course, this leaves individuals exposed to some risk. In the case of public insurance, the list of services and frequency with which they may be used can be regulated in order to contain the costs of socially ineffective tests and other medical procedures. However, determining what medical procedures should be included or excluded from the system is always a difficult decision, and so one can foresee many more problems arising due to increases in genetic information.

For many susceptibility genes, the difference between the probability of incurring the disease if tested positive and the perceived probability of disease before taking a genetic test is not striking, and so the financial cost of population-based screening may not be worthwhile, even if individuals would from private incentives opt for genetic testing with a subsequent increase in screening (i.e. conditional on receiving a positive test result).[26] Of course, there are scenarios in which, from a social perspective, individuals may opt for too little screening either in the presence or absence of information from genetic tests. Consider, for example, a scenario in which all individuals choose a relatively high level of surveillance in the absence of a genetic test. Suppose a genetic test becomes available, and those who test negative recognize the value of surveillance is not so high and so these individuals choose to reduce their level of surveillance (i.e. since their probability of onset of disease drops below the initially perceived probability of disease). This reduction in the level of surveillance may be welfare enhancing.[27] The capacity of a genetic test not only to induce higher surveillance for those who test positive, but also to reduce the costs of health provision and the personal inconvenience by identifying true negatives who switch to a lower level of surveillance, is emphasized in the case of colon cancer, especially when the test is targeted at individuals in a high risk category with a family background (Kievit *et al.* 2005). However, the probability of early detection will be lower for those engaging in a lower surveillance level. Since individuals do not internalize the additional financial

---

[26] Miller, *et al.* 2002 note this concern with possible repercussions of excessive screening costs if whole populations have access to genetic tests. Such might be the case for genetic testing for Alzheimer's disease, which has at least currently a rather low predictive power and there is no effective prevention or treatment for this disease. In this case, testing is recommended at most for symptomatic patients in order to aid in diagnosis and to avoid more severe impairments.

[27] Of course, private and social values of reduced screening for those who receive negative genetic test results may or may not be aligned. The factors leading to this result are essentially the opposite of those listed in Conditions 1 and 2 above.

cost of treating disease that is detected at a late, rather than early stage, from a social perspective the reduction of surveillance might be inefficient and the overall welfare implications of the genetic test may be negative, even though the individual finds it worthwhile to take the test and react accordingly.

Besides the potential improvements in health care, through more focused surveillance directed at early detection of disease, information derived from genetic tests for some diseases can lead to more effectively targeted prevention technologies and behaviours that can improve one's chances of avoiding the onset of disease altogether. An example would be the use of prophylactic treatments, such as the use of tamoxifen or double mastectomy for women found to be carrying one of the breast cancer genes *BRCA1/2*. Many of the same considerations as for changes in surveillance level arise and a similar reasoning can be applied to understand which factors enhance the private and social value of genetic tests, in regard to their informativeness and effect on prevention.

Preventive care will have psychic or personal non-pecuniary costs to the individual (e.g. effects of changes in lifestyle or effects of the preventive activities on the person's sense of well-being), as well, as in some cases (e.g. use of drugs or surgery), it will have costs on the insurance providers. The gain from a higher level of prevention is a reduced probability of onset of disease. To the individual, this is related to a reduced expected loss of health status and from a financial point of view the gain from a reduced probability of disease also includes the reduction of expected treatment costs. Thus, from the individual's (private) perspective, the trade-off of adopting a high versus a low level of prevention reflects the reduction of expected loss in health status versus the increase of personal non-pecuniary costs, while the social perspective also involves the trade-off between lower expected treatment costs and higher financial costs of providing prevention. The value of a genetic test will arise from the knowledge of person- or genome-specific differences in the extent to which the probability of disease is sensitive to the level of prevention that leads to differences in the effective use of preventive behaviours or treatments.[28] As before, in the case of surveillance, there is a divergence in the privately and socially optimal levels of preventive behaviour, and the sources of the difference can be seen to be almost precisely analogous.

Challenges for phase II of the genetic revolution: public and private insurance

We believe that the primary challenge for the health care system, whether shaped more by private insurance or public provision, is the determination of what genetic tests to include, the target population to make these available for, and what related medical procedures to include (e.g. surveillance levels and prophylactic measures). One can think of genetic tests as simply another diagnostic tool and the determination of whether a new diagnostic tool is worthwhile, as well as deciding on a target population for its application, is not a new type of decision problem. The same argument applies to the

---

[28] See Hoy 1989 for a description on how the relationship between preventive care and the probability of disease can vary between 'types' (i.e., genotypes). Also see Doherty and Posey 1998.

introduction of new drugs. However, it is possible that the next two or three decades will see a very substantial increase in the number of genetic technologies that will be candidates to be integrated into heath care systems. Moreover, the way that people perceive information from genetic tests can be qualitatively different from how they perceive other medical test results. Genetic information carries psychological qualities relating to individuals' psychic costs, family implications, insurance issues, and other characteristics that are often less important for 'standard' medical technologies. Therefore, determining individual reactions to this type of information is more challenging.

From our reasoning of the determinants of the value of genetic tests, we see that much of the incentive for genetic information at the individual level arises from purely subjective elements. We assumed implicitly that these items had the same impact on all individuals' subjective determination of well-being. This, of course, should not be expected to be the case. Therefore, one can expect different responses to and demand for information that will become increasingly available through genetic testing. This will complicate the fact that private insurance companies (or public systems for that matter) will have to cope with deciding which of these tests should be included in their policies and, if appropriate, what level of cost sharing to require from policy holders. What fraction of policy holders will avail themselves of genetic information? What will be the impact of obtaining the information on the demand for surveillance and precautionary services (e.g. mammograms, prophylactic drug treatments)? What impact will the change in use of surveillance and precautionary services have on the ability to detect disease earlier and, hence, create some savings in treatment costs? Should regulators require inclusion of some genetic tests (mandated coverage) to reduce cream-skimming and inefficiency in insurance markets due to adverse selection?

For countries that mostly rely on publicly provided health provision (or insurance), the same factors associated with genetic technologies as noted in the preceding paragraph must also be dealt with, albeit in a different manner. Public health care systems must ration the number of procedures covered, as well as drugs that are made available through the public system. What items should be covered? Should public systems apply user fees in relation to some aspects of genetic technologies? If so, how should these be decided upon in regards to genetic tests, surveillance procedures, precautionary approaches, etc? In cases in which adoption of genetic tests and subsequent higher surveillance levels for those who test positive is socially valuable due to high cost savings to the health care system, it doesn't necessarily follow that (all) individuals' interests will be aligned with societal interests. Individuals may not wish to voluntarily adopt higher surveillance levels in such situations. Are there viable policies to promote individuals to adopt 'best practices' in such situations? We have suggested a line of reasoning for focusing one's attention on the social versus private costs of these items. However, we do stress that any sort of formal cost-benefit analysis of genetic technologies will be difficult due to the newness and scale of the information, as well as the uncertainty of individual behavioural responses.

Conclusions

We hesitate to label this section 'conclusions', since mostly this chapter can be characterized as listing questions and challenges, while providing a methodology for addressing these. Perhaps the biggest question not yet brought up is whether genetic technologies will or should shift the balance between private and public aspects of health care systems. Public health care systems, such as that of Canada's, have a great deal of support from people because of their perceived equity benefits (see Davies and Hoy 2007). This can be argued from two perspectives:

> Such a system (as the Canadian health care system) embodies, in effect, two principles of distributive justice: (1) that ability to pay should govern contributions, not coverage, and (2) that we must share the burden of health risks and we are not entitled to benefit economically from having better health.
>
> (Daniels 2004, p. 132).[29]

Private health insurance regimes, on the other hand, typically allow for a broader range of co-payment systems that has the potential to correct for socially inefficient choices of individuals regarding various aspects of health care services.

We have argued that the growth in the use of genetic technologies has the potential to create challenges for health care systems from both equity and distributional perspectives. The relative impact of these two types of effects will depend in part on the balance of how health care costs are covered through private and public coverage. Most countries have mixed systems, even those typified as having primarily public provision such as Canada.[30] Insurance providers, whether private or public, will need to keep abreast of the developments in genetic technologies in order to decide which should be included within their policies or system. We have characterized the first phase of the genetic revolution as involving advancements in knowledge that will be relatively more important from a distributional or equity perspective. This will not provide so much of a challenge to public systems where the question of what is appropriate risk-rating behaviour of insurance providers is not an issue. Countries which rely more heavily on private insurance will need to grapple with decisions regarding appropriate regulation of the use of genetic information by insurers (see Hoy and Ruse 2005).[31]

In the second phase of the genetic revolution, which we have characterized by increases in genetic tests and related information or technologies that can be used to modify the likelihood or consequences of disease, the types of challenges to the health

---

[29] This second principle of redistributing from 'good risks' to 'bad risks' is sometimes argued to be achievable via private insurance that is compulsory and includes a community rating regulation.

[30] The move towards more private supplementary health insurance in conjunction with the growth in genetic information and technologies may lead to complex interactions in the arena of policy making for healthcare systems. For discussion on the extent to which private insurers use risk-rating, see (Cutler and Zeckhauser 2000, p. 627–629) and Van de Ven and Ellis 2000.

[31] Interestingly, up to writing of the penultimate version of this paper there was no federal legislation restricting the use of genetic test results for pricing of health insurance in the USA. However, on May 21, 2008, President Bush signed into law the so-called GINA bill (Genetic Information Nondiscrimination Act) which prohibits insurers from charging different prices for health insurance based on genetic information.

care system will change. Whether private or public, health care systems must make decisions about which genetic tests and related technologies are appropriate to include. We have outlined some of the factors that should influence such decisions, but there is no doubt that measuring the benefits and costs of such technologies will be difficult.

Acknowledgements

We thank the Brocher Foundation, LSE Health, and Geneva Association for sponsoring the conference at which this chapter was presented: 'Technology, innovation and change in health and healthcare.' We also thank participants at that conference and also at seminar presentations at Ryerson University, and especially Roland Eisen, Hristina Petkova, and Vincenzo Caponi for very helpful comments. The second author also thanks SSHRC for funding support. We are, of course, responsible for any errors, omissions, or other shortcomings of the chapter.

References

23andMe [homepage on the Internet]. Available at: https://www.23andme.com/ (accessed 22 July 2008).

Babul R, Adam S, Kremer B, Dufrasne S, Wiggins S, Huggins M, Theilmann J, Bloch M and Hayden MR (1993). Attitudes towards direct predictive testing for the Huntington's disease gene. *Journal of the American Medical Association*, **270**, 2321–5.

Barrett G and Conlon R (2001). Adverse selection and the decline in private health insurance coverage in Australia: 1989–1995. University of New South Wales discussion paper #2001/5.

Biesecker BB (2005). Genetic counseling: psychological issues. *Encyclopedia of Life Sciences*, 1–5.

Breast Cancer Care, UK [homepage on the Internet]. Available at: http://www.breastcancercare.org.uk (accessed 22 July 2008).

Butler J (2003). Adverse selection, genetic testing and life insurance—lessons from health insurance in Australia. *Agenda*, **10**, pp. 73–89.

Cowan RS (1994). Women's roles in the history of amniocentesis and chorionic villi sampling. In: KH Rothenberg and EJ Thomson (eds) *Women and prenatal testing: facing the challenges of genetic technology*, 35–48. Columbus, Ohio State university Press.

Cox S and McKellin W (1999). There's this thing in our family: predictive testing and the construction of risk for Huntington disease. *Sociology of Health and Illness*, **21**, 622–46.

Crocker KJ and Snow A (1986). The efficiency effects of categorical discrimination in the insurance industry. *Journal of Political Economy*, **94**, 321–44.

Cutler DM and Zeckhauser RJ (2000). The anatomy of health insurance. In: AJ Culyer and JP Newhouse (eds). *Handbook of health economics*, pp. 564–643. Amsterdam, North Holland, Elsevier.

Daniels N (2004). The functions of insurance and the fairness of genetic underwriting. In: MA Rothstein (ed.). *Genetics and life insurance: medical underwriting and social policy*, pp. 119–45. Cambridge, MIT Press.

Davies J and Hoy M (2007) Progressivity implications of public health insurance funding in Canada. *Research on Economic Inequality*, **15**, 145–82.

Doherty NA and Posey LL (1998). On the value of a checkup: adverse selection, moral hazard and the value of information. *Journal of Risk and Insurance*, **65**, 189–211.

Eddleman DA, Malone FD, Sullivan L, Dukes K, Berkowitz RL, Kharbutli Y, Porter TF, Luthy DA, Comstock CH, Saade GR, Klugman S, Dugoff L, Craigo SD, Timor-Tritsch IE, Carr SR, Wolfe HM, D'Alton ME (2006). Pregnancy loss rates after midtrimester amniocentesis. *Obstetrics and Gynecology*, **108**, 1067–72.

Gajilan AC. (2007). Mapping own DNA changes scientist's life, CNN 4 September 2007 [homepage on the Internet. Available at: http://edition.cnn.com/2007/HEALTH/09/04/dna.venter/index.html (accessed 22 July 2008).

GENETESTS [homepage on the Internet]. Available at: www.genetests.org (accessed 30 August 2007).

Hall MA (2005). Discrimination in insurance: experience in the United States. *Encyclopedia of Life Sciences*, 1–5.

Hoy M (1982). Categorizing risk in the insurance industry. *Quarterly Journal of Economics*, **97**, 321–36.

Hoy M (1984). The impact of imperfectly categorizing risk on income inequality and social welfare. *Canadian Journal of Economics*, **17**, 557–68.

Hoy M (1989). The value of screening mechanisms under alternative insurance possibilities. *Journal of Public Economics*, **39**, 177–206.

Hoy M (2006). Risk classification and social welfare. *Geneva Papers on Risk and Insurance: Issues and Practice*, **31**, 245–69.

Hoy M and Lambert PJ (2000). Genetic screening and price discrimination in insurance markets. *Geneva Papers on Risk and Insurance Theory*, **25**, 103–30.

Hoy M, Orsi F, Eisinger F and Moatti JP (2003). The impact of genetic testing on health care insurance. *Geneva Papers on Risk and Insurance: Issues and Practice*, **28**, 203–21.

Hoy M and Polborn M (2000). The value of genetic information in the life insurance market. *Journal of Public Economics*, **78**, 235–52.

Hoy M and Ruse M (2005). Regulating genetic information in insurance markets. *Risk Management and Insurance Review*, **8**, 211–37.

Hoy M and Witt J (2007). Welfare effects of banning genetic information in the life insurance market: the case of BRCA1/2 genes. *Journal of Risk and Insurance*, **74**, 523–46.

Kievit W, de Bruin JHFM, Adang EMM, Severens JL, Kleibeuker JH, Sijmons RH, *et al.* (2005). Cost effectiveness of a new strategy to identify HNPCC patients. *GUT*, **54**, 97–102.

Knoppers B, Godard B and Joly Y (2004). Life insurance and genetics: a comparative international overview. In: MA Rothstein (ed.) *Genetics and life insurance: medical underwriting and social policy*, pp. 173–94. Cambridge, MIT Press.

Lemmens T (2003). Genetics and insurance discrimination: a comparative analysis of legislative, regulatory and policy developments and Canadian options. *Health Law Journal*, Special Edition, 41–86.

Macdonald A (2000). Human genetics and insurance issues. In: I. Torrance (ed.) *Bio-ethics for the new millennium*. St Andrews: St Andrews Press.

Macdonald (2005). Genetic factors in life insurance: actuarial basis. *Encyclopedia of Life Sciences*, 1–5.

Machina M (1987). Choice under uncertainty: problems solved and unsolved. *Journal of Economic Perspectives*, **1**, 121–54.

Mansfield C, Hopfer S and Marteau TM (on behalf of a European concerted Action: DADA (Decision-making After the Diagnosis of a foetal Abnormality) (1999). Termination rates after prenatal diagnosis of Down syndrome, spina bifida, anencephaly, and

Turner and Klinefelter syndromes: a systematic literature review. *Prenatal Diagnosis*, **19**, 808–12.

Meiser, B. and S. Dunn (2000). "Psychological Impact of Genetic Testing for Huntington's Disease: An Update of the Literature," *Journal of Neurology, Neurosurgery and Psychiatry*, vol. **69**, pp. 574.

Miller F, Hurley J, Morgan S, Goeree R, Collins P, Blackhouse G, *et al.* (2002). Predictive genetic tests and health care costs: final report prepared for the Ontario Ministry of Health and Long Term Care. Available at: http://www.health.gov.on.ca/english/public/pub/ministry_reports/geneticsrep02/chepa.html (accessed 22 July 2008).

Picone G, Sloan F and Taylor D Jr (2004). Effects of risk and time preference and expected longevity on demand for medical tests. *Journal of Risk and Uncertainty*, **28**, 39–53.

Polborn M, Hoy M, and Sadanand A (2006). Advantageous effects of regulatory adverse selection in the life insurance market. *Economic Journal*, **116**, 327–54.

Procter A. (2006). Genetic testing of children. *Encyclopedia of Life Sciences*, 1–4.

Quaid KA and Morris M (1993). Reluctance to undergo predictive testing: the case of Huntington's disease. *American Journal of Medical Genetics*, **45**, pp. 41–5.

Rabin M and Thaler RH (2001). Anomalies: risk aversion. *Journal of Economic Perspectives*, **15**, 219–32.

Rothschild M and Stiglitz J (1976). Equilibrium in competitive insurance markets: an essay on the economics of imperfect information. *Quarterly Journal of Economics*, **90**, 629–49.

Subramanian K, Lemaire J, Hershey JC, Pauly MV, Armstrong K, and Asch DA (1999). Estimating adverse selection costs from genetic testing for breast and ovarian cancer: the case of life insurance. *Journal of Risk and Insurance*, **66**, 531–50.

Tabarrok A (1994). Genetic testing: an economic and contractarian analysis. *Journal of Health Economics*, **13**, 75–94.

Van de Ven WPMM and Ellis RP (2000). Risk adjustment in competitive health plan markets. In: AJ Culyer and JP Newhouse (eds). *Handbook of health economics*, vol. 1A, pp. 757–84. Amsterdam, North Holland, Elsevier.

Wagstaff A, van Doorslaer E, van der Burg H, Calonge S, Christiansen T, Citoni G, *et al.* (1999). Equity in the finance of health care: some further international comparisons. *Journal of Health Economics*, **18**, 263–90.

Wilson C (1977). A model of insurance with incomplete information. *Journal of Economic Theory*, **16**, 167–207.

Witt J (2007). The effect of information in the utilization of preventive health care strategies: an application to breast cancer. *Health Economics*, 17, 6, 721–731

Zhong H (2007). Equity in pharmaceutical utilization in Ontario: a cross section and over time analysis, EPRI Working paper No. 2007-1, University of Western Ontario. *Canadian Public Policy*, 33, 4, 487–507.

Zuckerman S. Lahad A Shmueli A, Zimran A, Peleg L, Orr-Urtreger A, Levy-Lahad E, Sagi M (2007). Carrier screening for Gaucher disease, lessons for low-penetrance, treatable diseases. *Journal of the American Medical Association*, **298**, 1281–90.

Part 4

Innovation, social demand, and valuation

Chapter 9

Ageing and pharmaceutical innovation

Roland Eisen and Yasemin Ilgin

Introduction

In almost all industrialized countries populations are 'greying'. On the one hand, average life expectancy—and also the further life expectancy of the 65 years old and older—is increasing. On the other hand, the fertility rate is lower than necessary to keep the population constant.[1] Therefore, the average age of the population is increasing. One reason behind this development is medico-technical progress. Pharmaceutical innovations can be seen as a driving force for this process, too.[2] However, this progress must be paid for.

A superficial investigation of available data reveals that overall, health care expenditures and, within these, expenditure on pharmaceuticals are increasing with age. One interpretation of this trend may be that the willingness to pay for health in general, but also for pharmaceuticals is increasing with age. Three arguments can be suggested for this relationship.

+ The general health status of elderly people combined with the Sisyphus syndrome (cf. Zweifel and Ferrari 1992) or the multi-morbidity hypothesis (cf. Kraemer 1996).

The Sisyphus syndrome describes the relationship that medico-pharmaceutical progress increases life expectancy, so that the increasing number of elderly persons demands more medico-pharmaceutical progress and so forth. The multi-morbidity hypothesis, on the other hand, stresses the following relationship: if, because of medico-pharmaceutical progress, the mortality rate is decreasing, then not only the fittest survive, and the pool of elderly increases. In other words, people grow older, but not healthier, and have to fight against other illnesses and so on. This relationship, however, is dampened by the findings, gained from recent research, that most health expenditures are made in the last (half) year before death.[3]

---

[1] For example, the fertility rate of Germany, i.e. the reproduction rate, is around 1.3; to keep the population constant, the fertility rate should be a little over 2 children per woman.

[2] See Lichtenberg and Virabhak (2002).

[3] Cf. Fuchs (1984), and empirical evidence in Lubitz and Riley (1993), Zweifel *et al.* (1996), and Busse *et al.* (2002).

- Elderly people do not have a long further life expectancy and, therefore, people want to make higher expenditures.
- Finally, surgery is marginal in old age, while pharmaceuticals 'lighten' the living of it.

Accompanying these ideas is the notion that social security (but also health care expenditures themselves) raise the value of a long life, hence inducing elderly people to increase their demand for health care (and also pharmaceuticals).

Therefore, it is interesting to ask whether elderly people only spend more on pharmaceuticals to have an easier life, or whether the pharmaceutical industry reacts to this trend of 'population greying' by directing research and development (R&D) of new pharmaceuticals in this direction.

The following sections outline a general way in which the process of innovation might be conceptualized, stressing the importance of 'induced innovations.' In the third part, we develop the main hypothesis we seek to support with empirical investigation, namely that as the proportion of elderly in a population rises, not only the share of pharmaceutical expenditure rises, but also the share of pharmaceutical R&D devoted to this part of the population. With the help of a simple econometric model, we shall attempt to test this hypothesis and present some results. The chapter closes with a summary and some conclusions.

The process of innovation

Progress is a complex process, which has been described by Joseph Schumpeter already in 1911 (1964) as a 'process of creative destruction.' Behind progress for Schumpeter was the notion of innovation. Progress and, therefore, innovation is a phase in the life cycle of a product—and the phase of invention occurs prior to innovation, which then is followed by the phase of imitation or diffusion. In other words, innovation is part of the process of innovation, starting with research and development (R&D), resulting in an invention [i.e. a new technological idea or a new molecular entity (NME), leading in most cases to a patent], followed by the construction of a prototype, etc., leading, if successful, to an innovation or a new drug. This process ends with the spreading of the innovation, used not only by the innovator, but other firms (imitators), called diffusion, or in the special case of pharmaceuticals to 'me-too products.'[4]

It is evident that new ideas or ideas for new products are not freely available as 'free goods.' There is no 'sea of inventions' from which the creative entrepreneur (or pioneer entrepreneur as Schumpeter has called him) can fish for those promising profits. This picture of the 'inventor,' who creates 'unselfishly' new ideas, best described by serendipity or spontaneity, is no longer valid. Inventions must be seen as the result of productive inputs and, therefore, as a strategic instrument of the entrepreneur, called R&D (cf. Muennich 2000, p. 119).

This picture is of particular importance in the R&D of the pharmaceutical industry (as also stressed by Stan Metcalf and Andrea Mina): here one sees a 'circular

---

[4] This process is aptly described by Consoli *et al.* in chapter 2 of this volume.

intertwined process,' with many interdependencies and much feed-back prior to product realization on the market. This idea comes very close to the ideas of technical progress as an evolutionary process developed by Nelson and Winter (cf. Dosi *et al.* 2003). This then posits two interesting problems: on the one hand, imitation itself can hardly be delimited from innovation (as in the so-called 'me-too products'), while on the other hand, the relationship between R&D and marketing can hardly be dissolved (cf. in particular, Brekke and Straume 2008).

Given this, the process of innovation can then be related to the context of demand and supply.[5] On the supply side, patent law, admission procedures, regulation of prices, R&D expenditures, number of researchers, and the size and structure of the industry are important factors. On the demand side, income, and needs and wants are relevant. Behind these needs and wants stands the population, its illnesses, income, size, and in particular age structure. For example, as Yoram Barzel (1968) argued, all innovations are induced, since they become more profitable with the expansion of output. However, if pharmaceutical progress is made, then besides the argument that it will be made only when profits are increasing or costs decreasing, one can also ask, in which direction such progress will be driven? In other words, other than profit motivation, what incentives exist for the specific direction of progress?

Traditionally, economics labels 'induced technical progress,' as a type of factor price-induced technical progress. Here, such progress includes the substitution of the more expensive production factor for the other production factor(s).[6] This induced technical progress operates through a reduction in production costs and, hence, motivates process innovations. In the pharmaceutical industry, however, progress pursues new products, or new chemical or molecular entities, and hence product innovations. The question then is what drives this technical progress?[7]

Competition—so goes the argument—forces enterprises to an ever quicker development of new products. It is competition that forces the pharmaceutical firm to allocate resources in those market segments where high profits can be expected. The research centre of gravity is orientated toward short-term profit interests. Given the production costs, the profit is determined by revenue or demand. Behind demand stands the (marginal) willingness to pay of individuals. Hence, we are back to the relationship raised in the introduction: expenditures for pharmaceuticals are increasing with age. Therefore, it seems evident to suggest that technical progress in the pharmaceutical industry is driven by demographic changes that provide the new market opportunities.

---

[5] See also Cassel (2004) who stressed that the pharmaceutical industry is a highly concentrated high-tech industry combining research, production, and service industry.

[6] This idea originated with Karl Marx, was taken up by Hicks (1963), and mathematically formulated by Drandakis and Phelps (1966); see for a new source Acemoglu (2002).

[7] Besides the factor price-induced technical progress, the economic literature also discusses research-induced technical progress (for a summary cf. Eisen 1971).

Research hypotheses

Proceeding from the argument that demographic changes and, in particular, the 'greying of societies' induce pharmaceutical progress, we propose three related research hypotheses we wish to pursue:

- *Hypothesis 1:* if the share of the 65 years old and older in the population (henceforth, share of 65+) and their (further) life expectancy increase, then the share of pharmaceuticals in total health expenditures increases.

- *Hypothesis 2:* the expenditures of the pharmaceutical industry for R&D increase, if the share of 65+ and their (further) life expectancy increase.

The notion is, that the pharmaceutical industry is especially interested in innovative pharmaceuticals for the dominant health problems of elderly people (chronic diseases, diseases of the body, heart, etc.), who also show a higher willingness to pay.

- *Hypothesis 3:* if the R&D expenditures of the pharmaceutical industry, the share of 65+ and their (further) life expectancy increase, then the pharmaceutical innovations/inventions increase (measured by the number of patent applications).

According to Scherer (2001), it is the relationship between profits and R&D expenditures, which drives the pharmaceutical innovation process. However, since we do not have data on expected profits, we formulate the third hypothesis by considering patents. We use patent applications instead of patents granted, because both series run almost parallel and we believe it to be the better proxy for research output.

A first impression for the patent applications of selected patents is given in Fig. 9.1.

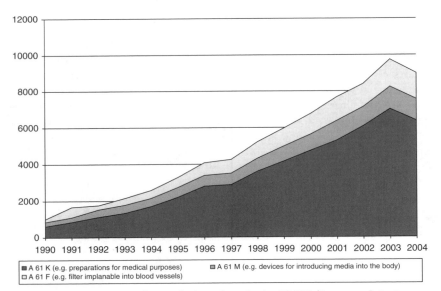

Fig. 9.1 Patent applications for medical products in the 30 EPC (European Patent Convention) states.

Econometric model[8]

The data set

Since the mid-1990s, the expenditure on prescribed pharmaceuticals has risen faster than all other relevant components of health care expenditures. Data for seven countries—Australia, Canada, Finland, France, Germany, Japan, and USA—over a period of 11 years (1991–2001) were taken for the analysis. OECD Health Data for 2005 are our main source. The research activity data are taken from the Yearbook 2005 of the WIPO PCT Statistical Indicators Report (2001).

Health Care Expenditures and the expenditures for prescribed pharmaceuticals increase (almost) monotonically for all the considered countries (cf. Fig. 9.2). Only for Germany and Finland do the data show some breaks in 1991, 1992 as well as in 1993. Figure 9.3 exhibits the data of expenditures for pharmaceuticals and other medical (non-durable) goods, for prescribed pharmaceuticals, and for non-prescribed pharmaceuticals. While France is leading in the first two categories, the USA takes over in the third category.

Methods and variables

For our analysis, three different methods were adopted: first, ordinary least-square method (OLS); secondly, the fixed effects estimator; and last, but not least, the generalized method of moments (GMM). The basic idea is to use ever more appropriate estimators to show clearly the improvements resulting from the different methods. The fixed effect estimator uses the idea that some of the regression coefficients vary between countries and time periods. The GMM (with first differences) is especially adapted for dynamic panel data. We have different observations for different countries, and we presume that past values of the variables determine or influence present values, thus adopting a dynamic approach. However, the small size of our data set must be taken into account in this respect.

The variables utilized in the model are defined as follows: Health Care Expenditures (HCE), population size (DEMO), share of population of 65 years and older (POP65 per cent), further life expectancy of women 65 years old (LIFEXP65), share of pharmaceutical expenditures in total health care expenditures (DRUG/HCE), doctor visits per thousand patients (DOC), production value (value added) of the pharmaceutical industry (PHARMAPROD), research and development expenditures of the pharmaceutical industry (PHARMA R&D), patent applications (PATENT), share of prescribed drugs in total health care expenditures (DRUGPRES/HCE).

Results

We report only the results with respect to the first-differenced GMM model, and these are presented in Table 9.1. This method uses a dynamic model and the lagged variables are found to be highly significant. For this model we did not use the share of pharmaceutical

---

[8] For a description of the model cf. Ilgin and Eisen (2006).

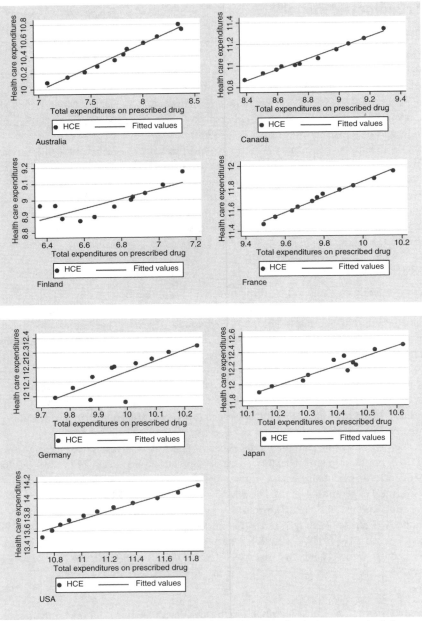

Fig. 9.2 Health care expenditure and expenditure for prescribed pharmaceuticals in Australia, Canada, Finland, France, Germany, Japan, and USA, 1991–2001 (in Mio US$, Purchasing Power Parity).

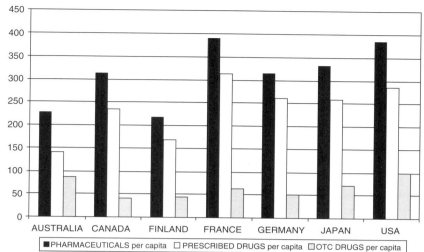

Fig. 9.3 Expenditures for pharmaceuticals and other medical (non-durable) goods, for prescribed and for non-prescribed (OTC) Drugs, 1991–2001.

expenditure as the dependent variable, but the nominal value of these expenditures. For all three hypotheses, either the share of 65+ or the further life expectancy of females 65+ are highly significant. Interestingly, the number of physician consultations is—if we consider our second hypothesis—only weakly significant (at the 5 per cent level), but negative. This result seems to contradict the popular hypothesis that physicians' create their

Table 9.1 First-differenced GMM estimations

Endogenous Regressor	H1	H2	H3.1	H3.2
HCE_{t-1}	1.024***			
HCE_{t-2}	-0.408***			
$DRUG_{t-1}$		0.646***		
$DRUG_{t-2}$		-0.017		
$PATENT_{t-1}$			0.451***	0.421***
$PATENT_{t-2}$			0.297***	0.250**
Predetermined Var				
Δ PHARAM_R&D	-0.002**	0.005*	0.166*	0.259**
$PHARAM\_R\&D_{\tau-1}$			-0.293**	- 0.315***
Regressor				
Δ POP65	0.005***	0.018**		
Δ LIFEP65			0.018***	-0.007
Δ DOC	0.010*	-0.024**		
Δ GDP				0.006*

own demand (physician-induced demand), at least with respect to pharmaceuticals. This result, however, might also reflect the effects of the public policy towards cost containment.

Summary and conclusions

The results relating to health care expenditures (HCE) and pharmaceutical expenditures (DRUG) are clear cut: both variables are highly significant with respect to the share of the elderly population (POP65 per cent) and the (further) life expectancy of elderly women (LIFEXP65). The negative sign on the number of physician visits is of noted interest.

R&D expenditures appear to be highly significant with respect to further (female) life expectancy. Patent applications are highly significant with respect to further life expectancy of women, and to R&D expenditures. Such results are in line with our research hypotheses: Pharmaceutical expenditures, as well as expenditures for R&D and the patent applications of the pharmaceutical industry are determined or induced by the 'effects of ageing', and the 'greying of society'.

However, the analysis is preliminary and requires confirmation using more countries and a longer time series. Also, different time intervals with respect to age should be taken into account. Health care expenditures and, therefore, also pharmaceutical expenditures can be expected to vary across different age groups, for example, they are likely to be different in terms of impact and motivation for the 60–64 age group, the 65–69 group, the 70–74 group, etc.

This would also allow testing of the aforementioned hypothesis relating to whether pharmaceutical expenditures can be used as a substitute for surgery interventions in older people. In other words, one could, in general, look at the effects of managed care with respect to changes in expenditures across hospital procedures and general pharmaceuticals. Furthermore, the data on patents could be more refined, in particular towards age-specific or chronic illnesses.

Acknowledgement

We thank the participants of the conference, and in particular the editors for valuable comments. However, the views are those entirely of the authors.

References

Acemoglu D (2002). Directed technical change. *Review of Economic Studies*, **69**, 781–810.

Barzel Y (1968). The optimal timing of innovations. *Review of Economics and Statistics*, **50**, 348–55.

Brekke KR and Straume OR (2008). Pharmaceutical patents: incentives for R&D or marketing? CESifo WP No. 243, Munich, Oct. Accessed on 13 December 2007.

Busse R, Krauth C and Schwartz FW (2002). Use of acute hospital beds does not increase as the population ages: results for a seven year cohort study in Germany. *Journal of Epidemiology and Community Health*, **56**, 289–93.

Cassel D (2004). Innovationshürden und Diffusionsbarrieren der Arzneimittelversorgung (Barriers to innovation in drug delivery). In: E Wille and MN Albring eds.

Paradigmawechsel im Gesundheitswesen durch neue Versorgungsstrukturen? pp. 275–87. Frankfurt, Peter Lang Publ.,

Dosi G, Malerba F and Teece D (2003). Twenty years after Nelson and Winter's 'An Evolutionary Theory of Economic Change'. *Industrial and Corporate Change*, **12**, 147–8.

Drandakis EM and Phelps ES (1966). A model of induced invention, growth and distribution. *Economic Journal*, **76**, 823–40.

Eisen R (1971). *Technischer Fortschritt und wirtschaftliches Wachstum. Beitraege zu einer Theorie des technischen Fortschritts (Technical Progress and Economic Growth)*. Dissertation, Muenchen.

Fuchs VR (1984). Though much is taken – reflections on aging, health, and medical care, *Working Paper*, NBER, Cambridge/MA. Available at: http://www.nber.org/papers/w1269 (accessed 13 June 2007).

Hicks JR (1963). *The theory of wages*, 2nd edn. London, Macmillan Press.

Ilgin Y and Eisen R (2006). Health care expenditures, ageing population and pharmaceutical innovation, *Working Paper*. Frankfurt, INEGES.

Krämer W (1996). Hippokrates and Sisyphus—die moderne Medizin als Opfer ihres eigenen Erfolgs (Hippocrates and Sisyphos—the modern medicine as victim of its own success). In: W Kirch and H Kliemt, eds. *Rationierung im Gesundheitswesen*, pp. 389–93. Regensburg, Roderer Press.

Lichtenberg FR and Virabhak S (2002). Pharmaceutical-embodied technical progress, longevity, and quality of life: drugs as 'Equipment for your Health', *Working Paper* No. 9351, NBER, Cambridge, MA. Available at: http://www.nber.org/papers/w9351, Accessed on 21 January 2009.

Lubitz JD and Riley GF (1993). Trends in medicare payments in the last year of life. *New England Journal of Medicine*, **328**, 1092–6.

Muennich FA (2000). Innovatorischer Wettbewerb auf dem Arzneimittelmarkt (Competition by innovation in the pharmaceutical market). In: J Klauber and J Bausch, eds. *Innovation im Arzneimittelmarkt*, pp. 107–29. Berlin, Springer Publ.

OECD (2005). *OECD Health Data 2005*. Paris, OECD.

Scherer FM (2001). The link between gross profitability and pharmaceutical R&D spending. *Health Affairs*, **20**(5), 216–20.

Schumpeter J (1964). *Theorie der wirtschaftlichen Entwicklung (Theory of economic development)*, 6th edn. Berlin, Duncker & Humblot Publ.

WIPO (2005). *PCT Statistical Indicators Report, Annual Statistics 1978–2004*. Available at: http://www.WIPO.int/ipstats, Accessed on 9 February 2008.

Zweifel P, Felder S and Meier M (1996). Demographische Alterung und Gesundheitskosten: Eine Fehlinterpretation (Demographic ageing and health care costs: a misinterpretation). In: P Oberender, ed. *Alter und Gesundheit*, pp. 29–46. Bade-Baden, Nomos Publ.

Zweifel P and Ferrari M (1992). Is there a Sisyphus syndrome in health care? In: P Zweifel and HE Frech, eds. *Health economics worldwide*, Developments in Health Economics and Public Policy series, vol. 1, pp. 311–30. Boston, Kluwer Publ.

Chapter 10

New approaches to health care innovation: information for the chronic patient

Manuel García-Goñi and Paul Windrum

Introduction

Our general aim is to obtain a better knowledge of health innovations, their key drivers, and dynamics. Developing a general model requires ongoing testing against different types of health service innovations. In this chapter, we focus on the interaction between two agents: health service providers and patients. The case study presented in this chapter highlights the importance of modifying the quantity and quality of the health information provided to patients, and *the way* in which that information is provided. With that aim, we have selected a case study consisting of the substitution of one educational programme for diabetes patients for a new programme.

We present the different approaches that have been developed and applied to innovation in services, specifically those built on the Lancaster characteristics approach: the Saviotti and Metcalfe (1984) model, and the Gallouj and Weinstein (1997) model. We then introduce a neo-Schumpeterian model of health services innovation proposed by the authors in an earlier work (Windrum and García-Goñi 2008). This differs from previous models in several aspects. One of its key features is its consideration of interactions between three different agents—health providers, patients, and health policy-makers. By contrast, earlier models only considered service providers. Hence, the model is a first step in the development of a general model of health service innovation, with the potential for application to other sectors.

The importance of education and information in healthcare need and provision has been analysed in the health economics literature. It has been found that patients using more information tend to accomplish more protective behaviours (Viscusi *et al.* 1986). Also, the literature has shown how there exists a strong correlation between education and health status (Kenkel 1991; deWalque 2007), and between income levels and health status (Sen 1999; Bloom and Canning 2000). As a consequence, individuals with a higher level of education/income, who better manage information, or both, make better health-related decisions. These health-related decisions are translated into a greater use of health services, because individuals with higher education realize sooner (or better) the marginal return of health services and, therefore, have a higher demand for health services (Kenkel 1990). However, in an ongoing project, we are analysing whether education interventions (specifically the development of a patient-centred education) have an impact, in terms of patients' seeking to improve their lifestyles and manage their condition, and hence on their health status. We are also interested on whether the effect of information might be different, depending on the type of health condition. Thus, while information plays a role in increasing demand for health services by patients with acute illnesses, in the case of chronic illnesses it may be that learning healthier lifestyles and habits results in a *reduction* of future demand, i.e. the substitution effect is greater than the income or educational effect (the decrease in the need of health services is greater than the increase in their demand given the educational or income effect). Hence, chronic patients may obtain greater benefits from detailed information than acute patients due to their greater capability to affect the demand (future need) for health services.

The way in which consumers demand health information has also been explored. It is found that the source of health information is changing, from physicians and/or health professionals to other sources such as the Internet (Wagner *et al.* 2001: Costa-Font *et al.* Chapter 16, this volume). As a consequence, not only are educational level and health information important, but also the means by which patients obtain the health-related information that they use. Therefore, education programmes and sources of information on health conditions can be included as an input in the health production function.

The selected case study examines the development of a novel patient-centred education for type 2 diabetics within the Salford Primary Care Trust (PCT)[1] between 2002 and 2005. This new programme replaced the previous didactic education programme. The new programme was developed by two public sector institutions: the Salford PCT Community Diabetes Team and a group of education experts from Manchester Metropolitan University. In the previous, didactic programme of healthcare education, the health care professional imparts information to a passive patient. By contrast, in the patient-centred education programme, patients are more active and the professional's role is one of a mediator. The health care professional mediates an open discussion with groups of patients, asks open questions, and helps patients consider alternative options for taking control of their diabetes, and considers the likely consequences.

This case study provides a number of important insights into the real impact of the interaction between health providers and patients on long-term health status. It also provides us with an opportunity to test whether our neo-Schumpeterian model of health innovations can capture these effects. The chapter therefore presents a new approach to understanding health service innovations, through the education and information provided to chronic patients in the public sector.

The model

This section introduces a number of Lancaster type models of innovation that have been proposed in the literature and their development, paying particular attention

---

[1] Salford is a district within the Greater Manchester region of England.

to the new features presented by each different model.[2] This culminates in the neo-Schumpeterian model of health services innovation, developed by Windrum and García-Goñi (2008), which will be tested in the remainder of this chapter.

The origin of the characteristics tradition of modelling innovation stems from the work of Lancaster (1966, 1971). He observed that all types of products (both material goods and immaterial services) can be described as a bundle of 'service characteristics' (or attributes) that goods or a service embodies. As a consequence, consumer choice does not depend on a product in itself, but on the particular bundle of service characteristics that it offers and its price. This insight was applied by Saviotti and Metcalfe (1984) and Saviotti (1996) to the study of innovation in manufacturing. In this model, firms compete by offering particular combinations of service characteristics that they believe will be more attractive to consumers than those of their rivals. In effect, they offer consumers distinct points within a multi-dimensional space of service characteristics.

The combination of 'service characteristics' of each product is directly related to a set of 'technical characteristics.' The latter include the underpinning product technologies that, together, generate the final consumer product. Hence, according to this model, improving the set of technical characteristics leads to an improvement in the service characteristics that consumers are interested in. In addition to product innovation, the Saviotti–Metcalfe model considers the impact of process innovation. The 'process characteristics' discussed by the model includes tangible assets (such as plant and equipment), intangible assets (such as brand name, copyright, and patents), human resources (such as education, training, experience, and skills of individual staff), and organizational resources (such as corporate culture, organizational structure, rules, and the procedures of the firm) that range from the design to production to marketing (also see Saviotti 1985, 1996). As a consequence, the vector of service characteristics changes over time as firms seek to improve their competitive position through a combination of product innovation (on the vector of technical characteristics) and process innovation (on the vector of process characteristics).

The Windrum–García-Goñi model builds on the Saviotti–Metcalfe model and the work of Gallouj and Weinstein (1997). The first notable difference is that the Windrum–García-Goñi model is a multi-agent framework, which includes policy-makers and public sector service providers, as well as service providers (firms) and consumers. This allows for interactions between economic, social, and political spheres. It captures the key groups involved in the health innovation process and who exerting an important influence on the evolution of innovations. This noticeably differs from the Saviotti–Metcalfe and Gallouj–Weinstein models, which focused almost exclusively on firms.

The second difference involves capturing the long-term co-evolution of agents' competences and interests, and innovation. Policy-makers, service providers, and end users (patients) each have a vector of competences and preferences, which is revealed

---

2 Note that the aim of this chapter is not to provide a complete and detailed revision of all such models, but to highlight the specific features of a number of important models, and researchers have developed these in their search for a general model of innovation - an ongoing research goal.

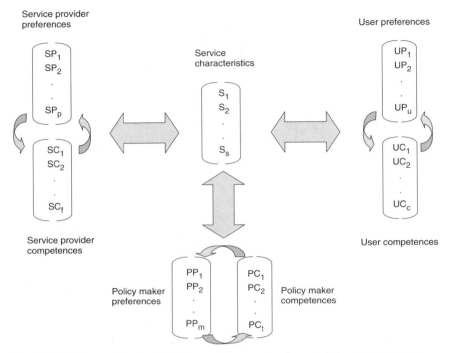

Fig. 10.1 Multi-agent framework of co-evolving service characteristics, competences, and preferences. Source: Windrum and García-Goñi (2008).

in their interests. Together, these make up the complex selection environment in which innovations succeed or fail. Over time, these competences and preferences, in turn, are altered as a consequence of the development and diffusion of radical innovations. Thirdly, the Windrum–García-Goñi model captures all five types of innovation discussed by Schumpeter (1934, 1943): organizational, product, market, process, and input. A radical innovation not only alters the dimensions of the service characteristics vector, but also the competences and preferences of the three agents. Thus, it captures the central neo-Schumpeterian message of long-term change. The framework is provided in Fig. 10.1.

Windrum (2007) observed that not all services require the active participation of users in their design, specification, or delivery. For example, there exist a number of health services that do not require patients' interactions, such as surgical operations, where the surgical team provide a service to an inactive patient under anaesthesia. This type of service is akin to the manufacturing of mass-produced artefacts. It does not involve interaction with patients in the design and delivery of the service, and the provider exploits opportunities for scale economies in production.

Note that the focus in this chapter is the interaction between health providers and users (or patients). Hence, we will not explore in detail here the interaction between the two institutions that together developed the patient-centred programme (i.e. MMU and Salford PCT). This allows us to make a number of theoretical simplifications to the original Windrum–García-Goñi model. Notably, we can simplify by treating the 'service provider' as a single, integrated producer. Hence, we do not need to consider the competences and preferences, or interaction, of different institutions that together delivered the final service. Also, for our current purposes, we will also treat policy-makers as a boundary group of actors: policy stimulated the development of a new service and influences some key parameters of the new service, but the development of the final set of service characteristics depends on the interaction between the service provider and patients.

Consequently, the simplified version of the Windrum–García-Goñi model we will use here focuses on innovation drivers that stem from the changing needs of health services provision (demand for health services by patients), which depend on demographic characteristics and preferences, and on the accumulated knowledge and preferences of the health provider. Thus, the key factors that drive changes in the vector of final service characteristics are competence and preference vectors of health providers and patients.

The vector of preferences and competences in the patient are in part privately determined, and in part socially influenced by the preferences and competences of his/her family and by the environment in which the patient lives. Hence, the demand for health services is determined in part by the patient but also by the family/social group to which patients belong.

As noted above, we are here considering patients who have a chronic illness. We argue that patients suffering chronic illness have a different composition in the vector of competences than patients that have an acute illness. There are several differences between acute and chronic conditions. For example, all the population is affected by acute conditions with the same probability, they usually come on suddenly with an identifiable cause and generally, after receiving the provision of health services, patients return to their previous health status after a normally short period. However, chronic conditions often begin gradually and rarely are cured, but patients suffer chronic conditions for an indefinite time. Therefore, different patients have different probabilities of suffering a chronic condition depending on their previous health status or other factors as the genetic component, lifestyle, or other environmental factors.

The key issue for our model is that, due to the different length of illness, and the different probabilities of suffering the condition, chronic patients may benefit more than acute patients of the knowledge regarding their illnesses. The idea behind this analysis relies on the fact that chronic patients need to learn how to live with their specific long-term conditions, while other patients basically need to promote normal healthy lifestyles. Therefore, the marginal utility provided by specific knowledge is greater for chronic than for acute patients, because they can prevent a more predictable need of healthcare provision. As a consequence, the competences vector of chronic patients is more technically developed in medical terms according to their health conditions than in the case of acute patients. Furthermore, because chronic patients need to learn with their condition, their lifestyle is more dependent on the health status and they will also have a different vector of preferences, on average, than acute patients, more orientated to prevent the need of health services provision because it means having a higher quality of life. As a consequence, the role of patients in the process of health innovations is also different. In the case of chronic patients, they will have a greater effect in the vector of service characteristics, while the role of acute patients is much more limited.

Note that, following Barras' (1986, 1990), a useful distinction is drawn between the user facing competences of service providers (which includes all the tangible and intangible skills, know-how, and technologies that are used to produce service characteristics), and back office competences (which includes the skills and administrative activities, such as payroll and patient booking systems) that support the user facing competences and activities.

The case study

In order to test the multi-agent model of health services innovation presented above, we consider an innovation that occurred in the Greater Manchester area. This involved the replacement of a 'traditional' didactic educational programme for type 2 diabetes patients by a new, patient-centred programme.[3]

Diabetes is a chronic long-term condition for which there is, as yet, no cure. It supposes a health condition for which we are interested in testing our model of health services innovation because it is a very common condition, and whose educational programmes are based on human capital. In order to understand the importance of this chronic condition it is relevant to note that diabetes mellitus supposes the fifth leading cause of death by disease in the USA (American Diabetes Association 2003), and also supposes an important proportion of the burden of disease in countries as Australia (Dixon 2005) or Canada (Ohinmaa et al. 2004). In England, there are 1.4 million people with diagnosed diabetes in England and its incidence is rising. This is a direct consequence of an ageing population (more than 10 per cent of people over 65 are diabetic) and an increasing incidence of obesity. The vast majority of those patients in England (85 per cent) living with the disease are diagnosed with type 2 diabetes. Patients with type 2 diabetes are able to produce some insulin, but the levels are not sufficient to properly control their blood sugar levels. However, it is estimated that 1 million people in the UK have the condition, but are currently undiagnosed due to a lack of screening. Type 2 diabetes tends to run in families and is particularly common amongst people of African, Caribbean, and Asian origin. At the moment, the average age for developing the disease is 52 years. Nevertheless, the average age is falling and some very overweight children are now affected.

Diabetes mellitus is an important example of chronic condition whose health service provision needs to be analysed because it contributes to higher rates of morbidity and to increase the demand of health services and the length of duration of that provision (Ramsey et al. 2002) and, therefore, an important amount of health expenditures. Complications associated with diabetes are very serious. They include blindness, heart disease, foot amputation, and (in men) erectile dysfunction. Through management of

---

[3] For more information, see the report by Windrum and Senyucel (2006).

their lifestyle and daily care control, type 2 patients can control and reduce the impact of complications. The key aspects are a healthy food regime, regular physical activity, the monitoring of blood sugar levels, and (if necessary) the use of drugs to control blood sugar levels. For some, changing exercise patterns may be all but impossible in practice (i.e. those who are badly overweight and suffering from arthritis), so the focus tends to fall on diet.

The literature has devoted efforts to different actions undertaken towards the provision of diabetes care, and to the relationship between the health status of diabetic patients and their need of health services provision. Thus, different clinical trials provide evidence, for example, of how lowering blood-glucose levels has a positive consequence, delaying the onset and slowing the progression of diabetic retinopathy, nephropathy, and neuropathy in patients with insulin-dependent diabetes mellitus (Diabetes Control and Complications Trial 1993), intensive diabetes therapy has long-term beneficial effects on the risk of cardiovascular disease in patients with type 1 diabetes (Nathan *et al.* 2005) or how intensive blood-glucose control for adult patients with type 2 diabetes decreases the risk of microvascular complications (UK Prospective Diabetes Study Group 1998). Beaulieu *et al.* (2007) review the cost-effective literature on different diabetes disease management programmes. They also analyse the fact that even if diabetes disease management programmes are potentially beneficial, less than 40 per cent of adults with diabetes achieve guideline-recommended levels of medical care with American data, finding evidence of adverse selection in the health provision of diabetes care given the payment system. Other literature reviews on economic analysis of intervention for diabetes are presented in Klonoff and Schwartz (2000) or Zhang *et al.* (2004).

Traditional and patient-centred educational models

The patient-centred diabetes education programme is one manifestation of the concept of patient-centred health. Patient-centred health is a new concept whose introduction and development marks a major departure from the traditional health care model. The traditional model has proved highly effective for the treatment of acute illness. Health professionals are in overall charge of care, which includes diagnosis, treatment decisions, and ensuring that treatment is carried out as prescribed. The person receiving treatment, meanwhile, is a passive patient who accepts medical decisions, complies with instructions, and is dependent on the health care professional. In other words, under the traditional model there is no interaction between the health provider and the patient.

Differently, in the patient-centred health model the patient is the central focus of health care, and engages in a partnership with the health care professional. In addition to the physical aspects of a condition, the knowledge and skills of the patient are important, as are their psychological, emotional, and behavioural states. Within the patient–practitioner partnership, each brings their knowledge and experience to the table, engages in negotiations, and makes decisions about areas for improvement in the patients' self-care and daily choices. Therefore, in the case of the patient-centred health model, interactions between health providers and patients become crucial in the development of the provision of health services.

With respect to the organization of the two different educational programmes, there is an important difference: the traditional educational programme used to take place in two sessions, while the patient-centred educational programme is scheduled for three sessions. Therefore, the innovation produces a higher quality in the education through an increase in the length and contents of the educational programme, but also increases the opportunity cost of time in patients.

In the case of the educational programme for diabetes patients, the health care professional brings knowledge about the illness, treatment options, preventative strategies, and prognosis. At the same time, the diabetes patient brings their knowledge and personal experience of living with the condition, their values and beliefs, their social circumstances, habits and behaviour, and attitudes towards risk taking (Coulter 1999). The professional adopts a facilitating role, asking open questions, helping individual patients to look at alternatives, and assisting in the setting of behaviour-based goals. It is argued that the patient-centred health model is more suitable than the traditional model for the treatment of chronic diseases such as diabetes (Hampson *et al.* 1990; World Health Organization 1998; Ashton and Rogers 2005). This is because diabetes patients need to self-manage their condition, i.e. by self-testing blood glucose, taking medication, eating healthily, caring for feet, and balancing medication against food intake and medical activity. Basically, the argument is that patient-centred health models are more useful for chronic patients whose condition last for a long period because they need to learn how to live with the condition, and the provision of the health service does not require a high degree of qualification. In the learning process of living with the condition, they can avoid the need of a higher level of health care provision by improving the healthiness of their habits and lifestyles. That is the reason why interactions between health provider and patients are potentially beneficial. Other health services provision, such as surgical operations, cannot benefit from the interaction between the health provider (the surgeon) and the patient, since they require highly skilled personnel, which cannot be substituted at any proportion by the patient.

The innovation

The particular programme that we analyse is the outcome of collaboration between two public sector institutions interested in experimenting with new models of diabetes education: the Salford PCT Diabetes Education Unit (hereafter 'SCDT') and a group of education specialists at Manchester Metropolitan University (hereafter 'MMU'). The SCDT comprises 8 staff members, 7 are medical practitioners (2 podiatrists, 2 dieticians, 3 specialist diabetes nurses), and there is 1 full-time administrator. They deliver diabetes education services for around 80 GP practices in Salford PCT. The education services are delivered at 4 venues within Salford: a local public library and 3 large GP practices to which patients have easy access.

The innovation consists of the substitution of the traditional model of education for type 2 diabetes patients for the patient-centred model of education. This substitution took place between 2003 and 2005. During that period, there was no clear sense of what a patient-centred diabetes education programme actually looked like. Rather, there were a set of experiments (of which the Salford PCT programme described here was one) that were exploring content, design, and delivery.

Two policy agencies determine the minimum standards of care and targets for diabetes education services to be delivered by Primary Care Trusts (PCTs) in the UK; National Service Framework (NSF) and the National Institute for Clinical Excellence (NICE). The NSF for diabetes contains 9 standards, ranging from screening, to education, to the detection of complications. The set of NSF standards and NICE guidelines issued in 2002, deliberately provided a window of opportunity for groups experimenting in the development of patient-centred educational programmes.

The programmes designing and delivering patient-centred diabetes education needed to address a set of fundamental conceptual issues and constraints. First, they need to operationalize a set of inter-related concepts as are patient-centred health, consumerization, and empowerment. The goal of the patient-centred education is the development of empowered and self-motivated patients. This goal is framed within a political and media discourse which proposes that users of health care services are now highly sophisticated and demanding (Cumbo 2001; Department of Health 2004). They are 'customers', rather than 'patients', and are likely to litigate when errors are made. The change is said to be driven by two factors. The first is a shift in attitude, partly driven by the influence of the USA, where litigation is now common practice. The second is the growth of the Internet as a source of medical information. This provides an opportunity for people to go beyond their GP, and gain information about conditions and treatments when they want, and from many sources.

Closely linked to consumerization is the notion of individual empowerment. This means that the individual is willing to take responsibility for the management of his/her health condition. Consecutive governments in the UK have been keen to place greater emphasis on the responsibility of individual 'health service consumers' to take greater care of their own health. The shift from 'passive patient' to 'empowered customer' is illustrated by the proposal, put forward in the late 1990s, that smokers should be refused cancer treatment if they failed to quit smoking (the public outcry that ensued meant that this proposal was never actually put into practice). As yet, there is no political consensus in the UK about the appropriate balance between societal and individual responsibility.

The second constraint for programmes delivering patient-centred diabetes education deals with the fundamental economic constraint that faces all health service providers—the opposing forces of scarce resources, on the one hand, and of unlimited users' wants, on the other. Any educational programme must deal with the fundamental economic trade-off that faces all health care providers (public and private). There is the goal of maximizing service quality. At the same time, public service providers must control the use of highly expensive, extremely scarce resources. This fundamental trade-off pervades all discussions within the NHS. The stated aim of NSF/ NICE is to develop patient-centred education in order to address NHS costs by reducing (or at the very least warding off for as long as possible) diabetes-related complications of heart disease, amputations, and liver damage. At the local level, the PCTs delivering diabetes education need to provide a high quality service within tight budgets.

Designers of patient-centred diabetes education programmes need to carefully negotiate these core concepts. By treating them differently, one will end up with very different looking programmes. Furthermore, one needs to carefully address the quality-cost trade-off. The success of a patient-centred programme, to a large extent, depends on how this trade-off is addressed.

Designers of patient-centred education programmes also need to address the significant problems faced by both health care professionals and patients in shifting to this new conceptual paradigm. For professionals, patient-centred education requires a radically different set of skills and knowledge to be developed in order to deliver patient-centred health. Skills and knowledge, developed over years of formulating and delivering directive education programmes become redundant. Patient-centred diabetes education requires a very different set of skills and knowledge on how to support self-motivation and empowerment. This helps explain the findings of Roisin *et al.* (1999). They found that practitioners had extreme difficulties changing their mode of interaction with type 2 patients, and continually fell back on directive education methods and practices where 'experts' engage with 'passive patients' in a one-way discourse to impart a maximum amount of medical information. People with diabetes can also find it difficult to change their behaviour and to buy in to the new paradigm. Not only do they typically lack the necessary skills and knowledge to be self-motivated, independent managers of their own disease, but the concept is alien to them. Their previous experience of interaction with professionals is invariably under the traditional medical model. Indeed, they continue to experience the traditional model in the majority of their interactions with the NHS, including aspects of their diabetes such as visits to hospitals for annual check-ups, visits to foot specialists, and surgery.

Applying the model to the change in the educational programme

We use the innovation of substituting the traditional model educational programme by the patient-centred educational programme for type 2 diabetes patients in the Salford area as a case study, in order to test the validity of our theoretical model of health innovations. Specifically, the test is valid for those health innovations in which the role of patients is crucial in terms of education and prevention activities, and also in order to highlight the importance of how the third agent, health policy-makers, need to realize about the effect of promoting healthier habits in the population with the aim of improving their health status. If the goal is obtained, a direct consequence is a decrease in the future need of health provision and, therefore, in health expenditures, helping to solve the problem of the inefficiency in the provision of health services.

Radical innovation

The simplified version of the Windrum and García-Goñi (2008) model presented above enables us to clearly classify this as a radical innovation. First, and perhaps most noticeably, a radical innovation involves a change to the dimensions of the service characteristics vector (S). This arises because a radical service innovation offers one or more new service characteristics that were unobtainable using the old service. In this case, a patient-centred health educational programme must, in addition to delivering the same basic content regarding the illness, its symptoms, and how to manage the condition, build additional competences in the patient, i.e. self-confidence, and the ability to engage in different searching for, and using effectively, different forms of information. These are new dimensions of service characteristics not available under the traditional educational programme.

There is an economic cost associated with this development. In order to deliver this extended set of service characteristics, the length of the educational programme needed to be increased from two to three sessions. In addition, a specially prepared set of supporting materials (taking the form of an 'education pack') needed to be developed, printed, and distributed.

In addition to altering the dimensions of the service characteristics vector (S), a radical medical innovation produces variations in the vectors of competences and preferences of the different agents; in this case study, the competences and preferences of providers and patients (SC, SP, UC, UP). We will discuss how the innovation modified these vectors in greater detail in the following subsections. The key point is that increased interaction between health providers and patients is the key driver of this radically new educational programme. A higher quality of patient knowledge and understanding of their condition, and how to pro-actively start to deal with its control is identified as the essential prerequisite for a change in patient lifestyle.

The model also enables us to identify and discuss second-order interactions between agents and their evolution over time. The analysis of these interactions leads to subsequent incremental improvements in the service characteristics vector, such as the realization by health providers of the needs of specific knowledge that patients have.

Changes in service characteristics

Here, we list the detailed the change in the vector of service characteristics (ΔS) that took place following the development and introduction of the patient-centred education model. Those changes are:

- The introduction of a direct contact with patients. Health professionals changes fundamentally. They are 'mediators' who manage discussions between groups of patients on key areas of diabetes and its control. Under the old programme, health professionals were 'teachers' who verbally imparted information to a passive recipient (the patient). In the patient-centred education model, in contrast, the health care professional mediates an open discussion, asks open questions, and helps patients to consider alternative options for taking control of their diabetes and the likely consequences. The most important feature of this innovation is the introduction of interaction between health providers and patients.

- The development of a specially designed 'Education Pack' comprising a number of 'sections' of education material. Each section of the pack relates to a different topic area covered by the course. Prior to an education session, patients are given the supporting material as a hand-out. This provides patients with the material they will discuss in the next education session. The course requires that patients read the relevant section of material before attending each session. In this way, key content and messages are imparted, through a combination of prior reading and discussion amongst fellow patients in the education sessions. As the patient proceeds through the course, so the material in the Education Pack is built up. The material is held in specially designed folder. The folder and all materials are provided to patients free of charge.

- Developing patient self-confidence and skills requires an increase in the time needed to deliver the new educational programme: it takes three sessions compared with the two sessions required to deliver the traditional programme.

- The increase in time required to deliver the new programme was reduced from what it would otherwise have been. This was achieved by increasing the number of 'learning points.' Together, the education sessions and the learning material containing in the Education Pack provide 6 'learning points.' This compares with just 2 separate learning points (the two 1-h sessions) under the old educational programme. Effectively supporting the three education sessions placed a great onus on the quality of the education material. Freely available hand-out materials were used in the old programme. These were leaflets and other printed materials published by the NHS, Diabetes UK, and other sources.

- Ongoing commitment—the education process does not end with the third education session. Patients return to their local GPs/diabetes nurses where they continue along their diabetes pathway. A patient contract, titled 'My Action Plan,' is drawn up between the SCDT and the patient at the end of the last education session. This establishes a link between the educational programme and the local GP practice. The contract is, in part, a certificate of achievement for having attended the course. More importantly, it is an agreement (of good intentions) on diet, exercise, etc., that the patient takes back to his/her local GP where the process of ongoing learning continues.

Changes in the preferences and competences of agents

Let us next consider the changes in preferences and competences that occurred as a consequence of the patient-centred education innovation.

Service providers

The health providers we consider in this innovation are the front line professionals who deliver the education programme. These are all members of the SCDT—a public sector institution. Patient-centred education requires a very different set of skills and knowledge to be developed in order to support self-motivated patient learning and patient empowerment. These skills are not taught during the training of NHS GPs and nurses, and therefore it was a difficulty observed during the process of adopting the innovation. Furthermore, because interaction between health provider and patient is important, health providers needed to adapt to the specific characteristics of the patients. Thus, even if Salford is predominantly a white, working class area, where the average educational background is low compared with the national average, interviews were conducted with Salford patients, and revealed a diversity of educational backgrounds and needs. The patient-centred educational programme needed to take this heterogeneity into account.

Our research found that both practitioners and patients experience difficulties engaging in this new mode of interaction and, therefore, designers of patient-centred educational programmes needed to address the significant problems faced as a consequence of the innovation process. Practitioners delivering patient-centred education needed to continually resist the temptation to revert back to a position (in which they have been trained) where they are the 'experts' who impart information to a 'passive patient.' They needed to develop a radically different set of skills and knowledge in order to deliver patient-centred health. Skills and knowledge, developed over years of formulating and delivering directive education programmes become redundant, and was not useful to support self-motivated patient learning and patient empowerment. This result confirms those shown in Roisin et al. (1999).

Therefore the innovation produced a change in the vector of service provider's competences (SC) through the inclusion not only of new skills and knowledge in practitioners providing the educational programme, but also through the inclusion of organizational measures and changes derived from as, for example, having three instead of two sessions in the programme, the new material delivered or when it is delivered. As a consequence, the innovation has brought both back and front office competences changes.

The organizational changes in the back office competences are clear, in the sense that health providers need to educate patients in three sessions instead of two. Unfortunately, we do not have data on the variation in the effort of health providers in the new educational programme. A signal that is used as a proxy of how health providers have modified their behaviour is the use given by patients to the new learning materials, compared with the traditional educational programme. In order to obtain that signal, patients were asked how often they had looked at the learning materials provided on their education course over the intervening 12 months.

Figure 10.2 shows the distribution of answers received from the control (patients involved in the traditional programme) and trial group (patients involved in the patient-centred programme) respondents. The average number of times that trial group respondents looked at their hand-out material is 4.85 times, compared with just 2.73 times by the control group. What is more, we see from Fig. 10.2 that the tail of the distribution for trial group respondents is much longer than for control group

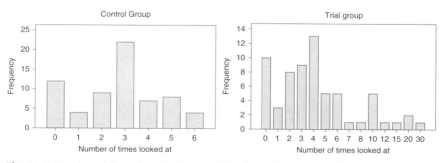

Fig. 10.2 Number of times hand-out material looked at in previous 12 months.

respondents, indicating that the specially designed Education Pack is referred to by more patients, much more frequently than the freely available leaflets produced by NHS and Diabetes UK that were given to the control group. Furthermore, both distributions present statistically different variance (the significance level of the estimated Levine statistic is 0.000, which is below the significance value of 0.10), and the mean difference between the means of the trial and control groups is statistically significant at the 95 per cent confidence level (obtaining a test value for 2-tailed significance of 0.003 lower than 0.05), as shown in Table 10.1.

With respect to the provider's preference vector (*SP*), it includes all the recommendations from the specialists involved in both public institutions. Although different criteria might be used in the management of a public health services institution, we assume that health providers always include in this vector the perceived quality by users, and having more patients looking at the learning material and more often, we conclude that health providers also modify their vector of preferences being more positive for the patient-centred educational model. As a consequence, the innovation has produced changes in both preferences and competences of service providers.

Because of the changes in the provider competences, the introduction of the patient-centred health provision model is considered as an organizational innovation. As noted, the potential benefits following this innovation are the better knowledge that patients have regarding their chronic illness, and therefore the change in the lifestyle and habits developed by patients. The ulterior consequence is that health providers will need to adapt to the new needs of patients given the healthier lifestyles, and will be able to devote funds to other health services different to the diabetes care and other co-morbidities related to diabetes. Thus, the model is able to predict future innovations in health provider's competences that will bring new changes in the vector of service characteristics.

Patients

Type 2 diabetes patients are the second agent in the model of health services innovation in this case study. As mentioned, under the traditional model patients behave as a passive agent accepting medical decisions, while the health providers are in charge of the overall charge of care, which includes diagnosis, treatment decisions, and ensuring that treatment is carried out as prescribed. Thus, there is no interaction between health providers and patients. Differently, under the patient-centred health model, the patient takes an active role in the provision of care, and engages in a partnership with the health care professional. This innovation involves changes in the users' competences and preferences vectors.

It is important to note that all the patients involved in our case study suffer diabetes and, therefore, belong to the set of chronic patients depicted in the simplified model in section 3. As a consequence, all the vectors referring to patients from now on are specifically referred to chronic patients. The patient competences vector (UC) changes because the educational programme is different and, with the new programme, patients obtain a better knowledge with respect to their chronic condition. In order to test whether the knowledge, and therefore the competences of patients, are better under the patient-centred with respect to the traditional model, 12 months after the

Table 10.1 Independent samples test for number of times hand-out material is looked at

	Levene's test for equality of variances		t-test for equality of means			Mean difference	SE difference	95 per cent CI Difference	
	F	Signif.	t	df	Signif. (2-tailed)			Lower	Upper
Equal variances assumed	15.199	0.000	−3.089	129	0.002	−2.119	0.686	−3.476	−0.762
Equal variances not assumed			−3.070	77.971	0.003	−2.119	0.690	−3.493	−0.745

educational programme patients received a questionnaire with aspects regarding the retained, long-term knowledge about diabetes and in the degree of self-confidence of patients.

Complete questionnaire data was collected for 129 of the total 235 patients that comprise the control (64 out of 120 patients, 53 per cent) and trial (65 out of 116 patients, 56 per cent) groups. This represents a sample of 55 per cent of the total population of the control and trial groups almost equally distributed between both populations. 47 per cent of all sample respondents are male and 53 per cent are female, while half of the patients belonged to each gender. Hence, the proportions of gender and respondents are representative of the true population of the control and trial groups.

The questionnaire tested long-term knowledge by means of 4 separate questions, each covering a different aspect of diabetes education. They are the causes of diabetes, symptoms, foot complications, and exercise. Sixty-eight per cent of trial group respondents correctly answered the question on the causes of diabetes compared with 47 per cent of control group respondents. Fifty-seven per cent of trial group respondents correctly answered the question on the symptoms of diabetes compared with 31 per cent of control group respondents. For the questions on foot complications and exercise, the scores for trial and control group respondents are almost the same—81 per cent of control group respondents and 82 per cent of trial group respondents answered the question on foot complications correctly. Finally, 91 per cent of control group respondents and 82 per cent of trial group respondents correctly answered the question on good exercise regimes that help control diabetes. Thus, the findings indicate a better long-term knowledge in the sample of patients who took the patient-centred educational programme with respect to those attending the traditional programme, and there has been a positive change in the vector of users' (patients) preferences.

A good indicator of self-confidence is whether individuals with diabetes are happy to provide information about diabetes to others. In doing so, a person is clearly stating to others that they have the illness. This requires a good degree of self-confidence in itself. An even greater degree of self-confidence is required for a person to be willing to share his/her knowledge of the condition in order to assist others. Two questions were used to probe this issue. The first asked whether respondents had provided information on diabetes to other people with diabetes in the last 12 months. 37 per cent of trial group respondents answered 'Yes,' compared with 12 per cent of control group respondents. The second question asked whether respondents had provided information on diabetes to family and friends in the last 12 months. Twenty-six per cent of trial group respondents answered 'Yes,' compared with just 9 per cent of control group respondents. Taken together, the findings indicate a higher level of self-confidence in the sample of patients who took the patient-centred educational programme, which is another signal for a positive change in the vector of patient competences.

In addition, there is a change in the vector of patients' preferences (UP). The reason is that during the educational programme there are aspects better treated as their psychological, emotional, and behavioural states. Thus, the idea of locally delivered patient-centred health challenges both health providers and patients because it breaks the traditional model of the 'passive patient,' and, instead, it supposes a model of the self-motivated, independent 'client' who manages their own disease. However, the adoption of this patient-centred model was found difficult to adapt to by patients used to following directions given by providers and were unable to manage their illness.

In order to test for the change in the vector of patients' preferences, we check the attendance of the patients to the different programmes. It is a signal of how involved they become under each of the educational programmes. Table 10.2 shows the results for the attendance. It shows how, under the patient-centred educational programme, the proportion of patients attending the first session (63 per cent) is significantly higher than under the traditional model (44 per cent), being equally important the increase in the attendance for men (from 46 to 59 per cent) than for women (from 52 to 67 per cent). It is important to note that the change in the attendance for the first session stems from the different learning packages sent to patients. Therefore, this increase is due to two effects: a change in the users' preferences with a better disposition to the educational programme with the new package, and to a change in the vector of provider's competences, derived properly from the different learning package.

However, patients' preferences for the different programmes are revealed unequivocally through the proportion of patients completing the educational programme (or the drop-out rate). Table 10.2 shows how this proportion increases from 80 to 96 per cent with the change from the traditional to the patient-centred model of education, this increase being consistent in both genders, but significantly higher for men (from 74 to 96 per cent in the case of men and from 87 to 95 per cent in the case of women). This increase is important because, under the traditional model, men presented a significantly lower attendance rate, while under the patient-centred model both men and women present a similar drop out rate.

It is important to note that, in this innovation process, the interaction between health providers and patients reports a better health provision, as is shown in the model. However, not all innovation processes work in the same way. When the health service has to be provided uniquely by the health professional and the interaction of the patient does not increase the utility of the service, then the model still works,

Table 10.2 Attendance at the different educational programmes

	Traditional programme			Patient-centred programme		
	Total	Men	Women	Total	Men	Women
No. patients contacted with appointment	244	141	103	184	88	96
No. patients who attend 1st session	119 (44%)	65 (46%)	54 (52%)	116 (63%)	52 (59%)	64 (67%)
No. patients who complete the course	95 (80%)	48 (74%)	47 (87%)	111 (96%)	50 (96%)	61 (95%)
Drop-out rate	20%	26%	13%	4%	4%	5%

simply eliminating the role of patients or assigning them null proportion of interaction. That would be a case more similar to an innovation process in manufacturing firms.

Interactions and evolution

The neo-Schumpeterian model of health service innovations that we have tested is a multi-agent model that highlights the importance of inter-agent interactions. In this section, we consider the differences in inter-agent interactions that occur following the replacement of the traditional educational programme by the patient-centred programme. Also we consider whether these interactions affected the adoption of the innovation and the dynamics, in terms of a mutual co-evolution of preferences and competences, around the innovation.

Interactions between health providers and patients is the most important feature of this innovation, fundamentally altering the vector of service characteristics that is provided. This interaction consists of a direct contact with mediated discussions between patients and health providers on key areas of diabetes. Thus, the health care professional mediates an open discussion, asks open questions, and helps patients to consider alternative options for taking control of their diabetes and the likely consequences. Therefore, the vector of (users) patients' competences (UC) is affected by health providers in the educational model, but also the vector of service provider' competences (SC) is affected by patients through the adaptation to the questions and need that they present. As mentioned, both agents affect the service characteristics vector (S).

Therefore, the model captures all the interactions between the different agents in this case study. The dynamics of the innovation process is also captured by the model. The innovation brings as a consequence a change in patients' preferences given by the improvement of their self-confidence and the long-term knowledge of their health condition. More importantly, it brings an improvement in healthier habits and lifestyles. We have two different tests for this hypothesis. The first is subjective in the sense that it is provided by the questionnaire sent to patients one year after the educational programme. They answer to the question 'Do you believe you have made a major change to your life in the last 12 months?' While only 34 per cent of patients following the traditional educational programme answered 'Yes,' this proportion was 70 per cent of patients following the patient-centred programme.

Because self-perception in habits needs to be treated with caution, we ran a second test, with objective data on the health status of patients: the HbA1c blood test data. The HbA1c blood test is the best biomedical indicator of whether patients have changed their lifestyles and brought their diabetes under control. It is the main test for diabetes control in the UK. The HbA1c test is conducted every 2–3 months by a patient's GP. The test score should be below 7 per cent. Data was collected on patients' HbA1c scores at 2 time points. The first recorded score is for the blood test immediately following the educational programme, and the second was conducted approximately 12 months after the programme. Together, these scores give us a good indication of how well patients in the trial and control groups are controlling their diabetes, and the scores of each group can be statistically compared. There is complete data for 108 of the 120 patients in the control group, and data for 94 of the 116 patients in the trial group (80 and 81 per cent of samples, respectively). Missing data is due to the death of patients, or patients relocating away from the area, or their local GPs not recording data on the central information system.

Table 10.3 presents the average mean scores and standard deviations of patients following both types of educational programmes at the time of the educational programme and 1 year later. The estimated mean of both groups is very similar at the time of the educational programme (the control group is 7.739 for patients following the traditional programme and 7.745 for patients in the centred-patient programme) with a standard deviation of 1.61 (both groups). This indicates patients in both groups are starting from the same base. However, 1 year after the educational programme, the results in the blood score have changed. The average blood score for patients following the traditional programme is of 7.172, while the average score for patients in the patient-centred programme is of 6.838. Therefore, the HbA1c blood data indicates a marked contrast in diabetes control between the two groups 1 year after the education intervention, with patients who attended the patient-centred educational programme presenting far better control of their diabetes than patients who attended the traditional educational programme. Running the test for equality of variances we confirm this result: immediately after the programme the distribution of the average blood scores for the pooled and separate populations is the same (the difference in the variance is not statistically significant). However, 1 year after the educational programme, conducting the same test we find that the distributions are different with the difference between their means being statistically significant as presented in Table 10.4.

The importance of this results stems from the fact that healthier patients need a different basket of health services provision. Therefore, the economic resources devoted to the provision of the health services needed under the traditional educational programme, but not needed after the adoption of the patient-centred educational programme supposes a saving for the public health sector. Given the concept of the opportunity cost, those funds can be used to finance other health services or investments, which can be selected by health policy-makers through a system as the cost-benefit analysis, obtaining a more efficient use of health expenditure.

In general, the adoption of the patient-centred educational programme for type 2 diabetes patients follows the stages predicted by Barras (1986, 1990) in the 'reverse life cycle.' In the first stage of the innovation, the primary focus is devoted to improve

Table 10.3 Statistical data on HbA1c scores

	Group	*n*	Mean	SD	SE of mean
bA1c score at the time of the programme	Traditional model	108	7.739	1.6165	0.1534
	Patient-centred model	94	7.745	1.6193	0.1661
bA1c score 1 year after the programme	Traditional model	108	7.172	1.0099	0.0972
	Patient-centred model	94	6.838	0.8599	0.0887

Table 10.4 Independent samples test for HbA1c scores

| | Levene's test for equality of variances | | t-test for equality of means | | | | | 95% CI | |
	F	Signif.	t	df	Signif. (2-tailed)	Mean difference	SE	Lower	Upper
HbA1c score month 1 — Equal variances assumed	0.317	0.574	−0.029	200	0.977	−0.0065	0.2261	−0.4524	0.4393
Equal variances not assumed			−2.029	199.014	0.977	−0.0065	0.2261	−0.4525	0.4394
HbA1c score month 12 — Equal variances assumed	2.780	.097	2.510	200	0.013	0.3339	0.1330	0.0716	0.5963
Equal variances not assumed			2.538	199.910	0.012	0.3339	0.1316	0.0745	0.5934

the educational programme with effects in health expenditures. The second stage corresponds to the standardization of the patient-centred model of education. After the adoption of this model, now we are in this second stage, although regulation is still flexible. Finally, the third stage will come with an adapted health budget and basket of services provided to the new needs of the population promoting further innovations. The model, therefore, is able to analyse the ways in which the innovation changes agents' preferences and competences, over time promoting new innovations that is a central part of the long-term evolutionary dynamics discussed by Schumpeter (1934, 1943).

Conclusions

This chapter has applied the Windrum–García-Goñi model to the case of a radical service innovation. The model has proved useful in terms of capturing the different dimensions that are relevant in this particular service innovation. The fact that it is an explicitly multi-agent model enabled us to consider the roles played by health service providers, patients, and policy-makers in the innovation process. Secondly, the model raises the need to consider the long-term co-evolution of agents' competences and preferences that occur as a consequence of the innovation process. Thirdly, the model makes one examine the different dimensions of innovation, providing a precise definition of radical and incremental innovation through service, competence, and preference characteristics.

In this chapter we have narrowed the focus in order to concentrate on the interactions between health providers and patients. It is crucial that type 2 diabetes patients take an active role in the provision of their healthcare, in education, prevention activities, and in the changing of lifestyles and habits in order to improve their health status. To this end it was important to assess whether the model could capture the key aspects of the provider-patient interaction within this innovation process. The case study that was selected involved the development of a new, patient-orientated education programme that replaced a traditional didactic programme. Essential differences between the two approaches are evidenced by the way in which the new educational programme is provided to type 2 diabetes patients. While under the traditional model the provision of healthcare depends entirely on the health providers, the patient-centred model allows for a more intensive interaction and collaboration between health providers and patients.

The application of the multi-agent innovation model to this case study provides a number of important insights. First, the model has confirmed that the interaction between the different agents and, in this innovation especially, between health providers and patients has a key role in the innovation processes. Thus, allowing for the interaction between those agents in the educational programme, we obtain a higher satisfaction with the programme by patients, an improvement in their learning process, and as a consequence, a healthier lifestyle or habits that are translated into a better health status. Secondly, it is important to understand that this analysis is feasible depending on the interests and relative power of different agents in the provision of healthcare. The multi-agent model of health innovations 'works' properly when there is any level of relative utility created by the interaction of their agents. Our case study presents one of the extremes in which that interaction produces a significant improvement in health provision, by the learning of healthier habits or lifestyles for patients of chronic conditions. However, there are other health services in which the interaction between different agents is not that useful (or not useful at all), such as those acute illnesses services, for example, occurring at a surgical theatre in which all the responsibility of the result depends on the health professional. Those innovations in their analysis similar to innovations in manufacturing industries. The multi-agent model still 'works' properly, but we would assign zero relative power for patients in modifying the vector of service characteristics or providers' competences or preferences. Thirdly, we have learned how this innovation is catalogued as a radical organizational innovation, and how radical innovations change the preferences and competences of the different agents in time. The model allows for the analysis of the evolutionary dynamics of innovations.

The benefits of patient-centred educational programmes presupposes a change in the need of health services provision in patients with better health status. A lower demand on health services in the future might be a positive consequence of this innovation process, and would permit the reassignment of health expenditures and health budgets according to the needs of the population, in order to provide more efficient healthcare.

To summarize, our findings point towards a key driver of a type of health innovations and the evolutionary dynamics. Thus, it predicts improvements in the health status of the population, allowing for the interaction between the different agents in the adoption of the patient-centred educational programme, and will promote further health innovations and a more efficient use of health expenditures.

Acknowledgements

The authors gratefully acknowledge funding received through the Public-Private Services Innovation (ServPPIN) project, funded through the Socio-Economic Sciences and Humanities Programme of the EU 7th Framework.

References

American Diabetes Association (2003). Economic Costs of Diabetes in the U.S. in 2002. *Diabetes Care*, **26**, 917–32.

Ashton H and Rogers J (2005). A health promoting empowerment approach to diabetes nursing. In: A Scriven, ed. *Health promoting practice: the contribution of nurses and allied health professionals*, pp. 45–56. Basingstoke, Palgrave Macmillan.

Barras R (1986). Towards a theory of innovation in services. *Research Policy*, **15**, 161–73.

Barras R (1990). Interactive innovation in financial and business services: the vanguard of the service revolution. *Research Policy*, **19**, 215–37.

Beaulieu N, Cutler DM, Ho K, Isham G, Lindquist T, Nelson A and O'Connor P (2006). The business case for diabetes disease management for managed care organizations. *Forum for Health Economics & Policy*, 9(1) Article 1. Frontiers in Health Policy Research.

Bloom DE and Canning D (2000). The health and wealth of nations. *Science*, **287**(5456), 1207–1209.

Costa-Font J, Rudisill C and Mossialos E (2009). Demand for health information on the Internet. In: JC Costa-Font, C Courbage and A. Mcguire, eds. Chapter 16.

Coulter A (1999). Paternalism or partnership? *British Medical Journal*, **319,** 719–20.

Cumbo J (2001). Better-informed patients question bedside manners. *Financial Times*, 21 February.

Department of Health (2004). *Choosing health: making healthier choices easier.* London, Stationary Office.

deWalque D (2007). Does education affect smoking behaviors? Evidence using the Vietnam draft as an instrument for college education. *Journal of Health Economics*, **26**, 877–95.

Diabetes Control and Complications Trial Research Group (1993). The effect of intensive treatment of diabetes on the development and progression of longterm complications in insulin-dependent diabetes mellitus. *New England Journal of Medicine*, **329**, 977–86.

Dixon T (2005). *Costs of diabetes in Australia, 2000–01*, Bulletin 26, Australian Institute of Health and Welfare, Cat. No. AUS 59. Canberra, AIHW.

Gallouj F and Weinstein O (1997). Innovation in services. *Research Policy*, **26**, 537–56.

Hampson SE, Glasgow R and Toobert DJ (1990). Personal models of diabetes and their relations to self-care activities. *Health Psychology*, **9**, 632–46.

Kenkel D (1990). Consumer health information and the demand for medical care. *Review of Economics and Statistics*, **72**, 587–95.

Kenkel D (1991). Health behavior, health knowledge, and schooling. *Journal of Political Economy*, **99**, 287–305.

Klonoff DC and Schwartz DM (2000). An economic analysis of interventions for diabetes. *Diabetes Care* **23**, 390–404.

Lancaster KJ (1966). A new approach to consumer theory. *Journal of Political Economy*, **14,** 133–46.

Lancaster KJ (1971). *Consumer theory: a new approach.* Columbia, Columbia University Press.

Nathan DM, Cleary PA, Backlund JY, *et al.* (2005). Intensive diabetes treatment and cardiovascular disease in patients with type 1 diabetes. *New England Journal of Medicine*, **353**, 2643–53.

Ohinmaa A, Jacobs P, Simpson S and Johnson J (2004). The projection of prevalence and cost of diabetes in Canada: 2000 to 2016. *Canadian Journal of Diabetes*, **28**(2), 1–8.

Ramsey S, Summers KH, Leong SA, Birnbaum HG, Kemner JE and Greenberg P. (2002) Productivity and medical costs of diabetes in a large employer population. *Diabetes Care*, **25**, 23–9.

Roisin P, Rees ME, Stott N and Rollnkick SR (1999). Can nurses learn to let go? Issues arising from an intervention designed to improve patients' involvement in their own care. *Journal of Advanced Nursing*, **29**, 1492–9.

Saviotti PP (1985). An approach to the measurement of technology based on the hedonic price method and related methods. *Technological Forecasting and Change*, **29**, 309–34.

Saviotti PP and Metcalfe JS (1984) A theoretical approach to the construction of technological output indicators. *Research Policy*, **13**, 141–51.

Saviotti PP (1996). *Technological evolution, variety and the economy.* Cheltenham, Edward Elgar.

Schumpeter JA (1934). *The theory of economic development: an inquiry into profits, capital, credit, interest and the business cycle.* Cambridge, MA, Harvard University Press.

Schumpeter JA (1943). *Capitalism, socialism and democracy.* New York, Harper and Row.

Sen AK (1999). *Development as freedom.* Oxford, Oxford University Press.

UK Prospective Diabetes Study (UKPDS) Group (1998) Intensive blood-glucose control with sulphonylureas or insulin compared with conventional treatment and risk of complications in patients with type 2 diabetes (UKPDS 33). *Lancet*, **352**, 837–53.

Viscusi WK, Magat WA and Huber J (1986). Informational regulation of consumer health risks: an empirical evaluation of hazard warnings. *Rand Journal of Economics*, l7, 35l–65.

Wagner TH, Hu T and Hibbard JH (2001). The demand for consumer health information. *Journal of Health Economics*, **20**, 1059–75.

Windrum P (2007). Services innovation. In: H Hanusch and A Pyka, eds. *The Edward Elgar Companion to Neo-Schumpeterian Economics*, pp. 633–46. Cheltenham, Edward Elgar.

Windrum P and Garcia-Goñi M (2008). A neo-Schumpetenan model of health senices innovation. *Research policy*, **37**, 649–672.

Windrum P and Senyucel Z (2006). *Salford PCT patient-centred diabetes education programme*, 2006 report. Manchester Metropolitan University Business School.

World Health Organization (1998). *Health promotion glossary*. Geneva, WHO.

Zhang P, Engelgau MM, Norris SL, Gregg EW and Venkat Narayan KM. (2004). Application of economic analysis to diabetes and diabetes care. *Annals of Internal Medicine*, **140**, 972–7.

Chapter 11

The convergence of nano-, bio-, and information technologies in healthcare

Nicola Pangher

Introduction

The responsibility as Business Development director of a company offering clinical engineering services[1] for the successful management of technologies in the healthcare environment is becoming ever more challenging. The impact of electronics has resulted in the creation of more complex diagnostic devices, from different types of diagnostic imaging systems (CAT, MRI, PET, angiography) to endoscopes and clinical laboratory instruments: managing a medical institution means managing growing technological investments, the introduction of technology assessment procedures, and the need of correct usage and maintenance procedures in order to assure the safety of the patient. The Information and Communication Technology (ICT) revolution has lead to the creation of storage, and analysis procedures of medical data and signals, up to the introduction of electronic medical records: managing technologies means managing the software systems that are used to look at diagnostic data, plan therapeutic interventions, and organize therapeutic protocols.

This challenge is today becoming ever more complex due to a set of factors:

◆ Implantable devices such as pacemakers and defibrillators are 'talking' to the outside world, and can be programmed. More are developed and becoming smarter: brain stimulators, pain pacemakers, insulin-release pumps are the fathers of a whole generation of systems that will be able to monitor the physiological and biochemical environment in the body, to release drugs directly and possibly to manufacture them.[2]

◆ Genomics and, in general, molecular medicine are leading the path to personalized medicine, therapy and real lifestyle management. Yesterday's high level research technologies (DNA chips, protein chips, MALDI-TOF spectrometers, and many others), which were the exclusive domain of very advanced research groups, are entering into the normal healthcare arena and will flood healthcare operators with

---

[1] See http://www.italtbs.com for a description of the clinical engineering services of ITALTBS.
[2] LETI, Annual Report 2006. Available at: http://www.leti.fr

very extensive and detailed information, where personalized prevention and therapy protocol will have to be developed, evaluated, and distributed.

◆ Minimally-invasive surgery is becoming the gold standard of the day: moving to smart surgery, where surgical instrumentation will be functionalized in order to monitor the environment in the body during surgery, and the spreading of the robotic system will have a major impact in the operating theatre, where software and hardware system will take over some (or many) of the 'mechanical skills' from the surgeons, but will need more advanced technological support and know-how.

◆ Home and wearable monitoring system are becoming part of the management of assisted living conditions for the elderly and of chronic diseases. The measurement of ECG, blood pressure, saturimetry, blood sugar, and other physiological parameters is becoming part of disease management programmes for ailments such as congestive heart failure, chronic obstructive pulmonary disease, diabetes, arrhythmia and hypertension.[3]

These are just some features that characterize the present innovation drive in the healthcare sector. However, in order to choose the right R&D projects, but also to design the general development scenarios, many of these different trends have to be taken into consideration and choices have to be made, taking into account the resources available to the company, the timing for different innovations to impact on the day-to-day healthcare services, and the availability of the right professional competences. What is clear is that the old disciplinary boundaries are not up to this challenge: medicine, engineering (biomedical, mechanical, electronic, telecommunication), informatics, physics, mathematics are mixing up and converging in the development of solutions that include bits and pieces from different background. Multidisciplinary working groups will become the order of the day, not only to develop a new solution, but also to use and maintain it successfully. In parallel with technological advances, it is necessary to look also at organizational and financial innovation: how are we going to introduce and use the new technologies in the standard healthcare environment? The multidisciplinary approach will need to include management competences and will need to have access to a 'clinical' environment, to test not only the single technology, but the new medical process that incorporates it.

The bathroom-centred healthcare scenario

While many scientific publications are dealing with particular innovation pathways, presenting new molecules and prototypes, companies and investors have to build innovation scenarios that present a complete picture, in order to decide where to invest human and economic resources. Inspired by a very interesting series of essays on the future of healthcare,[4] in particular by the essay from

---

[3] See for example the Healthcare/Pharma market description at CSEM. Available at http://www.csem.ch/fs/healthcare.htm

[4] The Great Essays for Change from the Faster Cures/Center for Accelerating Medical Solutions

R. Merkin,[5] a sketchy scenario of a possible future for healthcare can be centred on the bathroom. Going to the bathroom after waking up will become the key to the successful management of health conditions: a mass spectrometer will analyse the breath, through a set of microneedles a blood sample will be extracted from the hand resting on the washbasin, the toothbrush will complete a screening of saliva, and the hand will be placed on the wall to look at heart frequency, oxygen saturation, and blood pressure. The whole set of information will be elaborated in order to design the diet for the day, and communicated it to the smart kitchen and the canteen, a fitness programme for the day will be scheduled on the smart phone and directly to the gym, possibly some drug molecules will be added to the food intake in order to prevent or cure some ailment, and an appointment with the doctor and some more extensive diagnostic tests could be also booked. This science fiction picture may sound very futuristic, but almost all components presented here are present today, at least as prototypes:

- The use of breath testing through mass spectrometry and other techniques to detect the presence of *Helicobacter pylori* is a well known technique (Kannath and Rutt 2007).

- The use of microneedles to painlessly collect blood samples and deliver drugs directly to the blood stream has been studied extensively in the past years (Gardeniers *et al.* 2007).

- Microsystems for the analysis of biochemical samples have been under development in the past 10 years (Hogan 2006).

- Microsystems for the manufacturing of drug molecules are under test by the pharmaceutical industry.

- Disease management services, based on cell phones and mobile technologies, are already available on the market (Whitten *et al.* 2002).

Even if several prototypes are at a very advanced stage, it is obvious that such an integrated picture will take decades to become reality and there might be some revolutionary technology that could modify the path that is being envisioned today. On the one hand, it is important to understand fundamental technologies that are part of the picture, and look at their impact in the future years and how they could change medical practice. The ever decreasing cost of analytical tools for genomics, proteomics, metabolomics, and 'all other -omics', is going to affect how medical services are delivered around the world. However, a major question arising is also about how this future of healthcare will fit into everyday's reality. Who is going to pay for the 'clinical bathroom'? Is it an out-of-pocket expense for the patient? Will it be provided by the private health insurance or is it financed by the state within a public system? Who is going to take responsibility for the correct functioning of the technologies? Who is going to check that the diagnostic tests are valid and able to detect dangerous situation and, on the other hand, that it is not generating unnecessary additional testing? How is the system going to be maintained as state-of-the-art? If a new biomarker is discovered, how is the system going to know that there is a new molecule that needs to be checked?

---

[5] A vision about the future? Richard Merkin, MD, in http://www.fastercures.org/sec/great_essays

Trend 1: assisted living and home-based disease management

It is worth to look at how technologies are already changing today healthcare services: the impact of home monitoring technologies is already starting to change how chronic diseases are managed today (Pare *et al.* 2007; Stachura *et al.* 2007; Barlow *et al.* 2007.[6]

The needs of the ageing population are one of the main drivers behind the development of monitoring technologies—the decrease in physical and mental abilities and the need to prevent and manage chronic ailments pose new requests.

The goals of home-based disease management are:

◆ *Ageing independently:* elderly citizen want to continue to live safely and with an appropriate standard of quality in their own homes.

◆ *Control care costs:* the burden of care often falls on the family, creating explicit and implicit costs that add to those generated by the social and health services. Controlling these cost means also reaching efficiency and efficacy targets.

◆ *Create an ICT network* that supports citizens, families, and caregivers.

◆ *Avoid isolation and promote socialization.*

◆ *Develop 'usable' technologies.*

The complexity of the care organization and of the ICT services are depicted in Fig. 11.1. The need to communicate, store data, and organize processes poses challenges in terms of innovation of work practices and technology infrastructures. This infrastructure is the back office for all implementations of domotics. A key role in the organization is represented by the Multimedia E-health centre, which supports all information exchange and is the human factor behind the continuity of the care process. The E-health centre maintains all communications channels, as depicted in Fig. 11.2.

The multimedia E-health centre acts as the receiving node also for all information generated by the domotics systems installed at home.

The personal and environmental alarms let the citizen manage unexpected crisis events, using devices such as:

◆ The personal alarm system, a panic button plus microphone used to send an alarm and allowing communication from every room in the house.

◆ A fall detection system, plus an audio system, which identifies situations where sudden accelerations have been taking place.

◆ Flood, fire, and gas sensors, detecting anomalies in the environment.

◆ Motion detectors that can indicate that particular rooms in the house are not being used, such as the bathroom and the kitchen, suggesting a situation of inability to fulfil the most basic needs.

---

6 'Personalized medicines: hopes and realities', Study by The Royal Society, 2005

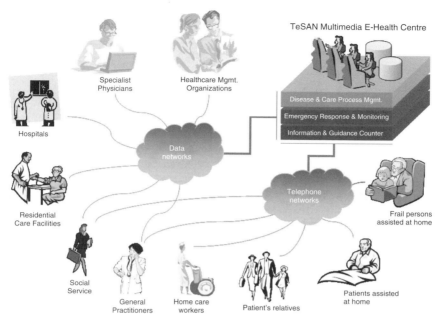

Fig. 11.1 The ICT network for social and health care services.

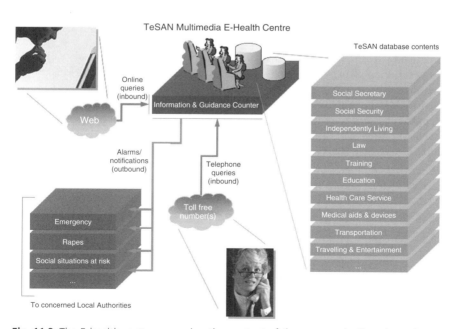

Fig. 11.2 The E-health centre managing the content of the communication channels.

- Door-opening sensors, indicating that the person is leaving.
- Anti-burglary devices and alarms, which can be implements in order to avoid unfriendly intrusions when the person is at home.

The multimedia E-health centre can filter these alarms, activating the proper response.

In addition to the alarm systems, there are systems that support people with reduced physical abilities, such as electromechanic blinds, motorized beds and armchairs, air conditioning, and so on. These devices are moving from a 'non-networked' situation to a 'networked' status: in this case, the E-health centre will collect also information from these devices, increasing the alarm detection capability.

The management of alarms represents the first layer of service for the elderly, but technologies now allow the first implementations of lifestyle management, both for disease prevention and disease management. Biomedical devices can be installed at home, measuring signals such as:

- Blood pressure.
- Pulse.
- Oxysaturation.
- Weight.
- Body mass index.
- Blood sugar levels.
- 1–12-lead ECG.
- Peak expiratory flow.
- Coagulation time, etc.

The most common chronic diseases can be monitored through this approach, thanks to the ICT network linking the patients to nurses and doctors, as depicted in Fig. 11.3.

Moving from an alarm management system to full time lifestyle management is the step that poses the most dramatic questions. Healthcare today is organized in order to deliver the services in *ad-hoc* environments, such as hospitals, policlinics and practices, and all related organizational, economic, and billing procedures are organized accordingly. There is space for home care services, which at the moment consist either of specialized nursing or social worker support, which is available for very precise 'atomic' services, or on the presence of a 'continuous' caregiver, who often has no specific professional background. The only solution that is available today when the level of disability increases is represented by the nursing home, where the patient often spends the remaining part of its life.

Trend 2: molecular medicine at the bedside

The most recent advances in molecular biology, genomics, proteomics, and the other –omics are paving the way to a 'molecular approach' to medicine. The advancement of technologies and the reduction in costs are making these devices available to many

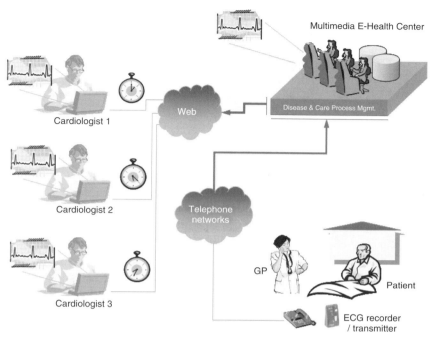

Fig. 11.3 Health management network.

healthcare providers. These tools will enable personalized medicine, where it will be possible to identify predispositions to certain diseases and to provide preventive medicine, giving guidance on the choice of preventive treatments and models of behaviour aimed at reducing the risk. Molecular information will also describe how the very personal 'molecular set-up and mechanism' responds to specific therapeutic molecules: the aim will be to choose the drug targeted at the biochemical response of the individual.[7]

The large scale applications of these technologies will result in the identification of new biomarkers, diagnostic indicators that show the risk or the onset of particular pathologies, but will also provide new drug targets, therefore amplifying the 'hunting territory' for pharmaceutical research.

The question is how to move from basic research to potential clinical applications. Multidisciplinary research teams need the access to patients, and medical professionals need to understand new technologies and to use them. Research hospitals are playing an important role in this development, since they unite the clinical competence with the scientists studying the basic mechanisms of diseases.

[7] Biobanks: accelerating molecular medicine - Challenges Facing the Global Biobanking Community", a study by IDC, http://www.idc.com, 2004

These institutions face a double challenge. First, the research challenge—the development of molecular tools for fighting diseases requires intense research activities based on the availability of a vast amount of detailed clinical data. Secondly, the so-called translational challenge: the fast and effective translation of research results, and all related innovation to the bedside of the patient. It is easy to understand how these two issues represent the two sides of a single coin—only by advancing research it will be possible to cure more patients and only by collecting data at the bedside it will be possible to perform effective medical research.

Hence, one might speculate that the smart research hospital in the future will include some of the following features (see Fig. 11.4):

◆ Sample collection, processing, and storage, with extensive biobank infrastructure.[8]

◆ Clinical trials management organizations, for Phases 1 and 2 smaller scale studies, including the know-how on analysis and prediction of toxicity of new molecules.

◆ Bioinformatics and medical informatics facilities and staff, to integrate electronic patient records and molecular research data.

◆ IT and pharmaceutical departments organized for personalized therapy.

◆ Advisory organization for risk management to prevent the onset of diseases with a higher genetic predisposition.

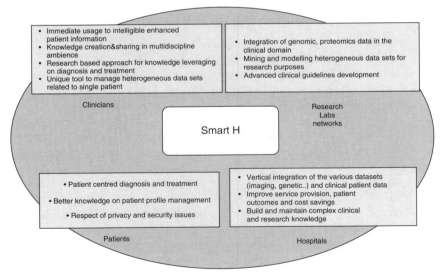

Fig. 11.4 The smart research hospital.

8 Information Technology Enabling Clinical Research", Findings and Recommendations from a Conference Sponsored by the Association of American Medical Colleges with Funding from the National Science Foundation

Similarly, personalized medicine will be information-based,[9] and the IT infrastructure will have to include the following capabilities:

- Integration of heterogeneous data from diverse sources (patient health care records, laboratory test results, medical images, genetic, genomic, and proteomic data, pathological data, etc.) belonging to hospitals and research laboratory networks
- Knowledge sharing and collaboration in a multidisciplinary ambience.
- Disease mining, modelling and targeted treatments among hospitals and research laboratory networks.
- Increased use of electronic medical records, connecting patient's clinical data with research data to create the basis for personalized healthcare diagnosis and treatment.
- An integrated information system (within the whole organization), linking stand-alone applications present in different departments.

Again, the change will be dramatic—the hospital becomes the real 'knowledge hub', since it will be the preferred meeting venue for the interdisciplinary team, in order to design research and therapeutic protocols. A huge amount of data will have to be managed and interpreted, which the different medical specialist will have to discuss with the scientific and technological staff in order to understand the medical meaning of the data. A critical mass of specialists will be needed in order to exploit successfully the potential for research and delivery of effective treatment.

Further questions

The examples that have been explored pose certain questions.

The first question posed by the contrast between the features of present healthcare systems and the scenarios depicted in the two trends is represented by the issue of prevention. Molecular medicine will allow the medical practitioners to identify new personal risk factors that will contribute to form a large and complex set, together with the known 'classical' and environmental risk factors. It sounds obvious to say that preventing the onset of disease is the most effective way of keeping the costs of health-care under control; therefore, prevention should be the keyword for all future developments in healthcare organization. It is easy to see how an E-health network could be of paramount importance to a prevention policy: phone and videocalls, easy to use software interfaces, and the results from molecular mapping and monitoring with medical devices are the bricks for collecting information, helping the patient to plan their everyday life in terms of diet, physical exercise, use of selected drugs, and reminders of specialized medical examinations. The huge hurdle is that, at present, the healthcare service is financed in order to treat existing diseases. How much would it cost to

---

9   Response to the request of information by the US Dept. of Health and Human Services on "Improving Health and Accelerating Personalized Health Care through Health Information Technology and Genomic Information in Population- and Community-based Health Care Delivery Systems" by The Harvard Medical School-Partners HealthCare Center for Genetics and Genomics (HPCGG), 2007

finance such detailed lifestyle support strategies, where professional advice and monitoring services could be available in a continuity of prevention mechanism? How would it be possible to finance a system designed to treat the healthy population? Currently, financing is left to the individual and this is not leading to satisfactory results. In many cases, the onset of a chronic disease is not seen as a real and immediate health threat, and the efficacy of individual strategies are often very closely connected to the economic and educational status of that individual. Is there any possible insurance policy that could result in the effective financing of prevention? There are some experiences that are linking health policies to lifestyle targets, offering services like gyms, dieticians, and medical check-ups at reduced prices, and trying to link insurance premiums discounts to the real achievements of these targets. Managing a chronic disease poses a similar question: avoiding complications requires a very strict adherence to a specific lifestyle, and continuous support is a complex and expensive organizational task.

The patient, informal caregivers, non-medical caregivers, nurses, primary care organizations and medical specialists—all these represent individuals that are now being grouped into multidisciplinary teams under the control of case managers who are responsible for single individuals. While this organization is, in many regions, still a future goal and not a present reality, the real challenge is represented by the design and implementation of care processes that are effective and efficient. Modern communication technologies allow almost immediate good quality audio and video communication between the patient and any operator in the care chain, while the standards in health information exchange allow the set-up of 'continuity of care' systems, but what are the relevant information and the effective care delivery processes?

The real challenge lies in identifying the pathways to manage the disease, to set up a framework to introduce and evaluate all possible medical and technological innovations, to distribute the information to all players from the patients themselves, to family, to all social and medical caregivers: the choice and the use of technologies has to find a place within a well-defined picture. The technology assessment project has to be based on scenarios that are partly based on evidence, but also accommodate the rules to introduce new steps and new technologies: small scale pilots are not significant in this respect, but statistically significant approaches have to be put to the test.

Conclusions

Healthcare services are at the centre of political discussions all over the world: soaring costs are starting to represent a problem both for state/public systems and for systems based on private insurances. There is no such thing as an ideal model: often public systems are moving towards the privatization of both provider institutions and the reimbursement organizations, while one big issue in the USA is the increased public role in healthcare. Moreover, one of the main features of the healthcare market is the very strong 'offer' drive: as soon as a new technology or treatment is available on the market, the population will want to have access to it, based on the 'right' to the best existing treatment, escaping in many cases all evidence-based guidelines.

Tomorrow's healthcare is promising to be more expensive, to open a large scale prevention scenario, to expose the need of collecting huge amount of molecular data in order to set up personalized therapies. How is it going to be possible to escape from this spiralling pathway? It is probably time to look also at the other side of the coin: these costs also mean that there is a growing body of industries, providers, and management organizations that are delivering the products and services that are needed. The healthcare market already has all characteristics of the 'Lead Market', where there are many chances to introduce and test innovation. All this value will be created and will have to be measured against the cost of the healthcare service: in a situation of uncertainty, where several revolutionary innovations may take place in the next year, the entrepreneur will find it a challenge to sailing these new oceans.

Healthier people, innovative industries: could this be the result in the age of convergence?

Acknowledgment

Nicola Pangher wishes to thank G. Pangher, his partners and his team at ITALTBS and TESAN for the collaboration in setting up the innovation 'engine' that is providing the right solutions for the 'Healthcare of the Future'.

References

Association of American Medical Colleges (2003). *Information technology enabling clinical research*, with funding from the National Science Foundation.

Barlow J, *et al.* (2007). A systematic review of the benefits of home telecare for frail elderly people and those with long term conditions. *JTT*, **13**, 172.

Gardeniers HJGE, Luttge R, Berenschot EJW, de Boer MJ, Yeshurun SY, Hefetz M, Vanapos T, Oever R, van den Berg A (2003). Silicon micromachined hollow microneedles for transdermal liquid transport. *Journal of Microelectromechanical Systems*, **12**, 855–862.

Harvard Medical School-Partners HealthCare Center for Genetics and Genomics (2007). Response to the request of information by the US Dept. of Health and Human Services on 'Improving Health and Accelerating Personalized Health Care through Health Information Technology and Genomic Information in Population- and Community-based Health Care Delivery Systems'. HPCGG. Accessed at http://www.hpcgg.org/News/HPCGG_RFI_Response_1_0.pdf, on 1 Feb 2009.

Hogan J (2006). A little goes a long way. *Nature*, **442**.

IDC (2004). Biobanks: accelerating molecular medicine—challenges facing the global biobanking community. Available at: http://www.idc.com. Study sponsored by IBM, available at http://www-03.ibm.com/industries/global/files/Biobanks_Accelerating_Molecular_Medicine.pdf, Accessed on 1 Feb 2009.

Kannath A and Rutt HN (2007). Development of low cost instrumentation for non-invasive detection of *Helicobacter pylori*. *Proceedings of SPIE*, **6430**.

Merkin R. A vision about the future? Available at: in http://www.fastercures.org/sec/great_essays, Accessed on 1 Feb 2009.

Pare G, *et al.* (2007). Systematic review of home telemonitoring for chronic diseases: the evidence base. *JAMIA* **14**, 3, 269.

Personalized medicines: hopes and realities. Study by The Royal Society, 2005.

Stachura ME, *et al.* (2007). Telehomecare and remote monitoring: an outcomes review. Prepared by the Medical College of Georgia for the Advanced Medical Technology Association.

The Great Essays for Change from the Faster Cures. Center for Accelerating Medical Solutions.

Whitten PS, *et al.* (2002). Systematic review of cost effectiveness studies of telemedicine interventions. *British Medical Journal*, **324**, 1434.

Chapter 12

Treatment uncertainty and irreversibility in medical care: implications for cost-effectiveness analysis*

Joshua Graff Zivin, Matthew Neidell and Lauri Feldman

Introduction

Over the past 20 years, the global policy environment that governs the approval and price-setting process for new pharmaceuticals has shifted its orientation from an almost exclusive focus on safety to one that is increasingly preoccupied with the 'value' of new products. As a result, we have witnessed the rise of cost-effectiveness analysis (CEA) and other economic valuation techniques as important tools in the evaluation of new medical interventions. In resource-constrained environments, this emphasis on value is an important step for achieving more efficient outcomes.

However, the metrics employed for determining the value of new medical technologies often produce measures that do not accurately capture its full costs or benefits, and thus its true contribution to social welfare. For example, some relatively inexpensive and effective interventions are neither covered by insurance nor provided by national health care systems, while other more expensive, but less effective treatments are regularly covered and provided. These inconsistencies may reflect the fact that economic evaluation methods in health care, as they are currently implemented, do not include all the dimensions germane to making a welfare-improving decision. The divergences between cost-effectiveness criteria and actual decision-making are often attributed to ignorance, politics, financial constraints, and equity concerns about the distribution of outcomes (Birch and Donaldson 1987; Gold *et al.* 1996). This divergence, however, may also be a consequence of important elements missing from the analysis as currently performed.

In determining the value of any new medical technology, it is essential to weigh the treatment's immediate benefits against any potential impact on the set of future treatment options. The influence of current medical technology on the effectiveness of future potential interventions is often overlooked in adoption and

* Financial support for this study was provided in part by grants from Pfizer Inc.

coverage decisions.[1] There are often large degrees of uncertainty about both the current costs and benefits of technology adoption, and/or coverage. Moreover, some health interventions, once exercised, restrict future potential interventions for both related and unrelated medical conditions.

Since actions taken today may involve some irreversible transformation of the set of available interventions in the future, this phenomenon has become known as the irreversibility problem. The benefit associated with actions that preserve treatment choices in the future, above and beyond the direct value associated with those actions, is referred to as the option value of the intervention. Investment rules that ignore this option value can be grossly in error.[2]

Incorporating option values in medical technology evaluations is potentially important for several reasons. First, this setting is one where there is tremendous uncertainty about the demand for future products. When we begin treating a population of individuals, we do not know what additional conditions they will develop in the future. Since new diseases are constantly emerging, we do not even necessarily know the nature of these future conditions. Moreover, recent improvements in life expectancy, which increase the opportunity for new conditions to arise—especially those associated with aging such as cancer and dementia—make option values in this context an especially important piece of the valuation equation. Secondly, despite brisk growth over the past several decades in the number of treatments available for a wide range of conditions, treatments generally share a fairly small set of common mechanisms of action, making inter-dependencies especially likely. Since the choice of a given present treatment would probably preclude some future treatment option, this implies particularly high option values. Finally, unlike many private investment decisions, those taken by national governments may be effectively irreversible for political reasons. Once medical technologies have been authorized for public consumption, it is extremely difficult to limit their use, such as ongoing concerns regarding antibiotic over-use and the resulting development of antibiotic-resistant bacteria.

Irreversibility, intertemporal uncertainty, and decision making

Certain interventions, once exercised, may restrict the set of future potential interventions available to treat future medical conditions that may arise. For example,

---

[1] The general point that current treatment decisions affect the *likelihood* of developing future medical conditions has received considerable attention in the health technology assessment literature (see, for example, Weinstein *et al.* 1980; Meltzer 1987). Here we focus on the 'irreversible' influence of current treatment decisions on the *effectiveness* of treatment for future diseases, and thus the value associated with preserving treatment options in the future.

[2] See McDonald and Siegel (1985) and Pindyck (1988), for empirical evidence about firm's operating decisions.

treatment of certain types of cancer patients with a bone marrow transplant and massive doses of chemotherapy will reduce the patient's ability to tolerate and respond to chemotherapy in the future, should some form of cancer recur (Messori *et al.* 1997; Schouten *et al.* 2000). Coverage and adoption of this course of treatment may be the best decision, but clearly its influence on the availability of future treatment protocols and the effectiveness of alternate, option-preserving treatments should be incorporated in the treatment decision.

Drugs that are subject to resistance are another example. Indeed, these concerns may help explain why there is still no consensus about when to start therapy in HIV patients (Cohen 2000; Harrington and Carpenter 2000). Some advocate the 'hit hard and hit early' approach, which suggests the initiation of complete treatment at the time of diagnosis in order to prevent the disease from progressing. Others are concerned that starting therapy at early stages, when T-cell counts are high and viral loads are low, may lead to the development of viral resistance to these drugs and related compounds. These clinicians advocate waiting until the disease reaches a more advanced stage to initiate therapy so that future therapeutic options can be preserved, although the disease may progress to an advanced stage more rapidly. While either approach may be appropriate, clinical and coverage decisions about when to initiate therapy should clearly weigh the benefits and costs of starting early versus waiting over the entire potential treatment time horizon.

This problem of current actions influencing the availability of future potential actions has received considerable attention in the environmental economics literature (Arrow and Fisher 1974; Hanneman 1989; Kolstad 1996) and, more recently, in the economic investment literature (for a good review, see Pindyck 1991). This literature suggests that if more information about the costs and benefits of these future potential interventions will become available over time, it may be optimal to delay investment in the 'irreversible' technology. The value of preserving options by delaying decisions until a future time when more information is available is called the quasi-option value of the decision.

Several recent studies suggest that investment and environmental development rules that ignore this value can be grossly in error (e.g. Brennan and Schwartz, 1985; McDonald R and D Siegel 1985; Pindyck 1991). For example, Fisher and Hanneman (1986) analysed a land development decision, where the land being considered for development might contain valuable genetic material for commercial maize production. While the benefits were more than triple the costs of development, the quasi-option value to waiting 1 more year for additional information was almost half the expected benefit. When the costs of waiting are less than the benefits, current development would clearly be sub-optimal. Given the similarities between environmental protection decisions and healthcare coverage decisions, similar effects may undermine the value of current CEA practice.

Let us further examine the role that uncertainty and irreversibility can play in determining the value of a particular medical intervention. For simplicity, we suppose that people live for only two periods, the discount rate is zero, and all treatment costs are equal and negligible. Consider a chronic disease X, which first occurs in period 1 (and always lasts two periods). Suppose that there are two choices in treating disease X, denoted T_1 and T_2, respectively. Patients with disease X treated with T_1 gain

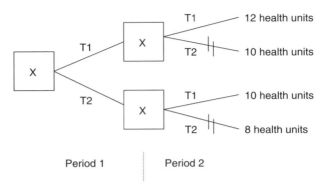

Fig. 12.1 Treatment for disease X.

6 health units in each period.[3] Patients treated with T_2 gain 4 health units each period. A traditional economic analysis would indicate that patients should be treated with T_1 in both periods, as illustrated in Fig. 12.1 (with purely dominated strategies demarcated by short parallel lines).

Now consider an acute disease, Y, which may occur in period 2. There is only one treatment (T_Y) for disease Y. Patients who contract Y lose 8 health units in the period in which the disease occurs. Patients who are treated with T_Y recover all of these units. Clearly, treatment with T_Y is strongly preferred to non-treatment for those patients with condition Y.

The problem of irreversibility occurs in circumstances when these two situations are combined and the treatments are inter-related. Suppose that patients who, in period 1, contracted disease X and were treated with T_1 cannot tolerate T_Y (i.e. T_Y is ineffective in treating Y) if they later develop disease Y. Let p denote the probability of developing disease Y, which we will assume is independent of developing (or treating) disease X. In this case, T_2 has two values associated with it—one due to its effectiveness in treating X and another due to it preserving the option to effectively treat Y. The treatment decision in this case is illustrated in Fig. 12.2. When patients are offered T_1 in the first period, it will always be optimal to offer T_1 again in the second period, although the overall benefit of this treatment strategy is clearly diminished for cases where disease Y develops. When patients are offered T_2 in the first period, the arrival of disease Y will dictate the second period protocol. If Y does not arrive, patients will switch to T_1 in the second period, since there is no benefit from option preservation at this point. If Y does arrive, then patients are treated with T_2 and T_Y.

The incremental value of T_2 (relative to the value of T_1) can be expressed as the difference in expected effectiveness between starting with T_2 and providing patients with T_1 in both periods:

---

[3] Note that we are being intentionally vague about our quality-of-life measure so as to abstract away from the specific assumptions associated with conventional outcome measures, such as the quality-adjusted-life-year.

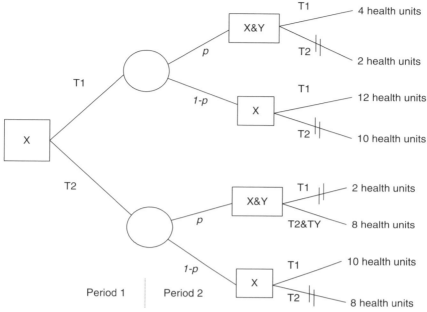

Fig. 12.2 Treatment for disease X and Y.

$$[p \cdot (8) + (1 - p) \cdot (10)] - [p \cdot (4) + (1 - p) \cdot (12)]$$

This value reflects both the direct treatment benefits of T_2 for condition X, as well as the value of preserving the option to use T_Y in period 2. This latter value is known as the option value associated with T_2. While this option value will always increase the value of T_2 relative to T_1, it will not always be the case that this 'extra' value is enough to justify its use. In this simple example, T_2, which is an inferior treatment for disease X alone, would only be the preferred treatment option if the probability of developing disease Y is greater than one-third. In general then, we see that the optimal treatment plan is contingent upon future expectations.

Modelling treatment values when actions are irreversible

Option values can be quantified and incorporated in analyses by explicitly formulating a multi-period, dynamic decision model that attends to uncertainty and the potential role of irreversibility. Generally speaking, there are three cases we must deal with complete irreversibility, partial irreversibility, and partial irreversibility with the possibility of learning more about the probability of future disease arrival (hereafter partial irreversibility with learning).

To illustrate these three cases, we again consider diseases X and Y, and the same set of treatment options as in our earlier model. We begin assuming that disease X is present in the first period. Disease Y will then arrive in the second period with some probability equal to p. Remember from the previous illustration that T_2 is an inferior treatment for condition X, but yields better results should it need to be combined with T_Y. Thus, there is an option value associated with using T_2, but that option comes at a cost.

First consider the case of complete irreversibility. Since the downstream impacts from ever receiving a given treatment are permanent, it will never make sense to switch from initial treatment regimens. Therefore, patients initiated on T_1 will receive that treatment in perpetuity and the same will be true for patients initiated on T_2.[4] As such, the decision-maker will use the forecast about the arrival rate of disease Y to calculate the expected present discounted value (PDV) of each treatment regime and select the one with the highest return.

The second case in need of consideration is that of partial irreversibility without learning. In this version of the model, we relax the assumption of complete irreversibility by assuming that the negative impacts of T_1 on the effectiveness of T_Y are temporary. In particular, we assume that after some time or cooling off period of duration n following treatment with T_1, T_Y can be fully effective once again. Since agents still cannot perform tests to update their knowledge about the arrival of Y, the least sophisticated treatment protocol would start patients on T_1 and switch them to T_2 when disease Y arrives. Under such a protocol, patients will pay a 'penalty' equal to n times the value of T_Y, which they forgo while they are waiting for the cooling off period to end.

Of course, decision-makers can use the information that they have about the expected arrival rate of disease Y to do better than simply waiting for it to arrive before switching to T_2. In this case, the optimal treatment strategy requires switching when the expected marginal benefit of one more period of treatment with T_1 is exactly equal to the expected present discounted value of adopting treatment with T_2.[5]

Now compare the value of T_2 under complete irreversibility to its value under partial irreversibility. When the cost of the cooling-off period is smaller than the relative value of the advantage of T_1 over T_2, the value of T_2 for those patients that would not receive it under complete irreversibility increases in a world of partial irreversibility. If the cooling off cost is larger than the benefits that would be received from introducing T_2, then the value of T_2 again decreases under partial irreversibility.[6] For those patients who would not have received T_2 under complete irreversibility, the move to partial irreversibility has an ambiguous effect on its value. The intuition for this result relies on the recognition that the introduction of partial irreversibility has two distinct effects. First, it reduces the amount of 'wasteful' T_2 that needs to be offered to patients to ensure that they can be effectively treated for condition Y when it arrives.

---

4 Unlike the two period example given in the previous section, the last period of the disease is unknown, so individuals who begin on T_2 will not switch to T_1.

5 Note this characterizes the optimal interior solution where both treatments are used. A corner solution where patients exclusively receive T_1 or T_2 could also arise when the probability-adjusted costs associated with the inferior treatment of Y is extremely high or low, respectively.

6 In this last case, the value of T_2 is going from negative under complete irreversibility to more negative under partial irreversibility. If we view the value of T_2 as bounded from below at zero, then the value of this treatment will be the same for these types of patients under both scenarios.

This yields changes on the intensive margin, since under partial irreversibility these individuals no longer need to initiate treatment (T_2) at time zero. Secondly, by reducing this 'wasteful' spending, the use of T_2 may become attractive for some patients who did not find it attractive when costs were higher. This yields changes on the extensive margin, since a subset of patients that would not have received any T_2 under complete irreversibility will receive some when irreversibility is partial. The first effect leads to reductions in the value of T_2, while the second effect leads to increases. The overall impact of a move to partial irreversibility on the value of T_2 will depend on the distribution of patients in each of these groups. Moreover, the value of T_2 largely depends on underlying economic and biologic parameter values, and the incident rate of disease Y.

Finally, we must consider the situation of complete irreversibility with possibility of learning more about the probability of disease Y occurring. Up to this point we have assumed that decision makers have basic knowledge about the population-level incidence of disease Y, but that they have no means of updating that knowledge with information about individual patients until the disease actually arrives. Now, consider the possibility of a test that can be performed to measure levels of the biologic indicator for Y within patients. The decision maker will perform the test precisely at the moment where the net benefits from waiting one more period to switch equal the costs of the test. If the test reveals that the biologic indicator is higher than expected, the decision-maker will switch earlier. If the test reveals that the biologic indicator is lower than expected, the decision-maker will wait. This process can be repeated indefinitely—thus, always ensuring that the treatment is optimal for the given period. The ability to increase knowledge about the probability of disease incidence in future greatly assists the present decision-maker in determining the optimal present treatment.

This test also significantly impacts on the value of T_2. The introduction of learning will lower the overall option value of T_2 for those that would have received it under partial irreversibility absent learning. Moreover, increases in the cost of the test make deviations from the expected protocol under partial reversibility without learning less likely and thus increase the value of T_2. The responsiveness of the value of T_2 with respect to underlying parameters remains qualitatively the same.

Conclusions

For many physicians, the observation that current medical treatment decisions have repercussions for the treatment of health conditions in the future, is an obvious one that often factors into their clinical decision-making, albeit heuristically. Yet, at present, such considerations form no part of health care technology assessment calculations at societal or sub-societal levels, leading to potentially significant mischaracterizations of treatment value. Growth in the availability of treatments for chronic diseases that require long-term interventions, along with general increases in life expectancy, suggest that the importance of this omission will only become larger.

It is thus essential to use a valuation model that attends to these inter-temporal dependencies—one that considers the uncertain arrivals of future diseases and the varying degrees of effectiveness with which they can be treated. More generally, there are several key insights that we can all consider. Irreversibility raises the value of the option-preserving treatment. The existence of an option value—that value above and beyond the direct value of treatment for the current condition—means that a treatment that is inferior to an alternative for its indicated use may be the superior choice when lifetime welfare is considered. Optimal decision-making requires a careful comparison of the 'costs' of a less effective treatment for a condition today with the 'benefits' of more effective treatments for conditions in the future. The size of the option value and thus the degree to which valuations that ignore it are miscalculated, depends critically on the relative effectiveness of treatments, the likelihood of diseases arriving in the future, the extent to which current interventions limit the ability to treat these future conditions, and the relevant discount rate.

Comparing treatment values under complete irreversibility to a scenario where irreversibility is only partial reveals a more nuanced role for option values. For those patients at high-risk for the future disease the value of the option-preserving treatment falls when irreversibility is incomplete, while the value increases for those at low-risk. In a world with patients that are heterogeneous in their risk for future diseases, the distribution of patient types will determine whether the option-preserving treatment is more valuable in an environment of partial or complete irreversibility. Each of these impacts is compounded when a test for future disease progression is introduced.

The intuition for these results is deepened when we recognize that one of the principal features driving our results is that health risks for future diseases increase with age, a characteristic that accurately describes the incidence profile for many diseases throughout the world. When patients are heterogeneous in early environmental exposures or their genetic predisposition to disease, older low-risk patients are conceptually akin to younger high-risk ones, since both have similar risks of developing disease in the coming years. The key distinction is that under complete or near-complete irreversibility, low-risk patients must begin the option-preserving treatment when they are young and it is precisely at this point that the treatment is least valuable. Only in the cases where future disease is both very likely and of significant consequence, i.e. when the option value is very large, will it make sense to place low-risk patients on this option-preserving regimen. As the 'costs' of reversing current treatment impacts fall, it becomes more feasible to provide the option-preserving treatment to these low-risk individuals at a later age, even if the impacts of future disease are modest.

This basic framework of option-valuation also highlights potentially important macro-level strategies to improve social welfare through medical technologies. Research investments that focus on transforming irreversibility from complete to partial could generate large social benefits. Clearly, investments in the development of alternative treatments for future diseases are also important, but the return to such investments will hinge critically on the degree of irreversibility in the system. Insofar as irreversibilities are a function of shared modes of actions among interventions, investment strategies that focus on a diversified portfolio of interventions in terms of these modes will also create social benefits. At a broader policy level, this argument points toward support for research that strengthens our understanding of disease and its evolution over time, which stands in contrast to approaches that focus on investing in disease treatments for the sole purpose of reducing the onset and severity of symptoms. Assessing the value of such strategies is an important area for future research.

Also essential is a revision of the CEA methodology itself. CEA is used to determine optimal funding and resource allocation for medical technologies, research, and treatment. As long as CEA fails to incorporate uncertainty and irreversibility, it will continue to miscalculate medical valuations with potentially severe consequences. Revision will take time and will come at a cost, but the option value of future policy gains is high.

References

Arrow K and Fisher A (1974). Environmental preservation, uncertainty, and irreversibility. *Quarterly Journal of Economics*, **88,** 312–19.

Birch S and Donaldson C (1985). Applications of cost-benefit analysis to health care: departures from Welfare Economic Theory. *Journal of Health Economics*, **6,** 211–25.

Brennan M and Schwartz E (1985). Evaluating natural resource investments. *Journal of Business*, **58,** 135–57.

Cohen O (2000). Antiretroviral therapy: time to think strategically. *Lancet* **132,** 320–2.

Fisher A and Hanneman M (1986). Option value and the extinction of species. In: V. Smith, ed. *Advance is applied micro-economics*. Greenwich, JAI Press.

Gold M, Siegel J, Russell L and Weinstein M, eds (1996). *Cost effectiveness in health and medicine*, pp. 9–21. Oxford, Oxford University Press.

Hanneman W (1989). Information and the concept of option value. *Journal of Environmental Economics and Management*, **16,** 23–37.

Harrington M and Carpenter C (2000). Hit HIV-1 hard, but only when necessary. *Lancet* **355,** 2147–52.

Kolstad C (1996). Fundamental irreversibilities in stock externalities. *Journal of Public Economics*, **60,** 221–33.

McDonald R and Siegel D (1985). Investment and the valuation of firms when there is an option to shut down. *International Economic Review*, **26,** 331–49.

Meltzer D (1997). Accounting for future costs in medical cost-effectiveness analysis. *Journal of Health Economics*, **16,** 33–64.

Messori A, Bonistalli L, Costantini M, *et al.* (1997). Cost-effectiveness of autologous bone marrow transplantation in patients with relapsed non-Hodgkin's lymphoma. *Bone Marrow Transplant*, **19,** 275–81.

Pindyck R (1988). Irreversible investment, capacity choice, and the value of the firm. *American Economic Review*, **78,** 969–85.

Pindyck R (1991). Irreversibility, uncertainty, and investment. *Journal of Economic Literature*, **29,** 1110–48.

Schouten HC, Kvaloy S, Sydes M, *et al.* (2000). The CUP trial: a randomized study analyzing the efficacy of high dose therapy and purging in low-grade non-Hodgkin's lymphoma (NHL). *Annals of Oncology*, **11,** 91–4.

Weinstein M, Fineberg H, Elstein A, Frazier H, Newhauser D, Neutra R and McNeil B (1980). *Clinical decision analysis*. Philadelphia, Saunders.

Chapter 13

The limits and challenges to the economic evaluation of health technologies

Adam Oliver and Corinna Sorenson

Introduction

In most countries in the world there are increasing pressures on health care resources. These pressures are caused by a multitude of factors, including population ageing, the detection of 'new' illnesses, rising public expectations about what health care systems 'ought' to deliver, and the development of new medical interventions and pharmaceutical products. With the global economic downturn, these pressures are only likely to increase. Governments internationally are therefore increasingly aware of the fact that rationing health care technologies, as a means of controlling health care expenditure growth, is inevitable.

The method of rationing can take many forms, such as, rationing by price and rationing by waits. In many countries over the past 20 years, rationing by value for money, by using health economic evaluation, has come to occupy an increasingly prominent place in the discourse on priority setting in health care. At face value, the ethos underlying health economic evaluation, i.e. the allocation of health care resources so as to maximise health from each unit of health care expenditure, appears quite sensible. Indeed, if one assumes, as many do, that the production of 'health' is the only relevant outcome of 'health care', then one may argue that it is an ethical requirement to allocate health care resources to those who can benefit most, in terms of health gain, from them. Allocating it otherwise would mean that decision maker are denying the rights of those who have greater claims.

However, many legitimate challenges can be made to the notion that 'health' from 'health care' ought to be maximised. Indeed, stakeholders from virtually every sector of the health care community have raised concerns against the use of economic evaluation in the decision-making process. This chapter will briefly review some of these concerns from a wide range of disciplinary and stakeholder perspectives, and will then offer some reflections on the National Institute for Health and Clinical Excellence (NICE), which uses health economic evaluation to assess whether health care interventions ought to be made available in the National Health Service (NHS) in England and Wales. In terms of considering cost-effectiveness information across a wide range of interventions in the health policy process, NICE is perhaps the most developed health technology assessment (HTA) agency in the world, and thus some attention will be directed towards the extent to which it addresses stakeholder concerns.

Before moving on to the various stakeholder views, however, it seems apt to outline some of the methodological limitations of cost-utility analysis (CUA). Although CUA is the most often recommended form of health economic evaluation by HTA agencies,[1] it would be possible to devote a whole book to its limitations. Here, however, just three of them will be described, the first two of which relate to the perhaps erroneous assumption that one should always aim to maximise health from health care, and the last of which appears to represent an intractable flaw in cost-effectiveness analysis, even if the health maximization assumption were valid.

Methodological limitations

For the first limitation, consider a person (or people) with a chronic or debilitating condition; for example, a wheelchair-bound person. Most people would no doubt prefer to be fully able than disabled, and therefore a fully able person would experience more quality-adjusted life years (QALYs) than a disabled person over a specified time period, *ceteris paribus*.[2] Thus, an otherwise fully able person would be assigned more post-treatment QALYs than the disabled (and thus be prioritized over the disabled), purely by virtue of being free from disability. Nord (2001) has argued that, in these circumstances, QALYs should not be used in choosing between fully abled and disabled people for life-extending interventions, because when deciding who should live longest, we are implicitly placing a value on people's *lives*. We are thus making a moral judgment on how much their life is worth to them, i.e. on how much they *value* their life, for which no simple measure of health can account, and indeed, there is some limited empirical evidence to suggest that Nord's objections may be widely supported (Oliver 2004, 2006).

Following the above logic, CUA, via QALY maximization, can therefore discriminate unjustly against the chronically ill and disabled, an argument that has been termed 'double jeopardy' (Harris 1987). In other words, the chronically ill and disabled are not only disadvantaged by their illnesses and disabilities, but also by their relative prospects of receiving treatments for unrelated conditions. To counter, Nord *et al.* (1999) have recommended that life years gained should always be given a weight equal to one, irrespective of the health state of the individual. Johannesson (2001) has proposed an alternative 'rule' to resolve the potential problem of discrimination against the chronically ill and disabled, which would generate identical *weighted* QALY gains, where the same *relative* change in expected QALYs has occurred, irrespective of the total number of expected *unweighted* QALYs on offer. The weights to be attached to the QALY gains are calculated by:

(Average expected number of QALYs for the group)/(Expected number of QALYs for the individual)

---

[1] CUA is a specific form of cost-effectiveness analysis (CEA) that uses quality-adjusted life years (QALYs) as the health outcome measure.

[2] As indicated in footnote 1, QALYs are a measure of health.

The weighted QALY gains for an equal extension of life would, with all else being equal, be identical for the fully able, and chronically ill or disabled.[3] Williams (1997, 2001) advocated a very different line of reasoning to deal with the 'discrimination' problem, by arguing that 'society' may choose to compensate the chronically ill and disabled for their misfortunes. He relates this explicitly to the 'fair innings' argument, which requires the consideration and redress of lifetime inequalities in health to be a main driver in health care priority setting,[4] and allows those who have always been in a state of relative poor health to be given priority over those who have always been in better health, *ceteris paribus*.

All in all, although there are varying opinions on how to deal with the double jeopardy problem in QALY maximization, a problem nevertheless remains, specifically because it is rarely, if ever, seriously addressed in applied CUA. It may well be the case that social preferences call for QALY maximization to be traded off against providing equal access to health care interventions in some health care contexts (as is implicitly indicated by Nord), and for QALY maximization to be traded off against a more equal distribution of lifetime QALYs in other contexts (as is indicated by Williams). In other contexts—for example, when comparing the relative costs and outcomes of alternative treatments for the same patient group—simple QALY maximization might best match population preferences, but the important point to note is that the preferred priority setting decision 'rule' may vary across and be driven by context, which might, in part, explain the almost intractable disagreements that arise between different specialists working in this area. Identifying where which rule is 'best' is a key area for health economists to address.

A second possible problem with the QALY maximization approach relates to the issue of 'security'; that is, the feeling that one is secure in the knowledge that the health care system will be available, if at all possible, if one were to fall ill. This does not necessarily mean that interventions of very marginal benefit ought to be provided at all costs, but it does mean that, in some circumstances, the maximization of QALYs can be legitimately traded off to ensure that more people have access to the health care service.

For instance, hypothetically assume that there is currently no available treatment for, say, multiple sclerosis, but there is a treatment available for angina pectoris. Further assume that new treatments for each of these conditions are developed, but that the decision-maker is placed in the difficult position of having sufficient resources to fund only one of them. The decision maker is informed that the new

---

[3] For example, consider a 'group' of two individuals, A and B. Assume that A and B will live for three more years without treatment. For those three years, A will be in full health and B will be in a condition with a health state value of 0.5 (i.e. half as good as full health). The average number of expected QALYs for the group is therefore 2.25. Thus, the weight for A = 2.25/3 = 0.75; for B, 2.25/1.5 = 1.5. Now assume that if A or B take a health care treatment, their lives would be extended by six years, but their state of health remains the same. The weighted QALY gain for A = 6 × 0.75 = 4.5; and for B = 6 × 0.5 × 1.5 = 4.5. Thus, the weighted QALY gain is the same for both individuals.

[4] The fair innings argument can be concerned with life-expectancy, or it can be concerned with quality-adjusted life expectancy. In this chapter, the term is equated with the latter.

angina intervention produces more QALYs per additional required unit of resource than the multiple sclerosis intervention, and that therefore, following the rules of CUA, where health is the only relevant outcome of health care, the angina intervention ought to take priority.

In theory, following the above logic, CUA could require 'society' to devote, for example, 90 per cent of its health care resources to 10 per cent of all therapeutic areas, a point that Adam Oliver posed to the late Alan Williams in early 2005. Williams replied that, in his view, health is the only relevant outcome of health care and that, therefore, the above scenario would be perfectly acceptable if it led to the maximization of health outcomes from available resources. Williams' view is surely contentious, as a health care system that serves only 10 per cent of all illness categories is likely to garner little public and political support.

Returning to the multiple sclerosis and angina example, it is possible that all members of society could, either now or at some point in the future, suffer from either or both of these illnesses. Therefore, it may well be the case that most people would prefer the multiple sclerosis intervention to take priority, even if the new angina treatment can produce more QALYs per unit of expenditure, in order to provide the security of knowing that some form of public sector intervention will be provided if one were to suffer from either of these conditions. In these circumstances, broadening access may thus take precedence over QALY maximization. In other words, people may place a value on interventions even if they do not require them yet or even if they may never require them, due to the realization that they *might* require them at some point. Such preferences are not captured in applied CUA.

The final methodological limitation highlighted here would remain pertinent even if QALY maximization were always the appropriate prioritization rule to pursue. The limitation, which relates directly to the non-consideration of potentially substantial opportunity costs, was first presented by Birch and Gafni in 1992, but has thus far been largely overlooked by those who conduct CUA. The limitation can best be described with the following hypothetical example.

Consider a situation where there is a new intervention and an existing intervention for the prevention of hip fractures, and call these interventions A and B, respectively. In very basic terms, the cost-utility of the new intervention A is calculated by:

$$(C_A - C_B)/(Q_A - Q_B)$$

where C_A and C_B are, respectively, the cost of A and B, and Q_A and Q_B are the number of QALYs that each intervention produces.

For example, assume that $C_A = £2.5$ million, $C_B = £2$ million, $Q_A = 1500$ QALYs gained, and $Q_B = 1000$ QALYs gained. The new intervention is both more costly and more effective, a common occurrence in reality, and its cost-utility ratio is calculated at £1000 per QALY gained (i.e. £500,000/500 QALYs). Such a ratio would be deemed highly cost-effective, yet no account has been taken of the opportunity costs of the cost-increasing aspect of intervention A (i.e. £500,000) in the calculation of the ratio.

The non-inclusion of potentially substantial opportunity costs in CUA can – and, in England and Wales at least, does – pose serious difficulties for regional health care purchasers if they are required to purchase interventions on the basis of cost-effectiveness guidance. The purchasers may find themselves in the position of having to consider cut backs in existing services to finance new interventions, although such a step could be so unpopular with existing service users that it would be politically very difficult for the purchasers to put into practice. Moreover, although not assessed in terms of their relative costs and benefits, the existing services may actually represent better value for money than the 'cost-effective' intervention A, and thus the provision of A could lead to an overall decrease in efficiency, if efficiency is defined in terms of health production per unit of health care expenditure.

Aside from the above-mentioned methodological limitations of CUA, a large number of stakeholders from different academic disciplines, medicine, industry, and other sectors of society have expressed particular points of contention with this form of analysis. It is to some of these points that we now briefly turn.

Stakeholder challenges

The stakeholder perspectives presented in this section are, of course, only a 'snapshot' of the concerns presented in the literature, and the arguments cited here from particular commentators may not be a perfect representation of each of their disciplines. Nonetheless, it is hoped that they do at least provide a feel for the range of criticisms that have been directed at the use of economic evaluation in health care decision making.

From the perspective of political science, Chinitz (2004) argues that the uptake of HTA broadly, and economic evaluation specifically, has been high because policy makers harbour a technocratic wish to liberate them from difficult decisions. However, he further asserts that as this form of analysis is used increasingly in explicit policy-making scenarios, it will come under greater scrutiny, and policy makers who utilise these methods will face increasing political accountability to justify their use.

Webster (2004), a sociologist, refers to 'responsibility' and 'reflexivity' as being the primary social discourse running through institutions, with responsibility being a scientific, economic account of the application and implications of new technologies, and reflexivity being the need to emphasise the provisional status of any such account, and make transparent any claim of 'value' for the new technology. Webster argues that reflexivity makes it difficult to standardise the requirements for health economic evaluation internationally at a single point in time or nationally over time, because organizations, institutions, and cultures differ across time and place. For instance, in some countries, such as Sweden, local purchasers compete with one another to provide the latest interventions, which may undermine any scope to implement national HTA guidelines and guidance. Webster makes the further interesting point that governments may use economic analysis as a symbolic device to give the impression that they are showing cost-awareness, or to further legitimate decisions that have already been made, in much the same way as the government in England appeared to use the recommendations of the Wanless Review to justify previously made decisions to increase NHS expenditure (Wanless 2002).

From an ethics perspective, ten Have (2004) points out that health care technologies potentially affect the health, lives, and deaths of a great many people, and therefore the articulation and consideration of the values of a wide range of stakeholders is ethically required in health care priority-setting decisions, a factor that is often seemingly overlooked in applied CUA. Moreover, deciding what constitutes a harm, and whether benefits outweigh harms, argues ten Have, is far from straightforward. He asserts that there needs to be a high level of engagement of patients and the public in policy debates so as to understand their values regarding priorities and rationing; for example, there is a need to better learn what people consider to be 'fair' in the distribution of health care resources and/or outcomes.

Coulter (2004), writing from the patient group perspective, also thinks that patients and the general public should have an important role to play in determining priorities for CUA, and speculates that the public would place a strong emphasis on assessing existing as opposed to new and emerging treatments, because existing interventions clearly affect them more at any point in time. Coulter also contends that patients and the public should be more heavily involved in evaluating the cost-utility of interventions. Ultimately, Coulter argues that the neglect of patient preferences is a fundamental mistake because, like ten Have, she emphasises that technology appraisal involves values and judgements, and that in a democratic society people should have a say in decisions that potentially affect their lives.[5] She does acknowledge, however, that pharmaceutical industry funding of particular patient groups can lead to an inappropriate balance of influence across the groups.

Perhaps unsurprisingly, Lothgren and Ratcliffe's (2004) pharmaceutical industry perspective does not make mention of the industry's inappropriate funding of patient groups, but does question why a large proportion of CUA effort is focused upon pharmaceutical products. In common with other commentators, although probably for different reasons, they argue that more thought ought to be given to the prioritization and selection of assessment topics. Additionally, they express concern that the differing requirements across countries for conducting health economic evaluation places an undue burden on the pharmaceutical companies, although if Webster's aforementioned reflexivity argument is valid, the multiple requirements across different jurisdictions is seemingly inevitable, and perhaps necessary to account for local circumstances and concerns.

Holland (2004), from public health, is also disappointed that HTA agencies have traditionally focused upon pharmaceutical and clinical interventions, overlooking, to a large extent, the wider determinants of health. Although this is not a problem with the methods of health economic evaluation *per se*, it does call into question the simplistic assumptions inherent in these forms of analyses. Indeed, Holland recognises that public health evaluation would probably call for greater complexity, given that these approaches traverse many sectors (e.g. health care, education, sanitation, etc.) and often entail a greater time lag to ascertain the benefits and costs of interventions. Holland also states that the formal assessment of many public health interventions can

---

5 Although see Sunstein (2005) for a discussion of how people are often poor judges of what is good for them, and for a perspective on how one might constrain their choices to improve their lives.

encounter powerful political opposition, such as the tobacco industry's aversion to illegalizing smoking advertising.

Further addressing the inherent complexity of economic evaluation, Heath (2004) argues that, in general practice, patients often present with ill-defined and confused symptoms, which standard forms of economic evaluation fail to take into account. Moreover, CUA does not adequately capture social and ethical concerns, as alluded to by ten Have, and with which general practitioners have to consider and manage in daily practice. Thus, Heath feels that nuanced case-by-case decision making is more appropriate than acting on HTA-informed guidelines. If guidelines are to be enforced, Heath feels that politicians rather than doctors ought to take explicit responsibility for them, because the general practitioners' focus is inevitably on the individual.

Finally, from a clinical perspective, Chantler (2004), like Heath, also argues that HTA guidelines should not be too deterministic or prescriptive, because they cannot appropriately address all the concerns that arise when making individual treatment decisions. However, Chantler maintains that economic evaluation can be useful at the broader priority-setting level regarding decisions on whether particular interventions ought to be made available in a health care service. At this level, Chantler believes that this appropriately places the burden of responsibility for making interventions available on the politician, a move he welcomes, as he has long felt uncomfortable about doctors having to take responsibility for 'hiding' the availability of interventions from patients. Generally, however, Chantler prefers a conservative approach to the use of HTA. He contends that it should not be used to search for infinite wisdom, but should be used, instead, to try to minimize error at the individual clinical level, a point of view that may disappoint many health economists.

Overall, there seems to be many reservations from a whole variety of stakeholders as to whether the 'science' of economic evaluation appropriately incorporates important political, social, and ethical considerations that are inherent to medical decision-making. In England and Wales, NICE has recognised at least some of these limitations, and has attempted to address (or at least consider) the limitations of the science in its appraisals process. Nonetheless, has NICE done enough in this regard, and how has it performed generally? It is to these questions that we now turn.

The National Institute for Health and Clinical Excellence[6]

In the late 1990s, the relatively newly-elected Labour Government established NICE to assess the clinical and cost-effectiveness of a number of selected health care products and services. As intimated above, NICE is considered by many as the most sophisticated HTA agency in the world, in that it combines both scientific assessment and policy appraisal into a single decision-making body (Stevens and Milne 2004).

---

[6] NICE was originally called the National Institute for Clinical Excellence, but on having its remit extended to include public health interventions, partly in response to criticism that its original remit did not include interventions that probably have a greater impact than clinical services on population health (Holland 2004 – see above), it is now called the National Institute for Health and Clinical Excellence.

It has also been lauded for its transparency (Drummond 2007) and deliberative process (Culyer 2006). Despite these strengths, its operations and procedures are not without controversy, as many of the methodological issues and stakeholder concerns previously discussed pose challenges for NICE.

As with the majority of HTA bodies, NICE recommends the use of CUA as the preferred method of economic evaluation. Reflecting some of the limitations previously discussed, many stakeholders have criticised the Institute for its seeming over-reliance on QALYs, or cost per QALY, as the principal measure of cost-effectiveness and product value. In particular, as asserted by Coulter and ten Have, such methods do not adequately account for the indirect and social benefits of technologies, or capture the range of values and preferences that are important to patients—at present and over time. Consequently, in the view of many stakeholders, health gain is just one source of evidence that should be considered as part of the decision-making process. Other factors, such as equity and patient preferences over, for example, ease of use, should be duly taken into account.

Similarly, the cost-effectiveness threshold employed by the Institute has been a source of contention. The threshold at which NICE deems interventions to be cost-effective, although implicit, appears to be somewhere between £20,000 and £30,000 per QALY gained (Williams *et al.* 2007), with the more generous end of this range being employed when an intervention has particular positive characteristics; for example, if the intervention is especially innovative (Birch and Gafni 2007). This threshold has been criticised as being too generous, arbitrary, and out of line with NHS products and services not assessed by NICE (Appleby *et al.* 2007), and Williams (2004) argued that the NHS should pay no more than the average per capita GDP of about £18,000 for each QALY gained. However, NICE faces significant media-driven public pressure when it rules against the provision of interventions, emphasised by past decisions vis-à-vis drug therapy for multiple sclerosis. Indeed, given the political difficulties of recommending against the use of treatments, NICE guidance often only goes so far as to advocate restricted use in certain patient categories (Williams *et al.* 2007). This, as demonstrated in the previous section, can upset physicians, many of whom believe that broad brush guidance, even when applied in relation to specific patient categories, tends to overlook the unique situation of many patients, including the presence of co-morbidities, particular socio-economic circumstances, etc. NICE seems almost destined to be damned for going 'too high' or 'too low' in its choice of a cost-effectiveness threshold, depending on the perspective of the particular critic. Regardless of the actual threshold, however, it is generally agreed that the rationale and method of its determination should be much more transparent.

Further concerns have been cited. For instance, some have written that NICE has insufficient capacity to assess a meaningful number of interventions, and that it has traditionally focused too heavily on new interventions, overlooking a potentially large number of cost-ineffective interventions in the NHS, resonating with Coulter's (2004) arguments presented earlier. In a recent study, Linden *et al* (2007) looked at 159 technologies reviewed from 88 appraisals between March 2000 and June 2006, and found that 84 (53 per cent) were new technologies and 75 (47 per cent) were existing technologies, from which they argued that this did not indicate a bias towards new technologies. It is worth bearing in mind, however, that the number of existing technologies far outnumbers the number of new interventions, and there-fore an approximately 50-50 split may still represent a significant bias towards assessing the newer products and services. The limited capacity of NICE may create legitimate cause for concern that its impact will inevitably be limited, although one could counter this concern by arguing that the producers of medical interventions face the risk that their products *may* be assessed and thus have an incentive to make their products more cost-effective than they would be otherwise.

Despite the transparency of many aspects of NICE, with its processes and assessment reports published in detail and available for expert and – in theory – public scrutiny, the level of technical sophistication now applied in measurements of costs and outcomes somewhat undermines any claim that HTA-based decision making affords greater transparency to the public (Coast 2004). This is particularly worrying when one keeps in mind that the methods of economic evaluation are far from perfect.

Another key concern regards the slow and variable implementation of NICE guidance to date (Sheldon *et al.* 2004). To address this issue, NICE guidance to the NHS was made mandatory in 2001,[7] and primary care trusts (PCTs), the local purchasers of health care, must not deny funds for treatments that have been recommended for use by NICE when more than 3 months have passed since the guidance was issued (Stevens and Milne 2004). Unfortunately, this may steer the NHS towards a sub-optimal focus upon those interventions that NICE assesses, and away from other possibly higher priority investments or cutbacks in other activities (Stevens and Milne 2004; Birch and Gafni 2007). Moreover, there is little evidence that these efforts have adequately improved the implementation of guidance and, therefore, remedied the 'post-code' prescribing that NICE was intended to rectify.

As a result of poor implementation, some have pondered whether NICE itself is cost-effective (Freemantle 2004). One could argue that it is an inefficient use of NHS resources to support an appraisal system that is not fully implemented or prioritized by local purchasers. It appears that NICE guidance is more likely to be effectively adopted and implemented when it runs parallel to the support of opinion leaders, professional bodies, and marketing efforts by pharmaceutical companies (Sheldon *et al.* 2004), and when NHS organizations have established structures and processes to manage implementation (Audit Commission 2005).

NICE can, however, be seen in a more positive light. Many of the problems discussed above are methodological or process-orientated, and it may be possible to address these adequately with time. Moreover, one has to consider NICE with respect to the pre-NICE era, when general practitioner and hospital prescribing were influ-enced heavily by pharmaceutical companies and powerful hospital consultants and interest groups (Stevens and Milne 2004; Drummond 2007). The political path of least resistance is to say 'yes' to powerful lobbies and 'no' to weaker ones, irrespective of the products and services on offer. NICE has thus far offered a more systematic, transparent, and evidence-based approach to ascertaining the value of health technologies and

---

[7] The mandate does not apply to clinical guidelines.

making subsequent recommendations. Moreover, while there are existing limitations to economic evaluation, the Institute has made efforts towards improving its methods and procedures. For instance, it has offered funding for methods development and attempts to address stakeholder concerns surrounding social judgements and the estimation of costs. To that end, the Institute is probably the one HTA body that formally involves a wide range of stakeholders in its process, such as its use of a Citizens Council;[8] although, there has been much debate regarding the influence of stakeholder input. Overall, although NICE is beset with challenges, its underlying motivation is largely honourable and, although the jury is still out, it may, with time and with the appropriate developments, positively benefit the populations of England and Wales.

Conclusion

With burgeoning health care costs, in part fuelled by innovations in health care technology, and increased scrutiny of decisions regarding health care policies and programmes, many argue that a more comprehensive and accountable approach is needed to help decision makers set priorities and improve benefit from constrained resources. Thus, health economic evaluation has been increasingly considered and, in some cases, employed by governments internationally to try to more effectively regulate the diffusion and utilization of health technologies. However, as discussed throughout this chapter, there are a number of limitations in employing these methods.

For example, deemed 'double jeopardy,' the use of QALYs can place individuals with long-term conditions at a disadvantage in the treatment of life-threatening conditions. Similarly, the elderly and disabled may also be at a disadvantage under a QALY maximization 'regime.' A second issue concerns the notion that patient preferences for access to health care services may supersede QALY maximization. In general, it might be argued that people will trade-off QALYs for the 'security' of having access to interventions—now and in the future—irrespective of whether they will ever need such services. The final issue regarding applied CUA that was presented in this chapter is the lack of consideration of all opportunity costs, which may lead to an inefficient allocation of public resources.

Several of these issues—and, indeed, several others—are echoed in stakeholder perspectives on the use of HTA in Europe. Reflecting a range of disciplinary lenses, stakeholders perceive a number of challenges to economic evaluation when applied in medical decision making. For example, from a sociologist perspective, the provisional, evolving status of determinations of value must be considered in the HTA process. It is the evolving nature of new technology, HTA institutions, and governmental priority-setting concerns that renders international, even national, requirements for and implementation of economic evaluation difficult, if not ineffective. Also captured in

---

[8] The Citizens Council, open to participation of the wider public, assists NICE decision making by offering views from the public on key issues informing the development of guidance, especially regarding social values and judgments in relation to equity and need.

several different viewpoints is the call for greater consideration of the values of a wide range of stakeholders, including patients and the general public. In so doing, HTA would more effectively account for social and ethical considerations (e.g. equity) and patient preferences, as well as result in a more transparent and relevant process. Finally, while HTA has been predominately applied to pharmaceuticals and, increasingly, other health technologies, economic evaluation might be extended to broader, population-based issues, although the nature of public health interventions introduces its additional challenges in employing these methods.

The example of NICE further illustrates the aforementioned concerns and challenges, but also highlights how some of these limitations have been addressed by a national HTA body. For instance, the Institute has updated and evolved its economic evaluation methods and requirements, and makes these guidelines available to stakeholders. Additionally, it has attempted to formally involve patients and the broader public in order to consider social and ethical considerations, alongside cost-effectiveness evidence, in its processes. NICE has also expanded its remit to include public health interventions, and conducts appraisals on other technologies, such as medical devices.

Economic evaluation assumes an increasingly important role in health care priority-setting, particularly with regards to health technologies. While limited by challenges in capturing important issues central to both the clinical and policy decision process, it does offer decision makers a mechanism to more systematically evaluate the costs and benefits of available interventions, with the hope that this may aid them in a more efficient allocation of limited resources. However, the assumptions and methods employed in economic evaluation should be continuously challenged and improved so as to better meet these aims.

References

Appleby J, Devlin N, Parkin D (2007). NICE's cost-effectiveness threshold. How high should it be? *British Medical Journal*, 2007; **335**, 358–9.

Audit Commission. *Managing the financial implications of NICE guidance*. London, Audit Commission.

Birch S, Gafni A (1992). Cost-effectiveness/utility analyses. Do current decision rules lead us to where we want to be? *Journal of Health Economics*, **11**, 279–96.

Birch S, Gafni A (2007). Economists' dream or nightmare? Maximizing health gains from available resources using the NICE guidelines. *Health Economics, Policy and Law*, **2**, 193–202.

Chantler A (2004). Health technology assessment: a clinical perspective. *International Journal of Technology Assessment in Health Care*, **20**, 87–91.

Chinitz D (2004). Health technology assessment in four countries: response from political science. *International Journal of Technology Assessment in Health Care*, **20**, 55–60.

Coast J (2004). Is economic evaluation in touch with society's health values? *British Medical Journal*, **329**, 1233–6.

Coulter A (2004). Perspectives on health technology assessment: response from the patient's perspective. *International Journal of Technology Assessment in Health Care*, **20**, 92–6.

Culyer AJ (2006). NICE's use of cost-effectiveness as an exemplar of a deliberative process. *Health Economics, Policy and Law*, **1**, 299–318.

Drummond M (2007). NICE: a nightmare worth having? *Health Economics, Policy and Law*, **2**, 203–8.

Freemantle N (2004). Commentary: is NICE delivering the goods? *British Medical Journal*, **329**, 1003–4.

Harris J (1987). QALYfying the value of life. *Journal of Medical Ethics*, **13**, 117–23.

Heath I (2004). View of health technology assessment from the swampy lowlands of general practice. *International Journal of Technology Assessment in Health Care*, **20**, 81–6.

Holland W (2004). Health technology assessment and public health: a commentary. *International Journal of Technology Assessment in Health Care*, **20**, 77–80.

Johannesson M (2001). Should we aggregate relative or absolute changes in QALYs? *Health Economics*, **10**, 573–7.

Linden L. Vondeling H, Parker C, Cook A (2007). Does the National Institute of Health and Clinical Excellence only appraise new pharmaceuticals? *International Journal of Technology Assessment in Health Care*, **23**, 349–53.

Lothgren M, Ratcliffe M (2004). Pharmaceutical industry's perspective on health technology assessment. *International Journal of Technology Assessment in Health Care*, **20**, 97–101.

Nord E (2001). The desirability of a condition versus the well being and worth of a person. *Health Economics*, **10**, 579–81.

Nord E, Pinto JL, Richardson J, Menzel P, Ubel P (1999). Incorporating societal concerns for fairness in numerical valuations of health programmes. *Health Economics*, **8**, 25–39.

Oliver A (2004). Prioritising health care: is 'health' always an appropriate maximand? *Medical Decision-making*, **24**, 272–80.

Oliver A (2006). Review of Layard R. Happiness: lessons from a new science. *Economics and Philosophy*, **22**, 299–307.

Sheldon TA, Cullum N, Dawson D, Lankshear A, Lowson K, Watt I, West P, Wright D, Wright J (2004). What's the evidence that NICE guidance has been implemented? Results from a national evaluation using time series analysis, audit of patients' notes, and interviews. *British Medical Journal*, **329**, 999–1003.

Stevens A, Milne R (2004). Health technology assessment in England and Wales. *International Journal of Technology Assessment in Health Care*, **20**, 11–24.

Sunstein CR (2005). *Laws of fear: beyond the precautionary principle*. New York, Cambridge University Press.

ten Have H (2004). Ethical perspectives in health technology assessment. *International Journal of Technology Assessment in Health Care*, **20**, 71–6.

Wanless D (2002). *Securing our future health: taking a long-term view*, final report. London, HM Treasury.

Webster A (2004). Health technology assessment: a sociological commentary on reflexive innovation. *International Journal of Technology Assessment in Health Care*, **20**, 61–6.

Williams A (1997). Intergenerational equity: an exploration of the 'fair innings' argument. *Health Economics*, **6**, 117–32.

Williams A (2001). The 'fair innings argument' deserves a fairer hearing! Comments by Alan Williams on Nord and Johannesson. *Health Economics*, **10**, 583–5.

Williams A (2004). *What could be nicer than NICE?* London, Office of Health Economics.

Williams I, Bryan S, McIver S (2007). How should cost-effectiveness analysis be used in health technology coverage decisions? Evidence from the National Institute for Health and Clinical Excellence approach. *Journal of Health Services Research and Policy*, **12**, 73–9.

Part 5

Incentives, mechanisms, and processes

Chapter 14

Intellectual property rights and pharmaceutical development

Joan Rovira

Introduction

Innovation is usually considered one of the main factors of economic development and of increasing societal well-being. However, there are fewer consensuses on what constitutes innovation, and on the appropriate incentive mechanisms required to attain the optimal rate and types of innovation. These general statements apply to the specific areas of pharmaceuticals and biomedicine. Economic analysis identifies innovation by its capacity to generate income and profits, which is assumed to derive from the consumer's willingness to pay for the innovation. However, health goods are characterised by information asymmetry, consumer ignorance, and moral hazard derived from third party financing. It is therefore questionable that the market provides an appropriate valuation mechanism of innovation.

Of course, the discussion of what type of health innovation is or should society be trying to attain is an important policy issue in itself. This debate is about societal priorities and values, and economic analysis has no specific legitimate role in assigning values and priorities. However, innovation is a value laden concept, which is often used without a clear specification of its intended meaning, for instance, in comparing the effectiveness and efficiency of alternative mechanisms to promote innovation. Without an explicit definition of what is meant by innovation, the analysis and debate on the efficiency of instruments to promote it is likely to become a debate on values, rather than on empirical evidence.

The purpose of this chapter is to clarify the concept of pharmaceutical innovation, how it is related to well-being and other social goals, and what the best way to promote it is.

The first section of the paper addresses the various interpretation of the term 'innovation', especially in the field of medicines and health services in general, and how they differ across different actors, such as innovators, patent offices, and pricing and reimbursement agencies. The second section highlights the public good characteristics of pharmaceutical innovation and how economic systems have addressed this market failure; it outlines the characteristics of intellectual property systems in pharmaceuticals, and the arguments for and against them. The third section addresses the problems of IP (intellectual property) systems in an increasingly globalized world and the negative effects of IP harmonisation for access to medicines in developing countries. The fourth section outlines some of the alternative options that have been advocated to reform, complement or substitute the present IP systems. The chapter ends with a review of the main findings and some concluding policy implications.

Conceptualizing and assessing innovation in the pharmaceutical field

Innovation is not easy to define. Some existing definitions include:

- The act of introducing something new.
- Something newly introduced.
- A new idea, method or device.
- The successful exploitation of new ideas.
- Change that creates a new dimension of performance.
- The process of making improvements by introducing something new.

Moreover, many types of innovation can be distinguished: business model, marketing, organisational, process, product, service, supply chain, substantial, financial, incremental, breakthrough, and disruptive or radical innovation, new technological systems, social innovation, etc. In broad terms, an innovation can be understood as the 'successful introduction of something new and useful, for example introducing new methods, techniques, or practices or new or altered products and services.'[1] Such a broad definition is likely to attain widespread consensus, but it also leaves a lot of room for interpretation. A potential conflict lies in whether innovation is identified with commercial success or with added value to society. These two effects can co-exist, but this is not always the case.

Innovation is clearly different from invention. From an economic perspective innovation implies the existence of a value or utility associated to the novelty. Therefore, an invention or a discovery becomes an innovation only when a useful application is given to the finding. It can also be argued that a technological development that does not reach the market at an affordable cost to the target users is not an innovation, because it does not imply an actual, but only a potential improvement. It is apparently obvious, as well, that a new product need not always constitute an innovation, for example 'me-too' pharmaceuticals can be defined as new products, but not necessarily innovations, as long as they do not offer any advantage over existing treatments.

From a public health perspective, the relevant aspect of innovation is its contribution to improving health outcomes and well-being, i.e. whether the new technology is bringing additional benefits for the health and well-being of a population in a given country, irrespective of where it originated and of the revenues it provides to its supplier. However, from an industrial policy perspective, the relevant innovation may be the one carried out in the specific country—preferably by nationally owned companies— as this is what results in increased investment, competitiveness, income, employment,

---

[1] http://en.wikipedia.org/wiki/Innovation

and exports for the country concerned, irrespective of whether or not the innovation implies an actual or potential health gain, or other benefits to the users.

In a perfectly competitive market, innovation can be assumed to simultaneously produce a higher well-being to the consumers and a commercial profit to the innovator, because rational, perfectly informed consumers would only be willing to pay a price higher than that of existing options if a new drug showed an additional net benefit that justified the price difference. However, consumers of medicines are seldom well informed about their needs or about the capacity of existing products to satisfy these needs. Moreover, they often do not directly pay—at least fully—for the drugs they take. In a publicly-funded health system, the payer and the consumer of a medicine are usually not the same person.

Such issues raise the question of who should assess the social value of health technology innovations. Should this value be determined by often uninformed consumers on the basis of their perceptions of the private benefit of the drug? Should it be valued by some collective decision-making process, involving expert review of the evidence, and a mixture of technical and value judgements by health managers? Moreover, the decision to use a medicine is normally taken by a prescriber with no economic responsibility for the decision or even worse, with perverse incentives to prescribe an unnecessarily expensive drug. This situation leads to a potential divergence between the positive commercial effects of an innovation, and its impact on the health and well-being of the consumers. For instance, a new locally developed and produced statin that does not add any efficacy, safety or convenience for the patient over that of existing products would not be a innovation in the first sense of the term, but it might fit to the second one, as long as it is able to gain a certain market share and yield profits to the manufacturer and intellectual property rights (IPR) holder. On the other hand, a new product might be able to produce health gains to a certain population, but might not necessarily have a high commercial value if it targets a neglected disease for which no effective demand exists.

In fact, economic evaluation of health care technologies has acknowledged this situation and has progressively turned to a 'extra-welfarist approach', which quantifies benefits in terms of some measure of health gains, such as Quality Adjusted Life Years (QALYs), rather than market value. When willingness to pay approaches are used for assessing health services, consumers are asked to value health improvements, rather than the health technologies that generate them. This debate can also be seen as a particular case of the more general 'needs versus demand debate' that lies behind many health policy controversies. In fact, some authors usually refer to needs-based or needs orientated innovation, to designate innovation that is aimed at addressing health problems as defined by expert judgment rather than by market demand (Nathan 2007)

In the pharmaceutical field the distinction between product innovation and process innovation is a very relevant one. Process innovation refers to new processes for producing either existing or new products. Process innovations might lead to a reduction of production costs, but can also be economically justified if it allows a producer to bypass existing patented processes. A pharmaceutical product innovation can be defined as any new product or technology entering the market that brings some added value to the existing drug supply. This definition includes different possibilities. It might refer, for instance, to a new drug that is effective in treating a disease for which no treatment was previously available. It can also refer to a new drug that has a higher effectiveness and safety—or a better risk-benefit ratio—than existing drugs in treating a certain condition, or even one that makes the treatment more convenient for the patient, e.g. allowing the patient to take only one instead of three pills per day. Finding a new indication for an existing drug should also be considered a form of innovation.

A particular issue that has also raised a hot debate is the relative merits of break-through versus incremental innovation. Some critics state that the present IP system distorts research and development (R&D) priorities towards the so-called 'me-toos' or follow-on drugs, i.e. products that are similar to some pre-existing product. Focusing on 'me-toos' is a rational private decision because they have lower R&D (research and development) costs and a lower risk of failure relative to new drugs developed for under-served diseases. However, the benefits of 'me-toos' for society are smaller or non-existent compared with those of breakthroughs.

Pharmaceutical innovations are formally assessed at different stages of their life cycle. First, when the innovator applies for a patent, later when it is subject to regulatory authorisation, and finally, when it enters the market and faces demand. The three assessments are usually done independently by different agencies with no or limited coordination.

A patent is assumed to require an innovative step. However, national IP legislations and agreements allow a broad range of interpretations of the concepts of innovation. IP offices usually grant patents to any new chemical entity that produces a certain health benefit, even if it operates according to a similar biological mechanism than other existing drugs and does not lead to improved health outcomes, cost reductions or other benefits to consumers. Some authors state that one of the main problems of the patent system is that the quality of patents has been steadily decreasing, meaning that patents are granted to alleged innovations that do not fully comply with the originally intended requirements of inventiveness and non-obviousness (Jaffe and Lerner 2004). It is also stated that patents are increasingly granted to things outside the traditional scope of patentability.

Drug regulation in most countries establishes high standards of safety and quality on new products seeking marketing authorisation. However, in few cases are new drugs required to show relative efficacy, i.e. that they are more efficacious than existing drugs. In most countries it is enough for new drugs to show that they are either better than placebo or not worse than some existing medicine. As a result, the registration of a new drug does not require nor guarantee any therapeutic innovation or added value.

In the past a market authorisation meant an almost automatic decision to reimburse a new product by health insurers. However, in most countries it has become customary to separate registration or market authorisation from the pricing and reim-bursement decisions that determine the commercial performance of a pharmaceutical product. Whereas market authorisation is based solely on criteria of efficacy, safety, and quality, pricing and reimbursement is often conditioned to the proof of effectiveness, relative effectiveness or value for money (cost-effectiveness)

Proof of therapeutic or economic added value is, however, requested in some countries at the time of pricing and reimbursement decisions. There is an increasing use of economic evaluation techniques in assessing the cost-effectiveness or efficiency of new drugs in comparison with existing treatments, and using the results as one of the criteria for setting the price and the reimbursement status of a new drug. A new drug is more likely to be publicly financed at a premium price over existing competitors if it is able to show some added value in terms of health or economic outcomes.

How does society pay for innovation? IPR in pharmaceutical development

Innovation is essentially knowledge and information, and hence normally has the characteristics of a 'public good'. Public goods are one of the forms of market failure that lead to a likely production of the good at a socially sub-optimal level in a competitive market, unless appropriate mechanisms, such as public financing, are established. Of course, some individuals and companies might devote resources to R&D and innovation motivated by curiosity, prestige, or altruism. However, it is obvious that few private investors would be prepared to invest the large amounts of money required to bring new medicines into the market if they could not expect to have an adequate chance of recovering the investment made and obtaining an appropriate profit because they faced competition from companies that could copy their products without having incurred in the corresponding R&D cost and were therefore able to supply the products at a much lower price. In order to address this market failure, society can pay for pharmaceutical innovation in several, non-exclusive ways:

- ◆ Direct public and non-profit financing of biomedical and pharmaceutical R&D. This includes R&D carried out in public and academic institutions as well as the grants, subsidies, contracts and tax deductions accorded to commercial firms for private R&D.

- ◆ Granting market exclusivity to innovations, thus allowing the IPR holder a higher price than it would obtain in a competitive market.

- ◆ Public financing of innovative products under exclusivity.

- ◆ Directly paying for innovations, for instance, in the form of prizes.

The four mechanisms are not mutually exclusive, but they can operate simultaneously and complement each other. The share of public and non-profit financing of medical and pharmaceutical R&D is similar to that of private financing [World Health Organisation (WHO) 2004]. However, private investment seems to have a dominant role in relation to public funding in the overall establishment of R&D priorities, while prizes have been only rarely used in that field. Public financing of pharmaceuticals is, for most products, the main mechanism for recovering R&D costs. Public financing amounts to between approximately 80 per cent of pharmaceutical expenditure in developed countries to 20 per cent or less in low income countries.

It is important to note that, although innovation is the expected outcome of a R&D process, the success of R&D activities is, by its very nature, an uncertain one. Therefore, any system aimed at promoting innovation has to accept and somehow cover the cost of failures.

In the case of public financing the potential innovator usually does not bear any financial risk, as it gets the resources *ex ante*, and the reward is usually not conditioned to a positive outcome of the R&D activity. The financial risk of a lack of success is born by the financing organisation (ultimately, by tax payers and donors).[2] The innovators might still have an indirect incentive to attain valuable results, such as academic prestige or because future funding is likely to depend on past R&D performance. With this modality of financing it is obvious that society will pay for both successful and unsuccessful R&D activities, as only a proportion of the R&D projects funded will attain success.

The private and public purchase of medicines under exclusivity at higher-than-competitive prices is an indirect, ex post form of financing R&D. In this particular case, successful innovators must get a sufficiently high reward to recover prior R&D costs of both successful and unsuccessful R&D activities, by charging higher prices than under competition and, hence, obtaining an extraordinary profit on successful products. This approach means that society has to pay for all R&D through the higher prices of successful innovations, while the products concerned are under exclusivity or enjoy some form of market power. Although public financing of pharmaceuticals is primarily motivated by a concern for equity and solidarity, it obviously becomes an additional incentive to innovation, as long as it increases the demand for on-patent products.

Finally, prizes imply a direct monetary reward for successful innovations. Once the innovator is rewarded for its effort, the innovation can be put into the public domain, or made available at a given royalty to any potential manufacturer under competitive conditions. As in previous cases, the size of the prizes must take into account a certain rate of failures of R&D projects.

The distinctions between the mechanisms outlined is not always as clear as the previous descriptions might suggest and real mechanisms might contain a mix of the former pure mechanisms. The IPR system can be conceptualized as a prize system where the prize is a monopoly or exclusivity right, instead of a monetary reward. On the other hand, price and reimbursement policies might counteract the market power of the IP holder, and turn the IPR system into something close to a prize system.

The available mechanisms for promoting innovation should be considered in relation to social goals and priorities, for instance, on the type of technologies and disease areas they are expected to address, or on the balance between innovation, access, and other social goals. A very relevant distinction is the one popularized by the WHO Commission on Macroeconomics and Health, as types 1, 2, and 3 diseases, which refer to whether a disease affects both developed and developing countries (type 1),

---

[2] Of course, public financing of private R&D might not cover the full amount of the investment, and hence the private investor bears part of the risk.

mainly developing countries (type 2), or predominantly or exclusively developing countries (type 3; WHO 2001). The IPR system is likely to produce sufficient R&D for type 1 diseases, although problems of access might arise in developing countries, especially while the products are under exclusivity. However, for type 2 and especially type 3 diseases, the main problem is that the IPR system is likely to generate an insufficient level of R&D.

The debate on the role of IPR as a tool to promote innovation is not new; on the contrary, it is as old as patents, which according to some experts first appeared in the legislation of the Republic of Venice in 1474, where for the first time royal privileges were associated with innovation. In England, exclusivity rights became associated to innovation only several centuries later. Kings often granted exclusive market right for things already invented, such as salt, vinegar or playing cards, in order to favour friends and supporters. The requisite of innovation was only introduced in 1603, as a result of the opposition of public opinion and parliament to such practices. In 1871 the Dutch General States debated the advantages and disadvantages of patents. Critics argued that patent evaluators devoted insufficient time to assessing the validity of the applications and often granted patents to already existing technologies, placing well established business at risk of unfounded litigation. From more radical positions, it was argued that patents offered real innovators a small advantage, and were harmful or even totally useless for the public. As a result of this debate, the patent system established in 1817 was abolished and was not reintroduced until 1910 (Jaffe and Lerner 2004).

In a schematic way three basic positions can be distinguished in the debate on IPR and incentives to innovation:

- *Maintaining the status quo.* It supports high IP standards. This means reinforcement of the present IPR system by making it universal, increasing the length of exclusivity periods, broadening the spectrum of patentability, introducing new rights, such as test data protection, etc. It also favours no regulation (mainly, no price control) of the market of innovative products, i.e. allowing temporary extraordinary profits for these products. Regarding access it is usually claimed that there is no clear link between high IP standards and access.

- *Reforming to the present system.* This would support the broad use of flexibilities and safeguards in IPR systems, and complementary policies, such as competition policies, selective financing, and price regulation, to reduce the negative effects of high IP standards on access. It is basically concerned by access-related problems, especially in developing countries (DCs). Another set of reformers point to the decreasing quality of patents, which leads to uncertainty and unnecessary high litigation costs.

- *Introducing competition-based alternatives to the present IP system.* Supporters propose incentive systems, such as prizes, which are not based on exclusivity rights. While criticising the access impact of high IP standards it also challenges the present system in terms of efficiency in fostering innovation.

Of course, this scheme is a simplification of reality. It is, nevertheless, a useful way of classifying the continuum of actual positions into a simple scheme.

The list of negative effects attributed to IPR by its critics is long. Some of them point to efficiency issues, some to equity issues and others to both simultaneously.

The efficiency dimension refers to whether the market can make a better allocation of R&D resources than a regulator, for instance, a committee of experts. Consumers might show a high willingness to pay for products and treatments that might rank low among the preferences of a committee of experts in public health, or have a poor cost-effectiveness ratio, and vice versa. Under an IPR system the demand of the final products is what determines the size of the monetary reward to an innovation. However, it is obvious that in the pharmaceutical market the usual characteristics of the demand make it a dubious tool to reflect the social value of innovations. The demand agents are usually ill-informed on the characteristics of the new products and demand agents do not face the usual budget constrains of the consumer in the theoretical market model. The asymmetry of information and the influence of suppliers on prescribers invalidate the assumption of independence between demand and supply agents that characterizes the theoretical market model.

The equity dimension points to the fact that if R&D priorities are set by the traditional IPR system, little attention will be paid to diseases that mainly affect either poor people or few people, because having exclusivity of a product for which there might be a need, but not an effective market demand is not an economic incentive for private investors. Of course, it is not clear that the establishment of a prize system or other alternative mechanisms to IPR would automatically result in a higher priority to R&D on neglected and rare diseases, because the prize mechanism might still allocate a higher priority to diseases that are likely to enjoy a high demand. On the other hand, a more equitable distribution of R&D could also be attained under the prevailing IPR system if the consumption of medicines by the poor was subsidised, e.g. by the establishment of a universal publicly-funded health system. Advanced purchasing commitments by donors has been also proposed as a way to increase the potential final demand of products for neglected diseases, which could provide an adequate incentive for R&D on diseases with an insufficient private demand.

The following section identifies and briefly discusses a number of the criticisms. Given that no one seems to support the position that innovation is not valuable to society or that it should be simply left to the market forces, criticisms of the present system should be made in relative terms, that is, comparing the performance of IPR with other available mechanisms for promoting innovation, for instance, contracts, prizes, etc. This is not an easy task, because it is hardly imaginable to conduct any form of comparative experiment or to derive conclusive results from actual experiences. The use of prizes and contracts, moreover, is rather limited, and the purposes and conditions under which they have been used make comparisons with the IPR system difficult. It must, therefore, be recognised that the arguments either for or against IPR and other mechanisms to induce innovation are largely theoretical and speculative.

Excessive market power

IPR grants the right holder a temporary exclusivity right to the innovation. This leads the markets away from the theoretical perfect competition model. If there are no close substitutes, the innovation will enjoy a pure monopoly. If there are other drugs or treatments for the same condition, the market will take the form of an oligopoly or of monopolistic competition, with product differentiation that might reflect both actual differences and the effects of advertising. In all these situations IPR are most likely to increase the price of the medicines above that of competitive equilibrium, thus out-pricing the consumers with lower ability (or willingness) to pay. This leads to the so-called deadweight loss of consumers' well-being. A prize system could theoretically bring prices close to the marginal cost of production, thus allowing a larger consumption and consequently eliminating or reducing the deadweight loss. However, it is not clear what amount of funds would be required by a prize system to produce an amount of innovation equivalent to what the IPR system would induce.

The higher prices associated with exclusivity rights have both efficiency and equity effects. The efficiency effect is the reduction of total consumption of the drug. In publicly funded systems with an open budget, higher prices might not lead to reduced utilisation, but to a higher expenditure for the same level of utilisation. The impact on equity will appear in settings where the consumer has to pay for the drugs, because the negative effects will be larger for population groups of lower income levels, both in developing and in developed countries

Excessive focus on 'me-toos'

'Me-toos', also known as similar or follow-on drugs, are products that have a similar chemical structure to an originator and also similar therapeutic effects. The differences (e.g. in efficacy or side effects) can affect all consumers or only some of them. It is often stated that IPR tend to induce too much R&D on 'me-toos' because there is less risk in this type of incremental, small step innovation, than aiming at breakthroughs or trying to innovate in areas where there are no satisfactory therapies available or no therapies at all. For instance, it is probably easier and requires a lower R&D investment to find a new lipid modulator than to find a cure for Parkinson disease. However, industry representatives claim that pharmaceutical innovation is usually incremental; meaning that progress is made by small steps on previous advances. Of course, there is nothing wrong with incremental innovations per se. The inefficiencies might arise from the possible divergence between social and private benefits, leading to a too high R&D investment in trying to develop 'me-toos' at the expense of less R&D aimed at more innovative goals. For instance, Morgan et al. (2005) found that between 1996 and 2003 the cost of prescription drugs per person doubled (from $141 to $316) in Canada.

The Patented Medicines Pricing Review Board's (PMPRB) classified 68 (5.9 per cent) of the new products as 'breakthroughs'. The authors increased this figure to 142, (12.4 per cent), including all forms and new drugs of the same subgroup. For the remaining 1005 new products, the PMPRB did not find any evidence of therapeutic advantage over existing treatments and were classified as me-toos. Expenditure on 'breakthroughs' rose from 6 per cent in 1996 to 10 per cent in 2003, accounting for less than 15 per cent of expenditure increase between 1996 and 2003. The share of generics (INN and branded) came down from half to one third of the total expenditure.

The result was that the share of 'me-toos' increased from 41 per cent in 1996 to almost two thirds in 2003, accounting for about 80 per cent of the increase in expenditure, which seems a high price for society to pay for the social benefit added by these drugs.

It is however argued that usually innovators do not make a choice between breakthrough and follow-on innovation. In this view, innovation in similar products does not proceed sequentially—meaning that when an originator has been successfully marketed other companies try to replicate it—but as a race, where several innovators are simultaneously pursuing similar objectives to address a health problem; the one that succeeds in entering the market first, becomes the 'originator,' while the rest appear as follow-ons. In that view, there is no way of effectively discouraging me-toos without reducing overall incentives for innovation. Moreover, it is stated that drugs appearing after the first drug enters the market are often better that the first one, for all or for at least a subset of patients (Wertheimer *et al.* 2001).

Inducement of socially useless or questionable activities to expand demand

IPR provides an incentive for right holders (and sometimes, competitors, as well) not only to innovate, but it also allows them to spend the extraordinary profits on activities of questionable social value, such as advertising, lobbying and capturing regulators, influencing prescribers, patients, and other stakeholders, as well as academics and public opinion, and in rent-seeking in general. IPR give rights holders an incentive to promote the consumption of the innovation beyond clinically justified or efficient utilisation, as profits grow proportionally to the number of units sold. However, there are examples of innovation that society would highly value, but which widespread use is not desirable, such as new antibiotics to be used in case of resistance to existing ones. Reserve antibiotics should be available, but used only in cases where all others have failed. A generalised use of a reserve antibiotic would quickly generate resistant strains, thus reducing its usefulness. Gagnon and Lexchin (2008), on the basis of the systematic collection of data directly from the industry and doctors during 2004, estimated that the US pharmaceutical industry spent on promotion 24.4 per cent of its US$235.4 billion US domestic sales, versus 13.4 per cent for research and development.

It is argued that in the absence of exclusivity rights, the profitability of advertising and other questionable activities would be lower and companies would be more inclined to focus expenditure on R&D.

Low priority to R&D on neglected and rare diseases

It has also been argued that IPR only provide an incentive to innovate in products that are expected to have a market demand. They are therefore not effective in inducing enough research in neglected and rare diseases. Contracts, grants and prized would be an alternative to IPR for this purpose, as they allow the funding agency to set the type of diseases and technologies that will be rewarded.

Incentives to counterfeiting

Although supporters of high IP standards often associate generics with counterfeits, it is rather the opposite, namely that the high price of drugs makes them a preferred target for counterfeiting as it allows higher profits that compensate the risk of the illegal activity.

IPR and development

A clear definition of property rights is generally accepted to be a requisite for economic development and this principle is likely to hold in the case of intellectual property. But this does not imply that higher IPR standards are necessarily beneficial for development. The supporters of high IPR standards claim that they are beneficial not only for developed countries, but also for developing countries. The arguments are that developing countries that adopt high IPR standards will have more domestic and foreign investment in R&D and technology transfer than if they opt for a low protection of IP. High IP standards in developing countries should also raise the interest of innovators in diseases that mainly affect poor countries. These arguments have are not supported by convincing empirical evidence and an increasing number of experts tend to accept that the optimal strength of the IP system depends on the level of economic and industrial development of the country concerned (The World Bank 2002). Therefore, the present trends towards an upward harmonisation of IPR standards, as required by the TRIPS and by some bilateral trade agreements, is more likely to benefit developed countries than developing countries [Commission on Intellectual Property Rights (CIPR) 2002].

Compelling evidence on the effects of IPR changes on development is scarce. In order to assess causality between IP and innovation or development one would ideally want evidence from experimental or quasi-experimental designs. This type of evidence is difficult to obtain for economic and social phenomena. Most alleged evidence on the impact of stronger IPR standards on innovation and economic development is nothing else than statistical association based on cross-sectional data that does not allow to unambiguously state the sense of causation: do high IP standards provide incentives for R&D and innovation or, on the contrary, do countries with innovative capacity and IP assets rise IP standards in order to protect the national industry and increase the value of its assets? Mascus (2002) acknowledges these limitations, while providing one of best examples of that relationship. His analysis suggests that the relationship is not linear, but U-shaped. This could mean that countries with a very low level of development do not significantly benefit from low IP standards. Only when countries attain a minimum level of development might they be able to take advantage of low IP standards in order to support an emerging national industry. Beyond a certain level of income, IP strength and development show a positive association.

An alternative approach is to model a counterfactual. Scherer and Weinburst (1995) used this approach to assess the impact of the introduction of pharmaceutical product patent in Italy. The results suggested a negligible or non-existent impact on the innovative capacity of the Italian industry.

Negative impact of IPR on the rate of innovation

One of the most paradoxical negative effects attributed to the IPR system is that it reduces the dissemination and access of the overall research community to research results, as a result slowing the global process of innovation. Innovation is an inherently cumulative process, therefore, IPR on key discoveries are likely to increase the costs of R&D for researchers that could use these discoveries for their own research programmes and reduce the prospects of a future profit as they might not be able to get the benefits of their discoveries, which would also imply a lower incentive for R&D.

High costs of management and litigation of the IPR system

IPR are much more difficult to define and enforce than property rights on tangible assets. IPR do not operate in a spontaneous cost-free way, but require the establishment of a costly bureaucracy both within the companies and in the public sector that manages the recognition and enforcement of PI, and settles the disputes between stakeholders. Moreover, the high prices of new products under IPR systems usually lead countries to set up complex price and reimbursement mechanisms aimed at controlling expenditure that add regulations and administrative costs and distorts the allocation of resources in the pharmaceutical market.

According to Crovitz (2008)

> new empirical research by Boston University law professors James Bessen and Michael Meurer, reported in their book, 'Patent Failure,' found that the value of pharmaceutical patents outweighed the costs of pharmaceutical-patent litigation. But for all other industries combined, they estimate that since the mid-1990s, the cost of U.S. patent litigation to alleged infringers ($12 billion in legal and business costs in 1999) is greater than the global profits that companies earn from patents (less than $4 billion in 1999). Since the 1980s, patent litigation has tripled and the probability that a particular patent is litigated within four years has more than doubled. Small inventors feel the brunt of the uncertainty costs, since bigger companies only pay for rights they think the system will protect.

Of course, all mechanisms used to promote innovation will have management costs; the critics of the IPR system claim, however, that they would be lower.

Bias towards patentable solutions to health problems

If innovation in health technologies is mainly led by IPR, research on non-patentable knowledge and technologies, such as lifestyles, use of off-patent drugs, etc., will receive little attention even if it offers a high potential and a more efficient option for improving health. This leads to an increased drug-based medicalization of health and social problems and to an increasing dependency of the individuals from the health system.

Pharmaceuticals in a global economy

The problems posed by innovation as a public good have become an international issue with the globalization of the pharmaceutical market. Innovation is a global public good and countries with limited or no innovative capacity can benefit from low

IP standards, which allow them to free-ride innovation both as consumers and as non-innovating producers. The response of the multinational innovative companies has been to lobby their governments to establish a global IP system.

In the last decade of the 20th century, following the signature in 1994 of the TRIPS agreement as part of the set of WTO agreements, the debate on IPR has mainly become a North-South issue. Developing countries have been pressured to accept higher IPR standards as a condition to join the WTO, and enjoy lower tariffs and potentially improved access for their products to developed countries' markets. However, developing countries soon came to feel that the benefits of the TRIPS agreement were smaller than promised and the costs, higher. The debate became especially hot in the case of pharmaceuticals, and more specifically, of anti-retrovirals, because patent protection implied high prices that made them unaffordable to low income groups, often the majority of those in need in developing countries. In 1997 the South-African government adopted a TRIPS compliant amendment to its patent law enabling it to produce and import generic medicines. A pool of multinational pharmaceutical firms lodged a complaint against the government, which they withdrew in 2001, partly as the result of an international movement of developing countries and NGOs. The DOHA declaration of 2003, by stating the pre-eminence of public health goals over commercial interests, seemed to reinforce the position of the pro-access lobby (Centrale Sanitaire Suisse Romande 2006).

However, the confrontations are not over. IPR has been debated in the context of many bi-lateral trade agreements negotiated between developed countries, such as the USA and the EU, and developing countries. Developed countries are trying to incorporate in the trade agreements IPR provisions that strengthen the IPR protection beyond TRIPS standards, the so-called TRIPS-plus provisions. As recently as in 2006–2007, new conflicts appeared (Novartis versus India, Abbott versus Thailand, and MSD versus Brazil) that brought face to face multinational pharmaceutical companies with developing/emerging countries on pharmaceutical IPR issues (Rovira 2007).

Big pharmaceutical companies and their supporting governments claim (e.g. Abbott versus Thailand) that compulsory licensing, an accepted safeguard foreseen in TRIPS, is only aimed at exceptional situations. They similarly claim that the EU and other countries applying forms of market regulation are free-riding US and not making a fair contribution to pharmaceutical R&D costs. They therefore lobby for the removal or weakening of price control mechanisms (like in the US-Australia trade agreement). The debate on IPR and developing countries has been brought to international fora, such as WIPO's development agenda, and the CIPIH and IGWG initiatives, supported by WHO.

The position of big pharma is that high IPR standards in all countries is the only way to guarantee that private R&D and, hence, innovation will continue in the future. Access has to be achieved by increasing the resources allocated by countries to health and by increasing donations from the richer to the poorer countries. They claim that the industry is already doing its part with donation programmes and voluntary differential pricing. The pro-access lobby claims that, although this approach provides a certain partial relief to some population groups, it is not a global appropriate solution. Some of the proposals made with the objective of improving access in developing countries are described in the next section.

Alternatives to the present IPR system

In the second section of this paper three basic positions to promoting innovation and access were identified, which were labelled as (1) maintaining the status quo, those that claim that the system is fine or, even that the present traits should be generalised and reinforced; (2) reforming the present system, which includes proponents of changes and safeguards to the present systems; and (3) introducing new competition-based options, those that propose different arrangements either as an alternative or a complement of the present system.

The first group claims that the present IP system is the only mechanism that can ensure the continuity of the flow of pharmaceutical innovations in the future. They are therefore for higher standards—enlarging exclusivity times and the subject matter of patentability, introducing new IP rights, such as test data protection—and against any policies that might balance or weaken them, such as price controls and compulsory licences.

Within the second group, there are many proposals aiming at improving the performance of IPR, while maintaining its basic traits. These include improving the quality of patents, improving the demand price sensitiveness to added value of innovation, removing (some of) the negative effects of exclusivity, limiting IPR rights in the cases of public financing of the R&D process of a certain innovation (e.g. sharing royalties with a public research fund), and the like.

Improving the quality of patents

It is often argued that the quality of patents and other IPR can and should be improved, and that this does not necessarily mean strengthening IP standards in the usual sense of the term. Quality is associated to patents that protect actual innovations, but not spurious ones. Patent quality might be improved by setting higher requirements of novelty and non-obviousness, and by improving the examination process, for instance, by allowing prior opposition. Improving patent quality would reduce litigation and uncertainty to all stakeholders.

Setting stricter criteria for novelty and non-obviousness is, nevertheless, a contentious issue, and some argue that the result might be a removal of rewards for me-too (follow-on) drugs, which would ultimately increase the risk of failure and, hence, increase the costs of pharmaceutical innovation, which often is of an incremental nature.

Rewarding innovation according to therapeutic added value

Regulators and purchasers could use their cohesive and monopolistic powers to adjust the reward of new patent-protected products according to the therapeutic added value. This implies defining pharmaceutical innovation as 'improved effectiveness or safety over best available technology for a give use'. On one hand, drugs that are likely to make a substantial contribution are given priority in the registration process, which amounts to enlarging the effective duration of patent protection. Moreover, drugs that are considered truly innovative are often excluded from reference price systems, which would drive the price close to that of therapeutically equivalent drugs. However, the most sophisticated approach to rewarding actual innovation is the use of economic evaluation to inform pricing and reimbursement decisions.

Generic policies

Generic policies are often advocated as an alternative to IPR, but in a country with a well established, TRIPS compliant, IP system for pharmaceuticals, generic policies should be rather seen as a component of the IP system, a mechanism to balance the interests of innovators and society, by promoting competition once IP protection has expired and avoiding exclusivity to extend beyond expiration dates.

Improving transparency

Increasing the validity and transparency of information on efficacy and safety of medicines, is a condition for allowing regulators and users to assess the existence and magnitude of the therapeutic added-value of a new drug. It has been customary in the past that companies do not report all the clinical trials of a given product, but predominantly those that give favourable results for the new product. Moreover, the information of the published trials is not always sufficient for third parties to assess the efficacy and safety of the drugs. Part of the research is only disclosed to the regulatory agencies, but not to the scientific community and to the public. There is an increasing demand for innovators to fully disclose the results of the clinical research. It does not seem to be a compelling argument for keeping this type of information confidential once the product has obtained marketing authorisation. Ideally, all clinical trials should have been registered before start at a public domain register and the results (positive and negative) should be publicised in such a way that they can be checked, validated, and reproduced by third parties. Some authors (Baker 2007) argue that, in order to attain that level of transparency, clinical trials should be planned and financed by the public sector, and carried out by entities independent of the industry. In general, information on drugs, medical education, and guideline setting should be done by independent agents, with no control from the manufacturer. Transparency should also be promoted in other domains, such as prices, patent status, and on the decisions taken by patent offices and regulatory agencies.

Improving the demand price sensitiveness to added value of innovation

Prescribers and patients should have easy and free access to comparative information of the available treatments (both pharmaceutical and non-pharmaceutical) for a given condition, especially to effectiveness, price, and impact on total costs, and they should have economic incentives for cost-effective prescribing. In the case of consumers, cost-sharing mechanisms that limit total consumer payments in a period and relate that limit to the consumer income might make the consumer more cost-conscious, with minimal adverse effects on equity.

The more radical alternatives to the present IPR system challenge the outcomes of the present system, for instance, the orientation towards demand, i.e. towards diseases and problems for which there is a capacity and willingness to pay by either the private or the public sector. They assume market and regulatory failures in the present system and favour a needs-based approach; proposals range from substantial changes in the characteristics of present IPR—basically in the definition of the IP holder rights and in the meaning of exclusivity—to totally different types of incentives for innovation, such as prizes, and in the way pharmaceutical R&D is financed. Some of these proposals include setting the duration of the patent in relation to the added value of the innovation, granting a reward without exclusivity rights, i.e. with fixed (tiered) royalties, restricting the rights of the patent holder when the research of a new product has been funded by public institutions, open access research (as in the Human Genome project), etc. Nathan (2007) makes a useful review of recent proposals and pilot initiatives regarding needs-based pharmaceutical innovation.

Recent proposals point to the convenience to set up incentives to innovation, such as prizes, that do not lead to the monopolization of the markets. This approach is usually referred to as the separation of the innovation and the products markets (Weisbrod 2003). The rationale behind that approaches that research-based pharmaceutical companies carry out two separate activities: R&D and manufacturing. Under an IPR system there is, however, only one form of rewarding the two activities—the sale of the final products. A prize system allows the separate rewarding of the two activities and avoids the problems associated with the monopolization of the product market, thus avoiding the deadweight loss of the monopoly.

Stiglitz (2006), in a recent article, also advocates the use of prizes instead of IPR to promote pharmaceutical innovation. While acknowledging that innovation is at the heart of the success of a modern economy, he raises the question of how best to promote it, pointing at the negative effects of IPR and claiming that 'TRIPS imposed a system that was not optimally designed for an advanced industrial country, but was even more poorly suited to a poor country'. He proposes a prize fund paid for by industrialised nations that 'would provide large prizes for cures and vaccines for diseases such as AIDS and malaria that affect millions of people'. In his opinion this would provide appropriate incentives for research without the inefficiencies associated with monopolization.

Prize systems, nevertheless, face several challenges, such as determining the appropriate size of the budget and the reward to be given to each innovation. They require the design of explicit mechanisms to define what will be considered an innovation and what amount will to be paid to each innovation. It must set up clear and credible rules to obtain the prizes.

There are many options in designing a prize (Hubbard and Love 2007). They can be linked to a precise objective (a malaria vaccine of a given minimum effectiveness) or to a generic one, such as reducing mortality or improving health as measured by QALY. The prize can consist of a single payment or of a sequence of payments. The second option allows a more precise match between the prize and the reward, as the benefits of an innovation are not fully understood until it has been in the market for several years. The prize can be of the type 'one winner gets the whole prize' or it might be shared among several applicants submitting similar or different innovations. They can be a one-event model or a permanent, regular system (e.g. prizes awarded each year to the more cost-effective innovations). Under the second option the government (or a donor) sets up a annual fund for rewarding innovation in health, generally. Any innovator that has marketed a new product can apply. Each innovation is allocated an individual score (e.g. based on cost-effectiveness criteria) and will receive a reward from the fund over a number of years. The points accumulated by the innovation in a given year are the cost-effectiveness score times the number of treatments consumed in the year. The annual fund is distributed among innovators according to the points (scores) accumulated during the year by the products introduced in the current or in the previous X years. Such a fund turns out to be a fixed prospective budget for innovation.

Concrete proposals of the creation of a fund for pharmaceutical research where the prizes are determined with the help of economic evaluation analyses has been proposed by Hollis (2004), and by Hollis and Pogge (2008).

In order to make the introduction of a prize system more politically acceptable, some proposals suggest that it should be only applied to neglected diseases and other areas where the present system is not just inefficient, but ineffective. Another option is to make the fund a voluntary option, but not compatible with a patent. Innovators should go for one or the other system. Finally, prizes can be used as a complement of IPR or other mechanisms for inducing innovation (National Research Council 2007)

Most of the previous proposals are applicable to both developed and developing countries, but some proposals are specific to developing countries. For instance, in one of the earlier proposals to reducing the negative effects of IP globalization on developing countries, Lanjouw (2001) proposed that developed countries should modify its IP legislation, making the innovator choose between patenting either in developed or in developing countries, but not in both. Innovators are supposed to patent drugs in developed countries for which there is a market, which would allow these products to be available as generics in developing countries. However, this approach would not provide any additional incentive to R&D over the present system in diseases that mainly affect developing countries. Moreover, this approach should be voluntarily implemented by developed countries and there is no reason to believe that they would be willing to do so.

Hubbard and Love (2004) advocate a more radical proposal: a medical R&D treaty that would require countries to make a contribution proportional to its GNP or to a similar indicator of economic capacity. Countries would be allowed to choose how to fulfil their financial obligation. Some countries might choose to maintain the present IP system, while other might prefer to remove IPR on pharmaceuticals and directly invest its contribution in R&D programmes, whose results would be freely accessible to all countries in the treaty. The proposal does not require the existence of a central fund, but only the establishment of a system for monitoring and checking the compliance of countries with their obligations. The positive features of this proposal are that it would avoid free-riding on other countries R&D, and that the distribution of the contributions and benefits would be more equitable. Prices would come down and accessibility would improve in poorer countries as they could obtain all drugs at generic competition prices. Moreover, low income countries could invest their contributions in disease areas that mostly or exclusively affect them. The treaty would be only a long-term solution; in the short-term countries should rely on a broad policy of compulsory licenses and generic competition for existing on-patent drugs.

Conclusions

This chapter reviewed the debate on the existing and proposed methods of incentivizing innovation in pharmaceuticals. It offers a set of reflections that attempt to explore potential options to improving the efficiency of policies to induce pharmaceutical innovation. It is argued that that the main problem in incentivizing innovation lies in the growing perception that the present IP system is not working efficiently as an incentive to pharmaceutical innovation for developed countries and that it is still more detrimental to the needs of developing countries. The system is very costly and its focus is partly misplaced

The IP system is often interpreted as an implicit social contract between the innovator and society. The innovator invests resources and takes risks that might yield benefits to society and is rewarded with exclusivity/property rights on the innovation. However, some discussion is probably required in order to clarify and, perhaps, redefine this social contract. For instance, should the exclusivity right be understood as an unrestricted monopoly or just as a tool to avoid competitors unfairly free-riding the innovators' efforts, thus destroying the incentive to innovate? Would other forms of reward besides exclusivity rights—such as money prizes or patents with fixed royalties—not provide a sufficient incentive for potential innovators, while avoiding some of their negative effects?

There is often stated that higher IP standards favour innovation, even if at the expense of access. However, there is increasing evidence that this is not always so, especially when higher standards are interpreted as extending the spectrum of patentability, reducing the requirement of non-obviousness, or giving more advantages to rights holders. These options might, in fact, discourage actual innovation. An increase in the volume of patents granted might not be a reflection of more innovation, but of a sign of private appropriation of public knowledge. Inappropriate granting of IPR amounts to a theft to society's public domain.

Some countries are trying to address the effects of the IP system on pharmaceutical expenditure by means of the regulation of the drug market with pricing and reimbursement policies aimed at minimising the financial impact of IPR while trying to preserve the incentives for innovation. However, high IP standards, irrespective of their effects on innovation, also increase the market and negotiating power of innovators in front of price regulators, because the former are able to withhold or substantially delay the marketing of new, patent protected products. In the absence of patent protection not reaching a price agreement with national regulators often meant that domestic generic manufacturers might launch generic competitors at lower prices. There are also some experiences and proposals aimed at making the best possible use of the flexibilities and safeguards of the present system, e.g. improving the quality of patents, making widespread use of compulsory licenses, and so on.

Finally, there are proposals aimed at establishing new mechanisms to promote innovation that complement or substitute the present system. The focus of the debate lies in determining the role of the market versus other mechanisms of resource allocation in reimbursing IPR. Particularly, to what extent should needs and priorities in medical R&D be implicitly defined by the market or by alternative mechanisms, such as experts' committees? There are probably good arguments for and against the two options. Any form of retribution of the innovation has to determine how much to pay for a given innovation. Under an IPR system, this decision is assumedly left to the market forces. However, in practice, especially in countries with a publicly-financed health system, the price is constrained by a combination of regulatory and selective financing decisions and often is the result of a monopoly-monopsony type of negotiation.

As long as price setting and priorization has to be the result of market forces, i.e. of many individual decisions, one would certainly want much more transparency on many issues, especially on the characteristics (efficacy and safety) of the products, because the information on the characteristics of a new product is less than perfect. The supplier does usually have the best information on a given product (e.g. clinical trials), but the agents on the demand side (patients/consumers, prescribers, third party payers) and other stakeholders, such as the regulators, often have only access to a partial and often biased information on the characteristics of the product. Even assuming that consumers have perfect information on the characteristics of a new product; innovations would need to be available at a cost that consumers or insurers were willing to pay. However, in spite of its common sense and appeal, such an approach raises many question marks. How many consumers should be willing to pay for the new product at its market price in order to deserve the name of innovation? Should a single millionaire willing to pay a price unaffordable for the rest of the population make the product qualify as an innovation? There are also the problems of information asymmetry. How well informed on the characteristics of the product should the consumers willing to pay for it be? In the best case, it is usually health professionals (e.g. the prescribing doctors) who know about the characteristics of the product, and they often do not bear any economic responsibility on their decisions to prescribe a certain product.

As innovation is a global public good, a globally acceptable strategy, rather than a national one is required. In the past, each country was able to optimize its own national strategy with little restrictions. Countries with limited innovation capacity usually choose a low level of IPR protection as this is beneficial in terms of access and industrial policy. Countries with a high innovative capacity, pressured by their national industries, claimed that this was taking an unfair free-ride and a theft of intangible assets and lobbied for an upwards global harmonisation of IP standards. The result was the TRIPS Agreement. More recently, these standards are being often raised at the occasion of bilateral agreements. Most emerging and developing countries resent that trend as a new imperialism that hinders its development and threatens public health. What would be desirable is a mechanism ensuring a fair contribution of all countries to the cost of pharmaceutical innovation that is acceptable to all parties.

In designing alternative mechanisms to promote innovation more efficiently, account must be taken of the inherent uncertainty of innovation processes: the failure of a R&D programme does not always mean it was inadequate; society must somehow accept payment for unavoidable failures.

It is unlikely that a single approach is appropriate for efficiently addressing all health innovation needs and the failures of the IP system. Some mechanisms might be best suited to specific innovation areas or objectives, e.g. WHO´s disease types 1, 2, and 3. An efficient strategy is likely to require a mix of mechanisms.

When considering changes in IP policies and in incentives for innovation, it is important to acknowledge that they will not only affect future innovation, but usually also the value of existing assets, such as IP portfolios and investment in on-going R&D processes. If the latter are preserved, proposals for reform are likely to attain less opposition.

Accepting the limited evidence on the characteristics of the optimal mechanisms to promote the socially desirable evidence, it seems wise to recommend the development of research and pilot experiences on alternative approaches to being innovative in promoting innovation.

References

Baker D, Chatani N (2002). Promoting good ideas on drugs: are patents the best way? *The Relative Efficiency of Patent and Public Support for Bio-Medical Research, Center for Economic Policy and Policy Research*, October 11.

Baker D (2004). *Financing drug research: what are the issues?* Center for Economic Policy and Policy Research, September 22.

Centrale Sanitaire Suisse Romade (2006) Intellectual property and access to medicines.

Commission on Intellectual Property Rights (CIPR) (2002). *Integrating intellectual property rights and development policy*. London, September.

Crovitz LG (2008). Patent gridlock suppresses innovation. *Information Age*, July 14, A15. Available at: http://online.wsj.com/article/SB121599469382949593.html?mod=todays_ columnists

DiMasi JA, Hansen RW, Grabowski HG. (2003). The price of innovation: new estimates of drug development costs. *Journal of Health Economics*, **22**, 151–85.

Gagnon MA, Lexchin J (2008). The cost of pushing pills: a new estimate of pharmaceutical promotion expenditures in the United States. *PLoS Medicine* January 3.

Hollis A (2004). An efficient reward system for pharmaceutical innovation. Available at: http://www.econ.ucalgary.ca/hollis.

Hollis A and Pogge T (2008). *The Health Impact Fund: making new medicines accessible for all*, Incentives for Global Health. Available at: http://www.healthimpactfund.org

Hubbard T and Love J (2004). A new trade framework for global healthcare R&D. *PLoS Biology*, **2**, 147–50.

Hubbard T and Love J (2007) *The big Idea: prizes to stimulate R&D for new medicines*, KEI Research Paper, revised March 2007. Available at: http://www.keionline.org/misc-docs/big idea prizes.pdf

Jaffe BA and Lerner J (2004). *Innovation and its discontents*. Princeton University Press.

Lanjouw J (2001). *A patent policy proposal for global diseases*, Annual Bank Conference on Development Economics. Washington DC, World Bank.

Mascus K (2000). *Intellectual property rights in the global economy*. Washington, Institute for International Economics.

Morgan SG, Bassett KL, Wright JM, *et al.* (2005). 'Breakthrough' drugs and growth in expenditure on prescription drugs in Canada. *British Medical Journal*, **331**, 815–16.

Nathan C (2007). Aligning pharmaceutical innovation with medical need. *Nature Medicine*, **13**.

National Research Council (2007). *Innovation inducement prizes at the National Science Foundation*. Washington, National Academic Press.

Rovira J (2007). Innovación y acceso a los medicamentos: contradicciones y propuestas. *Revista Española de Economía de la Salud*, **6**, 222–7.

Scherer F and Weinsburst S (1995). Economic effects of strengthening pharmaceutical patent protection in Italy. *International Review of Industrial Property and Copyright Law*, 26.

Stiglitz J (2006). *A better way than patents*, New Scientist Print Edition.

Weisbrod B (2003). Solving the drug dilemma. *Washington Post*, Op. Ed., August 22, A21.l. Available at: http://www.northwestern.edu/ipr/publications/newsletter/iprn0312/weisbrod.html

Wertheimer A, Levy R, O'Connor T (2001). Too many drugs? The clinical and economic value of incremental innovations. *Investing in Health: The Social and Economic Benefits of Health Care Innovation*, **14**, 77–118.

World Health Organisation (2001). *Macroeconomics and health: investing in health for economic development*. Report of the Commission on Macroeconomics and Health.

World Health Organisation (2004). *The world medicines situation*. Geneva, WHO.

World Bank (2002). *Global economic prospects. Intellectual property: balancing incentives with competitive access*. Available at: http://go.worldbank.org/D9UNNEWG50

Chapter 15

Home or nursing home? The effect of medical innovation on the demand for long-term care

Frank R. Lichtenberg

Introduction

During the last few decades, the fraction of elderly Americans who live in nursing homes has declined. In 1985, 4.5% of Americans over the age of 65 lived in nursing homes. By 1999, this fraction had declined to 4.2%. This decline is particularly note-worthy because a growing share of the over-65 population is very old—over 80—and the tendency to live in a nursing home rises very rapidly with age. This means that the age-adjusted probability of nursing home residence declined even faster than the crude rate in the over-65 population. Using data on the age distribution of nursing home residents in 1985 and 1999 from the National Nursing Home Survey and on the age distribution of the entire population from the Census Bureau, I calculated age-specific nursing home residence rates in 1985 and 1999. Nursing-home residence rates in 1985 and 1999, by single year of age (age 65–95), are shown in Fig. 15.1.

I also calculated what the nursing home residence rate would have been in 1999, given the age distribution of the population in 1999, if age-specific nursing home residence rates had been equal to their 1985 values. The results are given in Table 15.1.

For people age 65 and over, the 1999 nursing home residence rate was 23% lower than the rate one would predict from the 1985 age-specific rates: 4.2 versus 5.5%. For people age 80 and over, the 1999 nursing home residence rate was 24% lower than the rate one would predict from the 1985 age-specific rates: 11.8 versus 15.6%. The age-adjusted rate of nursing home residence declined at a 1.7% annual rate during the period 1985–1999.

Living in a nursing home is considerably more expensive than living in the community. As shown in Table 15.2, according to the Consumer Expenditure Survey, per capita expenditure by community residents age 75 and over was $12,505 in 2002.

According to the National Nursing Home Survey, average annual charges to nursing home residents age 75 and over was $42,160 in 1999.[1] The cost of living in a nursing

---

[1] The government pays for about 60% of the cost of nursing home care. (http://www.cms.hhs.gov/statistics/nhe/historical/t7.asp)

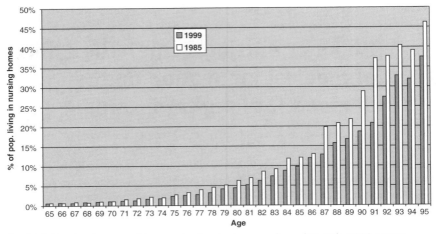

Fig. 15.1 Nursing home residence rates by single year of age (65–85): 1999 versus 1985.

Table 15.1 Age specific nursing home residence rates

Nursing-home residence rates	Age 65 and over	Age 80 and over
1985 actual	4.5%	14.8%
1999 predicted at 1985 age-specific rates	5.5%	15.6%
1999 actual	4.2%	11.8%

Table 15.2 Relative per capita expenditure of nursing home and community residents, by age group

1	2	3	4	5	6
		Community residents		Nursing home residents	5/4
Age of reference person	Average annual expenditures per household, 2002	Average no. of people in household	Average annual expenditures per person, 2002	Average annual charges, 1999	
65–74	$32,243	1.5	$21,495	$41,008	191%
75 and over	$23,759	1.9	$12,505	$42,160	337%

home was over three times as high as the cost of living in the community.[2] Reducing the rate of nursing home residence therefore reduces the average cost of living among the elderly. In 1999, there were 9.0 million Americans age 80 and over. As shown above, in 1999 the nursing home residence rate among people age 80 and over was

---

[2] Although nursing home charges may exceed nursing home costs.

3.8 percentage points ($= 15.6–11.8\%$) lower than it would have been if age-specific nursing home residence rates had remained at their 1985 levels. As a result of the decline in nursing home residence rates, 341,000 [$= (15.6 – 11.8\%) * 9.0$ million] fewer Americans age 80 and over resided in nursing homes in 1999. This may have reduced the total costs incurred by Americans age 80 and over by \$10.1 billion [$= 341,000 * (\$42,160 – \$12,505)$] in 1999.

The long-term decline in nursing home residence rates may be attributable to a number of economic and social factors. I hypothesize that improved health or functional status, among the elderly is an important contributing factor, and that the improvement in health is attributable, in part, to medical innovations: new medical goods and procedures.[3]

Economists believe that new goods generally account for a significant part of economic growth. In their book *The Economics of New Goods*, Bresnahan and Gordon argue that 'new goods are at the heart of economic progress.' Grossman and Helpman hypothesized that 'innovative goods are better than older products simply because they provide more 'product services' in relation to their cost of production' in their book, *Innovation and Growth in the Global Economy*. In a recent paper, *Measuring the Growth from Better and Better Goods*, Bils makes the case that 'much of economic growth occurs through growth in quality as new models of consumer goods replace older, sometimes inferior, models.'

Suppose that an elderly person needs to reside in a nursing home when his or her health status falls below a certain threshold (H_{min}) as given in Fig. 15.2. The fraction of elderly people residing in nursing homes is then equal to the area under the health density function to the left of H_{min}. Events that shift the health density function to the right reduce the nursing home residence rate.

Further suppose that the location of the health density function depends on the location of the vintage distribution of medical goods and services, where vintage is

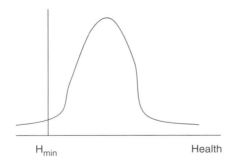

H_{min} Health

Fig. 15.2 A hypothetical distribution of health at the individual level.

---

[3] Poor health is the most frequent reason given by nursing home residents for their living arrangements.

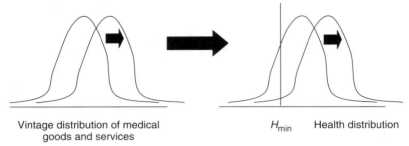

Vintage distribution of medical H_{min} Health distribution
goods and services

Fig. 15.3 A hypothetical shift in the distribution.

defined as the year of market introduction (e.g., the FDA approval year). In particular, a rightward shift of the vintage distribution results in a rightward shift of the health density function (Fig. 15.3).

The aim of this chapter is to test the hypothesis that medical innovation has reduced the age-adjusted nursing home residence rate, and estimate the contribution of medical innovation to the decline in the rate of nursing home residence during the period 1985–1999. This chapter investigates the effects of four types of medical innovation: drug innovation, and innovation in three types of procedures (therapeutic and preventive, diagnostic, and laboratory procedures).[4] Relative expenditure on prescribed medicines and on the three types of procedures during 1997–2002 is shown in Fig. 15.4.

Therapeutic and preventive procedures are the largest category, accounting for 43% of expenditure. Diagnostic procedures are the second largest, accounting for 28% of expenditure. Prescription drugs and laboratory procedures account for 22 and 7% of expenditure, respectively.

---

[4] These are the three types of "Health Care Activities"—"activities of or relating to the practice of medicine or involving the care of patients"—identified in the National Library of Medicine's Unified Medical Language System (UMLS) Semantic Network, one of three UMLS Knowledge Sources developed by the National Library of Medicine as part of the Unified Medical Language System project. The Network provides a consistent categorization of all concepts represented in the UMLS Metathesaurus. Therapeutic or Preventive Procedures are "procedures, methods, or techniques designed to prevent a disease or a disorder, or to improve physical function, or used in the process of treating a disease or injury." Diagnostic Procedures are "procedures, methods, or techniques used to determine the nature or identity of a disease or disorder. This excludes procedures which are primarily carried out on specimens in a laboratory." Laboratory Procedures are "procedures, methods, or techniques used to determine the composition, quantity, or concentration of a specimen, and which is carried out in a clinical laboratory. Included here are procedures which measure the times and rates of reactions."

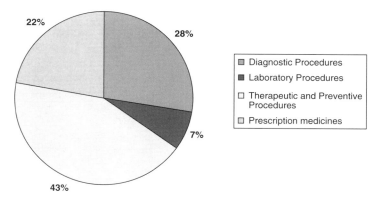

Fig. 15.4 Relative expenditures on prescription drugs and procedures, by type.

Methodology

I will use a longitudinal, disease-level,[5] difference-in-differences research design to investigate whether the rate of nursing home residence declined more rapidly for diseases with higher rates of medical innovation. The econometric model will be of the form:

$$\text{Prob}(NH_{it}) = \Phi[\Sigma_j \, \beta_j \, NEW\%_{ijt} + \alpha_i + \delta_t] + \varepsilon_{it} \qquad [1]$$

where Φ is the standard cumulative normal probability distribution; $\text{Prob}(NH_{it})$ is the probability that an elderly person with disease i in year t ($t = 1985, 1997, 1999$) resides in a nursing home (as opposed to the community); $NEW\%_{ijt}$ is the fraction of medical goods or procedures of type j used to treat disease i in year t that were introduced after 1985; α_i is a fixed effect for disease i; δ_t is a fixed effect for year t; and ε_{it} is a disturbance.

The fixed disease effects control for non-innovation determinants of nursing home residence that vary across diseases, but are constant (or change slowly) over time. The fixed year effects control for non-innovation determinants of nursing home residence that change over time (e.g. Medicaid policy), but do not vary across diseases. Of course, for estimates of β to be consistent, it must be the case that non-innovation determinants of nursing home residence not controlled for by the fixed disease and year effects be uncorrelated with the measures of medical innovation.

There are a number of possible ways to measure the shift in the vintage distribution of medical goods and services. An obvious way is to measure the change in the *mean* vintage. However, as indicated above, rather than the change in mean vintage, I will use the change in the percentage of medical goods and services whose vintage exceeds a certain value (1985). There are two good reasons for this, both related to incomplete data. First, vintage data are left-censored: for many procedures (and some drugs), we know only that their vintage is below a certain value. Second, we have good data on the

---

[5] In future research, I hope to investigate this hypothesis using individual-level data.

utilization of drugs and procedures since 1997, but not before that year. Hence, we can't determine the mean vintage of drugs and procedures used in 1985, but we know the % of drugs and procedures used in 1985 that were introduced after 1985: zero!

I will calculate the fraction of medical goods or procedures of type j used to treat *all people*, not just the elderly, with disease i in year t that were introduced after 1985. Most of the drug utilization data, and the vast majority of the procedure utilization data, I have are for people under age 65.[6]

Data

Nursing home residence rates

I computed nursing home residence rates as follows:

$$\text{Prob}(NH_{it}) = N\_NH_{it}/(N\_NH_{it} + N\_COMMUN_{it})$$

where N_NH_{it} is the number of nursing home residents (over age 65 or 80) with diagnosis i in year t, and N_COMMUN_{it} is the number of community residents (over age 65 or 80) with diagnosis i in year t.

No single survey covers both nursing home and community residents, so estimates of N_NH_{it} and N_COMMUN_{it} were obtained from two different surveys.

Nursing home residents

N_NH_{it} was computed from the National Nursing Home Survey (NNHS). The NNHS is a continuing series of national sample surveys of nursing homes, their residents, and their staff. Nursing home surveys have been conducted in 1973–74, 1977, 1985, 1995, 1997, and 1999. These surveys were preceded by a series of surveys from 1963 through 1969, called the 'residents places' surveys. Although each of these surveys emphasized different topics, they all provided some common basic information about nursing homes, their residents, and their staff. The most recent NNHS was conducted in 1999. All nursing homes included in this survey had at least three beds and were either certified (by Medicare or Medicaid), or had a State license to operate as a nursing home. The National Nursing Home Survey provides information on nursing homes from two perspectives: that of the provider of services and that of the recipient. Data about the facilities include characteristics such as size, ownership, Medicare/Medicaid certification, occupancy rate, number of days of care provided, and expenses. For recipients, data are obtained on demographic characteristics, health status, and services received. Data for the survey has been obtained through personal interviews with administrators and staff and occasionally with self-administered questionnaires in a sample of about 1500 facilities.

The NNHS collects information on the diagnoses of nursing home residents. For example, the 1999 survey reported that 279,000 residents suffered from diabetes and 232,000 suffered from Alzheimer's disease at the interview date (Jones 2002, Table 27).

---

[6] Less than 1% of the outpatient procedures captured in the MEDSTAT Commercial Claims & Encounters Database I will use were performed on people age 65 and over. MEDSTAT also has a Medicare Supplemental Database, but this was not available to me.

Although six nursing home surveys were conducted (in 1973–74, 1977, 1985, 1995, 1997, and 1999), I will use data only from the 1985, 1997, and 1999 surveys, since (as explained below) these are the years for which I can construct medical innovation measures. Moreover, the first two surveys did not use ICD9 codes to code diagnoses, and the 1973–74 survey was narrower in scope than subsequent surveys—it excluded facilities providing only personal care or domiciliary care. The number of nursing home residents sampled in the years used are 5238 (1985), 8138 (1997), and 8215 (1999).

Community residents

The number of community residents (over age 65 or 80) with diagnosis (condition) i in year t (N_COMMUN_{it}) was estimated from the 1987 National Medical Expenditure Survey (NMES)[7] and the 1997 and 1999 Medical Expenditure Panel Survey (MEPS) condition files. These surveys provide information on household-reported medical conditions collected on a nationally representative sample of the civilian non-institutionalized population of the United States. The number of community residents (including non-elderly residents) sampled in the years used are approximately 35,000 (1987), 34,441 (1997), and 34,618 (1999).

Measures of medical innovation

Measures of two main types of medical innovation were constructed: pharmaceutical innovation and innovation in medical procedures. The latter can be subdivided into several main categories, i.e. diagnostic procedures, laboratory procedures, and therapeutic/preventive procedures.

Pharmaceutical innovation

Data on prescribed medicines consumed in 1997 and 1999, by medical condition, were obtained from the MEPS Prescribed Medicines files.[8] The 1997 file contains data on 234,532 prescriptions, and the 1999 file contains data on 173,950 prescriptions. Each record in these files indicates the National Drug Code of the medicine and up to three ICD9 codes describing the condition for which the drug was taken. For the vast majority of prescriptions, only one ICD9 code is reported. The active ingredient(s) contained in each prescription were determined by using the NDC to link to *Multum's Lexicon* and the FDA approval year of each active ingredient from *Mosby's Drug Consult*. Let N_RX_{pit} = the number of prescriptions for product p used to treat condition i in year t. Let $POST1985_p = 1$, if product p's active ingredient was first approved after 1985 and $= 0$ otherwise.[9] Then:

$$NEW\_DRUG\%_{it} = \Sigma_p \, (POST1985_p \, {}^\star \, N\_RX_{pit})/\Sigma_p \, N\_RX_{pit}$$

---

[7] Because an appropriate community survey was not conducted in 1985 (the year of the NNHS survey), I will use the 1987 NMES data to estimate N_COMMUNit in 1985.

[8] See http://www.meps.ahrq.gov/Puf/PufDetail.asp?ID=24 and http://www.meps.ahrq.gov/Puf/PufDetail.asp?ID=91.

[9] In the case of combination drugs, let POST1985p = 1 if product p's *newest* active ingredient was first approved after 1985, and = 0 otherwise.

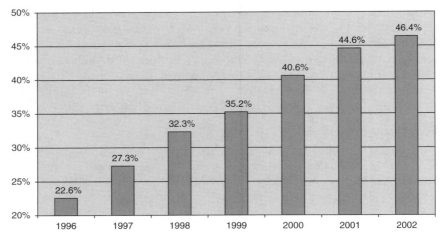

Fig. 15.5 Percentage of prescriptions that contained ingredients approved after 1985, by year, 1996–2002.

Because MEPS Prescribed Medicines files exist for each of the years 1996–2002, we can calculate NEW_DRUG%$_{it}$ in each of those seven years.[10] Figure 15.5 shows the percent of prescriptions for all conditions that contained ingredients approved after 1985 by year during 1996–2002.

The share of post-1985 drugs approximately doubled from 1996 to 2002. In 1999, the last year of the sample period we will analyse, post-1985 drugs accounted for 35.2 per cent of all prescriptions. The share of post-1985 drugs varied considerably across diseases in 1999. Table 15.3 shows some quantiles of the distribution of NEW_DRUG%$_{i,1999}$ across two-digit ICD9 codes ($n = 77$).

Medical procedure innovation

Data on outpatient and inpatient medical procedures used in 1997 and 1999, by medical condition, were obtained from *MEDSTAT MarketScan Data*. The MarketScan databases capture person-specific clinical utilization, expenditures, and enrolment

Tables 15.3 Quantiles of the distribution of NEW_DRUG%i,1999 across two-digit ICD9 codes ($n = 77$)

90%	51.9%
75% Q3	35.2%
50% Median	22.1%
25% Q1	11.8%
10%	0.0%

....

[10] Although a MEPS Prescribed Medicines files does not exist for the year 1985, it is safe to assume that NEW_DRUG%$_{i,1985 = 0}, \forall i$.

across inpatient, outpatient, prescription drug,[11] and carve-out services from approximately 45 large employers, health plans, and government and public organizations. The MarketScan databases link paid claims and encounter data to detailed patient information across sites and types of providers, and over time. The annual medical databases include private sector health data from approximately 100 payers. Historically, more than 500 million claim records are available in the MarketScan databases.

I used data contained in two types of MEDSTAT files: the outpatient and inpatient services files. The Outpatient Services file comprises encounters and claims for services that were rendered in a doctor's office, hospital outpatient facility, emergency room or other outpatient facility.[12] The inpatient services file contains the individual encounters and services that create the inpatient admission record (facility and professional claims). For example, claims for professional services rendered for an admission are found in the inpatient services table.

Each record in each of these files contains both ICD9 diagnosis codes and procedure codes. Up to two diagnosis codes are recorded on every outpatient and inpatient service record. The American Medical Association's CPT-4 (*Current Procedural Terminology*, 4th edn) coding system is the most frequently used system for classifying procedures.[13] There is space for one procedure code on each outpatient and inpatient service record. Since the claims in the database are processed by approximately 100 payers or administrators, the quality of the coding does vary. Every effort is made to select the entities with the best coding.[14] The diagnosis and procedure codes are validated and edited. If data contributors submit old codes, these codes are retained in the MarketScan data and reflect their original definition.

Determining the vintage of most medical procedures is much more challenging than determining the vintage of drugs, because unlike the introduction of new drugs, the introduction of new procedures is generally not regulated by the FDA. A noisy indicator of the vintage of a procedure is the date that the CPT code for that procedure was added to the Common Procedure Coding System established by the Centers for Medicare & Medicaid Services (CMS). This date is recorded in the *Version of Physicians' Current Procedural Terminology (CPT)* included in the Healthcare Common Procedure Coding System (HCPCS), 2005 produced by CMS.[15] Data on the 'HCPCS Code

---

[11] Unlike the MEPS prescription drug data, the MEDSTAT prescription drug data do not include ICD9 codes.

[12] A small percentage of claims in this table may represent inpatient services because the claim was not incorporated into an inpatient admission (i.e., no room and board charge was found); these generally have an "inpatient" Place of Service code.

[13] In 1997, 83% of MEDSTAT outpatient procedures and 77% of MEDSTAT inpatient procedures were coded using CPT-4 codes.

[14] See 1998 *MarketScan Research Databases User Guide and Database Dictionary*.

[15] Each year, in the United States, health care insurers process over 5 billion claims for payment. For Medicare and other health insurance programs to ensure that these claims are processed in an orderly and consistent manner, standardized coding systems are essential. The HCPCS was developed for this purpose. The HCPCS is divided into two principal subsystems, referred to as level I and level II of the HCPCS. Level I of the HCPCS is comprised

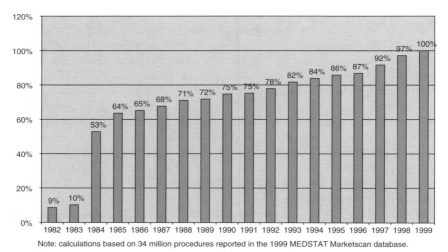

Note: calculations based on 34 million procedures reported in the 1999 MEDSTAT Marketscan database.

Fig. 15.6 Percentage of 1999 procedures whose CPT/HCPCS codes had been aided by given year.

Added Date'—the date the HCPCS code was added to the CMS Common Procedure Coding System—are included in the *Unified Medical Language System Metathesaurus* produced by the National Library of Medicine.[16]

Figure 15.6 shows the percentage of 1999 procedures whose HCPCS codes had been added up until each of the years 1982–1999.

These percentages are based on 34 million procedures reported in the 1999 MEDSTAT MarketScan database. Evidently, HCPCS was first established in 1982, but

of CPT-4, a numeric coding system maintained by the AMA. The CPT-4 is a uniform coding system consisting of descriptive terms and identifying codes that are used primarily to identify medical services and procedures furnished by physicians and other health care professionals. These health care professionals use the CPT-4 to identify services and procedures for which they bill public or private health insurance programs. Decisions regarding the addition, deletion, or modification of CPT-4 codes are made by the AMA. The CPT-4 codes are republished and updated annually by the AMA. Level I of the HCPCS, the CPT-4 codes, does not include codes needed to report medical items or services that are regularly billed by suppliers other than physicians. Level II of the HCPCS is a standardized coding system that is used primarily to identify products, supplies, and services not included in the CPT-4 codes, for example, ambulance services and durable medical equipment, prosthetics, orthotics, and supplies (DMEPOS) when used outside a physician's office. Because Medicare and other insurers cover a variety of services, supplies, and equipment that are not identified by CPT-4 codes, the level II HCPCS codes were established for submitting claims for these items. The development and use of level II of the HCPCS began in the 1980's. Level II codes are also referred to as alpha-numeric codes because they consist of a single alphabetical letter followed by 4 numeric digits, while CPT-4 codes are identified using 5 numeric digits. (http://www.cms.hhs.gov/medicare/hcpcs/codpayproc.asp)

[16] I corroborated the accuracy of these dates by consulting the AMA's CPT Assistant Archives 1990-2004, which identifies all CPT codes that have been introduced (or revised) since 1990.

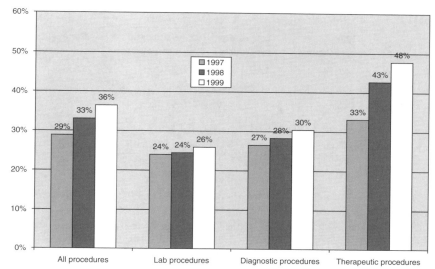

Fig. 15.7 Percentage of outpatient and inpatient procedures performed in 1997–1999, whose codes were added to HCPCS after 1985.

was not fully implemented until 1985. Most of the codes added during 1982–1985 were for procedures that had been introduced in earlier years. By the end of 1985, codes for 64 per cent of the procedures performed in 1999 had been added to HCPCS. In each year since 1985, codes for between 1 and 5 per cent of procedures performed in 1999 were added to HCPCS. This timing seems fortuitous to us, since it suggests that the fraction of procedures performed in 1997 and 1999, whose codes were added after 1985 (our 'baseline' year), is a meaningful measure of post-1985 innovation.

Figure 15.7 shows the fraction of outpatient and inpatient procedures performed in 1997–1999 whose codes were added to HCPCS after 1985.

The percentage of all procedures whose codes were added to HCPCS after 1985 is remarkably similar to the % of prescriptions that contained ingredients approved after 1985 (Table 15.4).

The percentage of post-1985 therapeutic procedures was higher, and increased more rapidly during 1997–1999, than the percentage of post-1985 laboratory and diagnostic procedures (Table 15.4).

Table 15.4 Percentage of procedures and prescription added after 1985

Year	% of all procedures whose codes were added to HCPCS after 1985	% of prescriptions that contained ingredients approved after 1985
1997	28.9%	27.3%
1998	33.1%	32.3%
1999	36.5%	35.2%

Table 15.5 Post-1985 procedures as % of total procedures

	All procedures	Laboratory procedures	Diagnostic procedures	Therapeutic procedures
90%	47.1%	43.6%	53.8%	57.0%
75% Q3	39.5%	32.4%	43.5%	40.8%
50% median	30.0%	25.7%	28.7%	25.0%
25% Q1	21.4%	21.1%	19.1%	16.6%
10%	15.0%	17.0%	12.4%	8.8%

As Table 15.5 shows, the % of post-1985 procedures in 1999, like the percentage of post-1985 drugs, varied considerably across diseases.

Closer inspection of the data on medical procedures reveals that some 'new' procedures are probably just relabelled or reclassified old procedures, rather than true innovations. For example, the three procedures whose codes were added in 1997, which were most frequently performed in 1997, were 98940, 98941, and 98942, which correspond to different types of chiropractic manipulative treatment of the spine. Undoubtedly, this type of treatment was performed well before 1997. A new CPT code should therefore be considered a necessary condition for a medical innovation, but not a sufficient condition: all innovations have new CPT codes, but some new CPT codes are not innovations. The fraction of procedures with new CPT codes exceeds the fraction of truly innovative procedures, perhaps by a significant amount, and the degree of overstatement varies across diseases. In the future, I hope to develop a reliable method of distinguishing between truly innovative procedures and old procedures with new CPT codes.[17] For now, I will include the fraction of procedures with new CPT codes, despite the limitations of this variable. Although the coefficient on this variable is difficult to interpret, including it may provide a robustness check on the drug coefficient.

I will now proceed to test the hypothesis that diseases with above-average rates of pharmaceutical innovation (i.e. above-average percentages of post-1985 drugs in 1997 and 1999) had above-average declines in nursing home residence rates during the period 1985–1999, conditional on (imperfect measures of) rates of other medical innovation.

Empirical estimates

Estimates of different versions of Eqn 1—probit models of the nursing home residence rates—are shown in Table 15.6.

---

[17] Perhaps this can be done by examining the trajectory of utilization following establishment of a new CPT code. One might expect truly innovative procedures to exhibit sustained growth after introduction, and old procedures with new CPT codes to show little growth after the transition period.

Table 15.6 Estimates of probit models of the nursing home residence rate

Model	1	2	3	4	5	6	7	8
Age group	65+	65+	65+	65+	80+	80+	80+	80+
Mean NH residence rate	3.6%	3.6%	3.6%	3.6%	9.8%	9.8%	9.8%	9.8%
No. of observations	109,072	109,072	109,072	109,072	28,324	28,324	28,324	28,324
Fixed disease effects?	No	Yes	Yes	Yes	No	Yes	Yes	Yes
Year 1985	0.0237	0.0491	−0.0763	−0.174	0.0947	0.1325	0.0069	−0.182
SE	0.0181	0.02	0.047	0.059	0.0263	0.0287	0.0675	0.084
Pr > χ^2	0.1913	0.0143	0.1044	0.003	0.0003	<.0001	0.919	0.029
Year 1997	−0.0145	−0.0077	−0.0358	−0.054	−0.0265	−0.0148	−0.0437	−0.079
SE	0.0171	0.0188	0.0211	0.022	0.0241	0.0262	0.0297	0.031
Pr > χ^2	0.3946	0.6822	0.0891	0.014	0.27	0.573	0.1412	0.011
Post−1985 drug %			−0.3803	−0.393			−0.3806	−0.396
SE			0.1286	0.129			0.1845	0.185
Pr > χ^2			0.0031	0.002			0.0392	0.032
Post−1985 procedure %				−0.300				−0.591
SE				0.109				0.153
Pr > χ^2				0.006				0.000
Intercept	−1.8019	−2.1766	−2.0469	−1.951	−1.3056	−1.8678	−1.7376	−1.552
SE	0.0125	0.0606	0.0749	0.083	0.0177	0.0774	0.0999	0.111
Pr > χ^2	<0.0001	<0.0001	<0.0001	<0.0001	<0.0001	<0.0001	<0.0001	<0.0001

Note: The 1999 year effect is normalized to zero.

I estimated models for two different age groups: people age 65 and over, and people age 80 and over. Estimates of models for the first age group are shown in columns 1–4. Model 1 includes just 2 year-dummy variables for the years 1985 and 1997, and an intercept, and the 1999 year effect is normalized to zero. The 1985 dummy is positive, indicating that the crude nursing home residence rate was higher in 1985 than it was in 1999, but it is not statistically significant. Model 2 also includes fixed disease effects (which are always jointly highly significant). Now the 1985 dummy is positive and significantly different from zero, indicating that, controlling for disease, the 1985 nursing home residence rate was significantly higher than the 1999 rate. In model 3, we add the drug innovation variable—the fraction of prescriptions for drugs approved after 1985. As expected, the coefficient on NEW_DRUG% is negative and highly significant (p-value = 0.003). This indicates that diseases with more rapid rates of pharmaceutical innovation had larger declines in the nursing home residence rate during the period 1985–1999. The 1985 dummy is not significantly different from zero in model 3, which implies that, holding constant NEW_DRUG% (i.e. in the absence of any pharmaceutical innovation), there would have been no decline in the nursing home residence rate.

We can evaluate the effect of pharmaceutical innovation on the nursing home residence rate as follows. In 1985, the sample mean nursing home residence rate among people age 65 and over was 3.6 per cent. The change in the nursing home residence rate attributable to pharmaceutical innovation is:

$$F[F^{-1}(3.6\%) + \beta_{drug} \text{ mean(NEW\_DRUG\%)}] - 3.6\%$$

where F is the standard normal cumulative distribution and F^{-1} is its inverse. The estimate of β_{drug} in column 3 is –0.3803, and the mean value of NEW_DRUG% in 1999 was 35.2 per cent, so the reduction in the nursing home residence rate attributable to pharmaceutical innovation is 0.9 per cent. In other words, in the absence of other trends (e.g. changing age distribution), pharmaceutical innovation would have reduced the nursing home residence rate from 3.6 per cent in 1985 to 2.7 per cent in 1999. We calculated earlier that the age-adjusted nursing home residence rate declined by 1.3 percentage points between 1985 and 1999. Hence, pharmaceutical innovation is estimated to account for almost three-quarters (73% = 0.9%/1.3%) of the total decline in the age-adjusted nursing home residence rate during the period 1985–1999.

We calculated above that the average annual cost of living in a nursing home exceeded the average annual cost of living in the community by $29,655. Thus, the value per person age 65 and over of the reduction in the 1999 nursing home residence rate attributable to pharmaceutical innovation might be estimated as $277 (= 0.9% * $29,655). (This does not account for the presumably greater utility from living in the community.) According to the Medical Expenditure Panel Survey, in 1999, average expenditure on prescription drugs by people age 65 and over was $948. I estimate that just over half (54 per cent) of this expenditure was on drugs approved after 1985, so average expenditure on new drugs was $508 (= 54% * $948). This implies that over half (55% = $277/$508) of expenditure on new drugs by people age 65 and over was offset by reduced expenditures on nursing home care.

Model 4 in Table 15.6 includes the procedure innovation variable (NEW_PROC%)—the fraction of procedures performed that had CPT/HCPCS codes added after 1985—as well as the drug innovation variable. Like the coefficient on NEW_DRUG%, the coefficient on NEW_PROC% is negative and highly significant, indicating that the introduction and use of both new procedures and new drugs reduced the nursing home residence rate. Controlling for NEW_PROC% has virtually no effect on the estimate of β_{drug} or its standard error. The change in the nursing home residence rate attributable to the combined impact of new drugs and procedures is

$$F[F^{-1}(3.6\%) + \beta_{drug} \text{ mean(NEW\_DRUG\%)} + \beta_{proc} \text{ mean(NEW\_PROC\%)}] - 3.6\%$$

The mean value of NEW_PROC% in 1999 was 36%, so the estimated reduction in the nursing home residence rate attributable to the combined impact of new drugs and procedures is 1.6%. In other words, in the absence of other trends (e.g. changing age distribution), pharmaceutical and procedure innovation would have reduced the nursing home residence rate from 3.6% in 1985 to 2.0% in 1999. This is greater than the 1.3 percentage point decline in the age-adjusted nursing home residence rate between 1985 and 1999. Moreover, when we replace the fraction of all procedures that are new by its three components—the fractions of laboratory, diagnostic, and therapeutic procedures that are new—the implied impact of procedure innovation becomes even larger. I suspect that the implied impact of procedure innovation is implausibly large due to our inability, at present, to distinguish between truly innovative procedures and old procedures with new CPT codes. Even though the procedure innovation measures are imperfect, it is reassuring that controlling for them has virtually no effect on estimates of the impact of drug innovation.

The last four columns of Table 15.6 show estimates of the same models as those in columns 1–4, but estimated on the group of people age 80 and over. This sample is less than one-third as large as the sample of people age 65 and over, but the nursing home residence rate is almost three times as high—9.8% versus 3.6%. Model 5 shows that the crude nursing home residence rate of people age 80 and over was significantly higher in 1985 than it was in 1999. Model 6 shows that the decline in the rate is even larger when we adjust for disease. In model 7, the drug innovation variable was added. As before, the coefficient on NEW_DRUG% is negative and highly significant (*p*-value = 0.030), and the 1985 dummy is not significantly different from zero, which implies that, in the absence of any pharmaceutical innovation, there would have been no decline in the nursing home residence rate of people age 80 and over.

Using the method described above to evaluate the effect of pharmaceutical innovation on the nursing home residence rate of people age 80 and over, it is estimated that the reduction in the nursing home residence rate attributable to pharmaceutical innovation is 2.1%. In other words, in the absence of other trends (e.g. changing age distribution), pharmaceutical innovation would have reduced the nursing home residence rate from 9.8% in 1985 to 7.7% in 1999. The age-adjusted nursing home residence rate of people age 80 and over declined by 3.8 percentage points between 1985 and 1999. Hence, pharmaceutical innovation is estimated to account for 56% = (2.1%/3.8%) of the total decline in the age-adjusted nursing home residence rate of people age 80 and over during the period 1985–1999.

The value per person age 80 and over of the reduction in the 1999 nursing home residence rate attributable to pharmaceutical innovation is estimated as $630 (= 2.1% * $29,655). In 1999, average expenditure on prescription drugs by people age 80 and over was $934.[18] It is estimated that just over half (54%) of this expenditure was on drugs approved after 1985, so average expenditure on new drugs was $501 (= 54% * $934). This implies that, among people age 80 and over, the reduction in expenditure on nursing home care due to the use of new drugs exceeded expenditure on new drugs by 26% [= ($630/$501) − 1].

Finally, in column 8 we include the procedure innovation variable, as well as the drug innovation variable. Once again, the coefficient on NEW_PROC% is negative and highly significant; indeed, its magnitude is twice as great as it was in model 4. As before, controlling for NEW_PROC% has virtually no effect on the estimate of β_{drug} or its standard error. These estimates imply that pharmaceutical and procedure innovation would have reduced the nursing home residence rate among people age 80 and over from 9.8% in 1985 to 5.0% in 1999. This is greater than the 3.8 percentage point decline in the age-adjusted nursing home residence rate of this group between 1985 and 1999. Our inability, at present, to distinguish between truly innovative procedures and old procedures with new CPT codes is presumably the reason for the implausibly large implied impact of procedure innovation. However, the drug innovation measure is not subject to this problem, the coefficient on it is essentially unaffected by inclusion of the procedure innovation measure, and the magnitude of its effect seems plausible.

Summary and conclusions

During the last few decades, the fraction of elderly Americans who live in nursing homes has declined. For people age 65 and over, the 1999 nursing home residence rate was 23 per cent lower than the rate one would predict from the 1985 age-specific rates: 4.2 versus 5.5 per cent. For people age 80 and over, the 1999 nursing home residence rate was 24 per cent lower than the rate one would predict from the 1985 age-specific rates: 11.8 versus 15.6 per cent. The age-adjusted rate of nursing home residence declined at a 1.7 per cent annual rate during the period 1985–1999. Living in a nursing home is considerably more expensive than living in the community, so the decline in nursing home residence rates reduced the total costs incurred by Americans age 80 and over by about $10 billion in 1999.

Improved health or functional status among the elderly may be an important factor contributing to the long-term decline in nursing home residence rates. In particular, an elderly person may need to reside in a nursing home when his or her health status falls below a certain threshold. Improvements in health may be attributable, in part, to medical innovations, new medical goods and procedures.

This chapter has tested the hypothesis that medical innovation has reduced the age-adjusted nursing home residence rate, and estimated the contribution of

---

[18] It is somewhat surprising that this is slightly *lower* than the average expenditure on prescription drugs by people age 65 and over ($934).

medical innovation to the decline in the rate of nursing home residence, during the period 1985–1999. It has investigated the effects of two main types of medical innovation: drug innovation and innovation in medical procedures and has used a longitudinal, disease-level, difference-in-differences research design to investigate whether the rate of nursing home residence declined more rapidly for diseases with higher rates of medical innovation. This research design controls for non-innovation determinants of nursing home residence that vary across diseases, but are constant (or change slowly) over time, and for non-innovation determinants of nursing home residence that change over time (e.g. Medicaid policy), but do not vary across diseases.

The dependent variable was the fraction of people with a given medical condition in a given year (1985, 1997, or 1999) who resided in a nursing home, rather than in the community. No single survey covers both nursing home and community residents, so estimates of this fraction were constructed using data from two different surveys: the National Nursing Home Survey, and the Medical Expenditure Panel Survey (MEPS). Disease-specific data on drug and procedure innovation were constructed from MEPS, MEDSTAT, and other sources.

Two models have been estimated: for people age 65 and over, and people age 80 and over. Estimates for both groups indicated that diseases with more rapid rates of pharmaceutical innovation had larger declines in the nursing home residence rate during the period 1985–1999. Pharmaceutical innovation is estimated to have accounted for almost three-quarters of the decline in the age-adjusted nursing home residence rate of people 65 and over, and 56% of the decline in the rate of people age 80 and over. I estimate that 55% of expenditure on new drugs by people age 65 and over was offset by reduced expenditures on nursing home care and that among people age 80 and over, the reduction in expenditure on nursing home care due to the use of new drugs exceeded expenditure on new drugs by 26 per cent.

Diseases with more rapid rates of medical procedure innovation, as well as drug innovation, experienced greater declines in the nursing home residence rate. However, the estimated impact of procedure innovation on nursing home utilization is implausibly large. This is probably attributable to our inability, at present, to distinguish between truly innovative procedures and old procedures with new procedure codes, a problem we hope to resolve in future research. Controlling for the (admittedly imperfect) procedure innovation measures has virtually no effect on estimates of the impact of drug innovation.

References

American Medical Association (2008). *CPT Assistant Archives 1990-2007* (CD-ROM). Chicago, IL: AMA.

Bils M (2004). *Measuring the growth from better and better goods*, NBER Working Paper 10606. Cambridge, MA: National Bureau of Economic Research, http://www.nber.org/papers/w10606.

Bresnahan T and Gordon R (1996). *The economics of new goods*. Chicago: University of Chicago Press, http://www.nber.org/books/bres96-1.

Center for Medicare and Medicaid Services (2009). *Alpha-Numeric HCPCS*, http://www.cms.hhs.gov/HCPCSReleaseCodeSets/ANHCPCS/list.asp.

Grossman, G and Helpman E (1993). *Innovation and growth in the global economy*. Cambridge, MA: MIT Press.

Jones A (2002). The National Nursing Home Survey: 1999 summary, National Center for Health Statistics. *Vital Health Statistics*, **13**, 152.

MEDSTAT Marketscan Data, http://www.medstatmarketscan.com/.

Mosby (2005). *Mosby's drug consult for health professions*. St. Louis, MO: Mosby Elsevier, http://www.elsevier.com/wps/find/bookdescription.cws_home/704078/description#description.

Multum Lexicon, http://www.multum.com/Lexicon.htm.

National Institutes of Health (1999). *Unified Medical Language System*. Bethesda, MD: National Institutes of Health. http://www.nlm.nih.gov/research/umls/.

Chapter 16

Knowledge, technology, and demand for online health information

Joan Costa-Font, Caroline Rudisill, and Elias Mossialos

Introduction

Information technologies can potentially impact on the way individuals update their health-related knowledge. Decision-making about one's own health presents an area pervasive with market failures, resulting from imperfect information on the side of individuals/patients. It is increasingly recognised that information (of a certain quality) about personal health and health care is costly to acquire, while the quality and quantity of health information required varies with individual context and an individual's prerequisite level of knowledge about a topic. However, information externalities appear as the ways in which we gather information expand and develop with social interactions (Helmstädlter 2003) and the use of new technologies, such as the Internet. The final effect of knowledge sharing is that knowledge grows when it is shared, and accordingly dissemination increases the value of knowledge. As a result, knowledge becomes a form of collective good, although its benefits depend very much on whether individuals end up learning and using the existing knowledge to improve their well-being.

In the production of services such as health information, individuals could employ a number of sources individually or simultaneously to update their health information, including medical doctors, family, and increasingly the Internet. The value and credibility individuals attach to each information source varies. However, little is known about the relationship between the demand for health information and determinants of whether individuals elect to use the Internet to fill their information gaps.

This chapter examines the process of knowledge sharing and use of information technologies in health care, drawing upon evidence from the use of the Internet for health purposes in the European Union. The Internet appears as a relatively new information with the potential to bring efficiency gains and health production benefits. However, little is known about the specific determinants of the search for information, especially under heterogeneous cultural and institutional settings, such as those of European Union member states.

Information and communication technologies

The process of generating practical knowledge results from a combination of previously known knowledge as well as new information. However, knowledge acquisition, far from being subject to no barriers, is often highly competitive (Hayek 1937), on the other hand, it is also an input for competition. Knowledge comes at costs such as search costs, when observed from an *ex ante* perspective, as well as standard transaction cost, when observed (Arrow 1968), namely the opportunity costs of spending the time and effort to acquire knowledge. The role of information and communication technologies (ICT) is to lower the costs of operating the system of sharing information and, accordingly, to indirectly expand the dissemination of knowledge of health and enhance the optimal combination of healthy inputs.

Increasingly, accessible information technology influences the use of health communication just as it has altered the dissemination of information on a variety of subjects. Having simultaneous access to both traditional information sources such as print, and new information sources, such as websites, has altered the way in which individuals keep their knowledge up-to-date. The Internet certainly has the potential for becoming a key tool in disseminating health information to the public (Cotton and Gupta 2004). However, the value individuals attach to information from the Internet depends not only on the credibility associated with information from the Internet, but also the value attached to information from alternative sources as substitutes or complimentary sources.

Although not substituting for medical care, online information channels may influence medical care utilization and overall health expenditure in a variety of ways. Patients using the Internet to access health information can alter traditional patterns of care, and relationships between patients and medical professionals. Better health information for patients provides the patient with an improved status from an information vantage in the patient–doctor relationship (McGuire 2000). No longer is the patient largely relying on the opaque body of information acquired by doctors upon receipt of a medical degree. As virtual medicine grows significantly, information-focused medical visits could be performed via the Internet. Greater access to health information through the web will probably also affect the physician-doctor relationship (Shackley and Ryan 1994) by empowering the patient with more complementary knowledge. Some evidence suggests that health information in general might substitute other forms of health care typically providing information to the consumer (Wagner *et al.* 2001a,b). Information gained through the Internet might also act as a supplementary information source to sources already used. Better health information could well induce more prevention and self-care, rather than reliance on health care resources. This would be especially true in health systems with waiting lists, where informed patients might be less likely to being willing to wait to see a medical professional if information becomes easily obtainable online. Wagner and Greenlick (2001) find that self-care information decreases paediatric utilization, although limited evidence was found in self-reported utilization.

In terms of a system impact, the use of Internet of health information could reduce health costs through decreased doctor visits, as well as reducing the costs of health information dissemination (Bundorf *et al.* 2004). Additionally, when possible, patients would be able to make more informed choices about treatment options or treatment locales through up-to-date online information sources displaying data about surgical success rates for procedures in general or even a specific hospital or physician.

The reasons behind why certain individuals seek health information are still not well understood. A 2001 US survey by the Centre for Studying Healthcare and Change found that only 38 per cent of respondents searched for health information themselves with only 16 per cent using the Internet (Tu and Hargraves 2003). Individuals might wish to prevent an illness' appearance (Patrick 2000) or search for information after experiencing a certain condition himself, or through some friend or relative. Little is known on the effects of the Internet as a tool for connecting less educated and low-income individuals (Zarcadoolas *et al.* 2002; Cotton and Gupta 2004). As health and income are well know to be associated (Kenkel 1990), if there is a socio-economic pattern explaining the likelihood of an individual searching for health information on the Internet, then access to the Internet and its use for obtaining information would either mitigate or exacerbate socio-economic inequalities in health.

Examining the determinants of individuals obtaining information through the web remains key to obtaining a better understanding of the potential impact of the Internet on individual and population health and healthcare systems. We conceptualize 'health information' as any messages conveyed by a variety of information channels that may have a potential impact on individual health by reducing the uncertainty regarding one's health status. Messages can be obtained from a variety of information channels categorised as traditional ones, such as the general practitioner (GP) and other health professionals, social networks or technology-related ones, such as the media and the Internet.

Limitations to the uptake of Internet as a source of health information hinge on questions of access. Access to the Internet can be a socio-economic or age-related issue, as well as language-related. However, as computer costs and connection costs continue to fall over the developed world, the growth of health-related health sites become more likely to improve the dissemination of health information across increasingly large swathes of society. Regardless, as computer and Internet use have been found to be linked with socio-economic position, these traits can still stand in the way of Internet-based health information use. Additionally, education and socio-economic position may also alter the capacity of an individual to find adequate health information, even if they have all the necessary technology. The dominant usage of English in medical and health-related research, and thus on many health-related websites might exacerbate the barriers of non-English speakers to access health information. The use of a computer is found to be linked with socio-economic position.

From rational learning to Bayesian updating

Health (care) information refers to the use of any device to gather information to prevent or cure a potential health condition. The Internet provides an extensive amount of information potentially useful to obtain medical advice and can be argued to substitute most traditional information sources (Goldsmith 2000). It provides individuals with anonymous, immediate access to a large amount of information and fosters the development of different viewpoints on a specific health condition (Cotton and Gupta 2004). However, Internet-based information could be regarded as being of questionable credibility. Evidence suggests that information can be dated and inaccurate (Impicciatore and Pandofini 1997). On the other hand, a study of the content of an online epilepsy support group was found to have only 6 per cent inaccurate material according to a panel of neurology specialists (Lester *et al.* 2004). Additionally, given the speed at which information can updated and edited on the Internet, incorrect postings can be altered quickly if the website is read often and/or well monitored. Websites operated or endorsed by medical school and hospitals also exist, and overcome some questions about credibility because of reputation risks. Therefore, the quality level of health information accessed via the Internet appears to occupy a wide spectrum of veracity depending on the particular webpage.

Gathering information online implies avoiding time and transport costs. However, there are still important search costs that, although they may be difficult to identify empirically, may be associated with knowledge and the capacity to process information (Kenkel 1990). Education and socio-economic position might determine the individual ability to discriminate between useful and not-useful information. Therefore, if we name the process of sifting through information to deem its usefulness as the primary transaction cost associated with seeking health information via the Internet, those individuals (less educated, lower socio-economic status) for whom this transaction cost becomes very high and time-consuming may not view the Internet as such a useful source of information. Education and socio-economic status might also pose a risk to individuals that have been shown to attach greater credibility to the Internet as compared with other sources (Cline and Haynes 2001), since what they believe to be correct might not actually be so.

Examining the demand for health information can be connected back to the demand for health model (Grossman 1972), where information is either an input in the health production function or a key variable influencing the production of health. Health is a stock that might be affected by individuals' behaviour, which in turn is dependent on their level of information, leading to the preventive behaviour of consuming certain health care, which may slow health depreciation. However, health information is largely heterogeneous. One might gather information on the best physician in town, the association between obesity and depression, or the impact of sexual behaviour on the likelihood of contracting AIDS. Heterogeneity might imply that the demand curve for those specific conditions would differ significantly. As is the case with any other service, information is affected by information costs and, in general, any barriers to access information (Coffey 1983; Cauley 1987). The Internet may be a 'cost-less' tool in terms of tangible costs per use, but fixed costs matter (e.g. buying or renting a computer, Internet connection, etc.). Individuals also face costs related to their own capacity for information-gathering. These costs constitute individual characteristics that are specific and non-observable, and thus subject to individuals' perceptions of these costs.

Individuals' demand for health as depicted by Grossman (1972) gives rise to a demand for health information, given the household nature of health production. Generally, individuals consume health by gaining utility from being healthy or invest in their production function by reducing the potential productivity loss from being unhealthy. Both reasons lead to the seeking of some form of health information aimed at preventing or curtailing ill health. The presence or lack of knowledge determines the capacity of individuals to consume or produce health efficiently. Individuals who are likely to benefit more immediately from health information are those of a poorer health status.

While doctors have a role in an individual's health production function, they cannot be fully informed about every aspect of an individual's status. Some studies suggest that patients have individually-specific information determining health production besides that of doctors, such as previous symptoms, personal history, preferences on treatment adherence (Haas-Wilson 2001). The impact of the physician on filling individual's knowledge gaps in order to maximize health varies as country-specific institutional and cultural differences are likely to influence the doctor-physician agency relationship (Hsieh and Lin 1997).

From rational learning to bounded learning

The rational learning literature assumes that individuals update information about health care interventions that may impact upon them and specific problems with their current or future health, following a Bayesian learning process. Yet, when individuals deviate from this pattern, they are either depicted as following a bounded learning process if constraints do not allow individuals to act as rational decision-makers. Individuals might simply follow some heuristics, but understanding the rationality of people's behaviour implies identifying their decision-making short cuts. The difference between rational and bounded learning lies in that with bounded learning, individuals rely on heuristics or short cuts in order to understand information that is otherwise unclear or about which there is uncertainty. They engage in information-gathering activity, but do not scan all the available information (Weyland 2002).

Social effects are expected to have an influence on information updating, and particularly the trust and credibility of particular information sources. Preference externalities exist in many settings whereupon an individual's choice can impact on those made by others. Consumers who are more prone to be influenced by preference externalities are less likely to be able to consume a product close to an ideal that is socially created; there is some evidence of this effect to explain pharmaceutical consumption (Waldfogel 2003).

New technologies bring generally large information costs that can be minimised by consumption externalities (seeing other people doing the same thing), or by personal use and experience. Generally, new technologies are considered credence goods as their utility cannot be evaluated immediately. Therefore, we expect it to be likely that access costs, represented by the likelihood of having Internet access at home, use of other information sources for health information and socio-demographic characteristics of individuals outside their particular their education level, will affect the demand for information from the Internet.

Estimating the potential influence of technology use for health purposes

Estimating the demand for health information implies examining how the probability of using the Internet to gain health information is influenced by the costs those individuals attach to Internet use. These costs can be associated with intrinsic socio-demographic characteristics of respondents, as well as their place of residence and income. Thus, we estimate an empirical model that examines the determinants of Internet use for seeking health-related information. Our model includes country-specific characteristics (C), individuals' income (Y), information costs that refer to Internet access among other variables (P'), specific social determinants of the demand for information (H), and other related variables, such as age and gender (Z) as follows:

$$DI_i = \beta_0 + \beta_1 C + \beta_2 Y_i + \beta_3 P_i^I + \beta_4 H_i + \sum \beta_5 Z_{i_i} + \varepsilon_i \qquad [1]$$

The price for health information depends on education and individuals' specific characteristics approximating ability. Additionally, education is normally seen as a proxy of health production efficiency (Kenkel 1990). The measure of Internet access used in this analysis was taken from 2007 Eurostat data on the percentage of house-holds with Internet access in each European member state (Smihily 2007). Therefore, we do not know if each individual respondent has Internet access, but use their country's percentage of households with Internet access instead to proxy individual access.

In order to take into account country-specific characteristics, control for the respondent's country of residence were included in each model by clustering the data by country. The clustering method meant that respondents were grouped according their country of residence, thus accounting for country-specific effects and treating clusters, rather than observations as independent (Williams 2000). In the same fashion as in multi-level modelling, we have overcome some deficiencies in existing datasets, such as the bias caused by using this clustering procedure.

The role of the Internet for health

If we examine the role of Internet as an element in individual's search efforts to solve their health-related decision-making problem, we can lay out the potential determinants of Internet use for this purpose. Search behaviour is likely to be influenced by need, namely whether the individual has experienced a specific health condition [e.g. the poorer the health status, the more likely to gather information (Bundorf *et al.* 2004)], social (interactions) and household learning (e.g. the closer one is to a sick person, the more likely to gather health information) and socio-economic characteristics. Education and affluence would particularly determine the capacity of an individual to cope with the price of health information. Socio-economic status can be expected also to impact the likelihood that an individual even has access to the Internet on the fist place. Hence, barriers in obtaining health information for a specific condition may come in the form of there actually being a lack of information online because of the novelty of a specific illness or the sheer percentage of the population who have it.

Previous studies indicate that education is likely to provide individuals with a stock of information acting as a starting point and a more advanced capacity to update that stock of information (Llera-Muney 2005). However, one channel that has not been yet properly investigated is the extent to which the demand for information is affected by education. If individuals who are more educated have the ability to access information on their own through mechanisms such as the Internet and without a medical profession's aid then this could explain why more informed individuals are less likely to use health care (Kenkel 1990; Hsieh and Lin 1997).

Empirical evidence draws upon data from the Eurobarometer 58.2, a survey collected for the EU-15 over the period October to December 2002. The survey contains questions on many topics including respondents' 'information behaviour' and, in particular, their use of information sources, including the Internet for information about matters pertaining to health and healthcare. Roughly 1000 respondents in each of the 15 countries surveyed were asked the same questions about their frequency of Internet use to find health information and which information sources are the mains ones they use for health information.

The Eurobarometer survey series is a social research tool of cross-national surveys designed to regularly monitor social and political attitudes of the EU public. Caveats (Inglehart 1990; Fuchs et al. 1995; Schmitt and Holmberg 1995) refer to the sampling procedure and the difficulties associated with measuring income and education among EU member states. Because the survey was conducted on a multi-stage random sampling basis rather than pure random sampling, it is a 'representative sample' of the national population over 15 years of age. Individual country population samples were taken on a random basis according to each country's distribution of metropolitan, urban, and rural residents. In the second stage, a cluster of addresses was selected from each primary sampling unit. Addresses were chosen systematically using standard random route procedures, beginning with an initial address selected at random.

Descriptive statistics indicate that Europeans use the Internet sparingly, if ever to receive health information. Table 16.1 highlights the lack of frequency with which respondents ever use the Internet to get information about health.

Only 28.7 per cent of respondents use the Internet on less than a monthly basis to access health information, while 33.7 per cent don't use the Internet at all, even for information about health.

Table 16.2 demonstrates that in comparison to other information sources, the Internet is the sixth most named main source of information about health behind doctors, television, newspapers, health or medical magazines, and friends, family and colleagues. The Internet was the main source of information about health for only 3.6 per cent of respondents.

30.8 per cent of respondents named the doctor as their main source of health information closely followed by the television at 29.2 per cent. Doctors and the television were described as the main source of health information in almost equal numbers.

Table 16.1 Frequency of health information on the Internet

Question: How often do you use the Internet to get information about health?

	n	%	% Accumulated
Once a day	279	1.72	1.72
Several times a week	848	5.22	6.94
Once a month	1060	6.53	13.48
Less often	2477	15.26	28.74
Never	5832	35.93	64.67
Don't use Internet (spontaneous)	5468	33.69	98.36
Don't know	266	1.64	100

These top two named sources of information are also both passive in form, as no searching is involved in getting information from a doctor or the television. On the other hand, less popular sources, such as books, newspapers, magazines, and the Internet require more effort on the part of the individual. This finding points to the importance of transaction costs in making decisions about information source use.

Country-specific findings displayed in Table 16.3 suggest that heterogeneity exists between how the populations of the EU-15 feel about the value of health information from the Internet.

Across all countries, at least one-fifth of the population (except in the Netherlands with 16.4 per cent) does not know if the Internet is a good means of getting health information. Germany has the highest percentage of respondents electing' 'don't know' with 40.3 per cent. This finding highlights the importance of value placed on

Table 16.2 What is your main source of information about health?

	n	%	% Accumulated
A doctor	4995	30.78	30.78
Television	4735	29.17	59.95
Newspapers	2128	13.11	73.06
Health or medical magazines	1551	9.56	82.62
Friends, family, colleagues	672	4.14	86.76
The Internet	590	3.64	90.40
Books	579	3.57	93.97
Other magazines	280	1.73	95.70
Radio	225	1.39	97.09
A chemist	144	0.89	97.98
Courses and lectures	134	0.83	98.81
Other sources (spontaneous)	105	0.65	99.46
Don't know	92	0.57	100

Table 16.3 Value of the Internet to gather health information

Question: In your opinion, is the Internet a good means of getting health information, or not?

	Yes	No	DK
Belgium	40.09	35.05	24.86
Denmark	45.90	32.90	21.20
Germany	37.56	18.22	44.22
Greece	49.15	24.83	26.02
Italy	41.97	28.92	29.11
Spain	44.60	24.50	30.90
France	45.71	28.06	26.23
Ireland	53.01	14.61	32.38
Netherlands	67.92	15.65	16.43
Portugal	44.21	20.26	35.53
UK	49.01	20.66	30.34
Finland	58.20	19.53	22.27
Sweden	36.40	43.60	20.00
Austria	48.88	24.54	26.59
Total	47.09	24.47	28.43

Source: Eurobarometer 58.2.

the Internet as a source of information. If individuals have no opinion on the value of Internet, then they would be less likely to deem information credible.

The Netherlands has the highest percentage of respondents expressing that the Internet is a good means of obtaining health information. Only Ireland and Finland have over half of respondents answering positively about the value of Internet-sourced health information. Sweden has the highest percentage of respondents stating that the Internet is not a good means of accessing health information with 43.6 per cent of respondents electing to answer 'no.' Belgium and Denmark are the only other two countries with over 30 per cent of respondents also attaching no value to health information from the Internet.

Results

Regression results using multiple model permutations further develop descriptive findings in order to understand their determinants. We run two sets of models with' 'frequency of Internet use to find health information' (Tables 16.4 and 16.5) as the dependent variable for one group and whether respondents think the Internet is a good means of getting health information. The diagnostic test of pseudo-R^2 indicates that the models predict a significant share of expected cases and the log likelihood test rejects the hypothesis of all variables being equal to zero. Furthermore, we tested for the existence of multi-colinearity as a result of interactions between explanatory variables and found that because the variance inflation factors (VIF) were systematically below ten, multi-colinearity is not an issue except in one model discussed below where the explanatory variable 'Internet access' was dropped because of multi-colinearity.

Table 16.4 provides evidence of respondent characteristics, as well as Internet access playing a role in the frequency of Internet use to find health information. Health status is negatively associated with an individual's likelihood of gathering health information on the Internet. Respondents living in a rural environment, age, and living alone also demonstrated a significant and negative relationship with frequency of using the Internet to access health information. Being male was found to be positively related to how often respondents use the Internet for health information. Education also appears to impact upon frequency of accessing online health information with those

Table 16.4 Regression results for frequency of Internet use to find health information

	Description	Mean	Frequency of Internet use (ordered probit)		
			Coeff.	SE	*t*
hea2	Good health status (HS)	0.427	−0.03	0.02	−1.42
hea3	Fair HS	0.242	−0.10	0.03	−2.95
hea4	Bad HS	0.051	−0.21	0.05	−4.24
hea5	Very bad HS	0.007	−0.10	0.07	−1.40
rural	Rural = 1	0.370	−0.10	0.04	−2.38
age1	>30	0.152	0.73	0.07	10.33
age2	30–45	0.276	0.69	0.05	12.93
age3	45–60	0.248	0.49	0.06	8.67
male	Male = 1	0.462	0.06	0.03	2.44
educ1	Finished education at 15 or below	0.259	−0.67	0.08	−8.42
educ2	Finished education at 16–19	0.391	−0.38	0.03	−11.58
educ4	Still studying	0.099	0.10	0.04	2.70
alone	Lives alone	0.181	−0.08	0.04	−1.73
Internet	Internet access in household	0.605	1.16	0.20	5.83
politic1	Self–identified as left wing	0.241	0.01	0.02	0.37
politic2	Self–identified as centre	0.345	−0.01	0.02	−0.46
Pseudo–R^2			0.081		
Log likelihood			−21001.0		

Note: All standard errors are robust.

Table 16.5 Multi-nomial logit regression results for frequency of Internet use to find health information

	Frequency of Internet use (never compared with less often than monthly)			Frequency of Internet use (never compared with monthly)			Frequency of Internet use (never compared with weekly)			Frequency of Internet use (never compared with daily)		
	Coeff	SE	t	Coeff	SE	t	Coeff	SE	t	Coeff	SE	t
hea2	-0.07	0.04	-1.76	0.02	0.07	0.32	-0.15	0.14	-1.08	0.08	0.17	0.48
hea3	-0.18	0.08	-2.15	0.03	0.16	0.18	-0.30	0.13	-2.30	0.06	0.19	0.34
hea4	-0.37	0.21	-1.79	-0.02	0.20	-0.12	-0.09	0.33	-0.28	0.07	0.42	0.15
hea5	-0.19	0.40	-0.47	-0.31	0.56	-0.55	0.56	0.30	1.88	1.21	0.58	2.07
rural	-0.26	0.09	-3.00	-0.17	0.12	-1.36	-0.27	0.16	-1.69	-0.40	0.14	-2.87
age1	1.00	0.19	5.27	1.02	0.21	4.77	1.25	0.18	7.01	1.77	0.32	5.51
age2	0.98	0.16	6.31	1.16	0.12	9.46	1.35	0.14	9.59	1.50	0.28	5.37
age3	0.77	0.15	5.29	0.81	0.16	5.20	1.00	0.11	9.15	1.31	0.31	4.27
male	0.07	0.05	1.31	-0.08	0.10	-0.80	0.02	0.09	0.17	0.48	0.19	2.57
educ1	-1.09	0.14	-7.58	-1.19	0.19	-6.39	-1.18	0.21	-5.55	-1.08	0.33	-3.27
educ2	-0.46	0.07	-6.54	-0.64	0.08	-7.70	-0.42	0.13	-3.31	-0.66	0.17	-3.91
educ4	0.02	0.11	0.19	0.04	0.16	0.23	0.01	0.15	0.04	-0.26	0.17	-1.57
alone	-0.10	0.07	-1.42	-0.23	0.11	-2.06	-0.25	0.14	-1.73	-0.17	0.21	-0.81
Internet	2.09	0.26	8.07	1.45	0.34	4.21	-0.41	0.61	-0.67	-0.43	0.44	-0.97
politic1	-0.06	0.08	-0.76	-0.10	0.08	-1.20	-0.18	0.12	-1.46	0.07	0.13	0.55
politic2	-0.05	0.07	-0.73	-0.14	0.10	-1.36	-0.04	0.13	-0.29	-0.14	0.20	-0.70
Pseudo-R^2	0.095											
Log Likelihood	-20671.4											

Note: All standard errors are robust.

respondents who stopped studying in their twenties being more likely to use the Internet for this reason. Therefore, education increases the likelihood of frequent Internet use for health information. Political affiliation did not emerge as a significant predictor in this model. On the other hand, living in a country with a higher percentage of households with Internet access was found to be positively related to frequency of Internet use for gathering health information.

In order to better understand how these determinants impact the different states of Internet use frequency, we employ a multinomial logit model to examine which determinants most influence the likelihood of electing one response versus another. In this instance, all responses are compared with respondents stating that they never use the Internet to access health information. Table 16.5 displays the results for comparing four responses to 'never using the Internet to find health information.' These four responses are 'less often than monthly,' 'monthly,' 'weekly,' and 'daily.'

Findings from this multi-nomial logit model are largely the same as for the ordered probit one in Table 16.4; however, we do see that being a male makes a respondent more likely to use the Internet daily to access health information, rather than never. On the other hand, gender does not make a significant difference when comparing the likelihood of less frequent usage patterns to never using the Internet for health information. Poor self-perceived health status appears to related to respondents being more likely to use the Internet for health information on a weekly or daily basis, rather than never. Results with regards to living alone also stand out when examining the determinants of differing responses to frequency of Internet use for health information. Those respondents who live alone are less likely to use the Internet monthly or weekly compared with never using the Internet for this purpose. The finding does not hold true for the 'never use' versus 'daily use' model. Percentage of households in a respondent's country with access to the Internet also seems to positively impact upon Internet use (less than monthly, monthly) versus never using the Internet, but there is no impact at a more consistent level of Internet use (weekly, daily) for obtaining health information.

Discussion

By looking at both the frequency with which individuals use online resources for health information we can understand which respondent characteristics translate into higher costs associated with using the Internet as a health resource. Our findings highlight that those respondents who live in a country where a higher percentage of households have Internet access, are more likely to use the Internet to meet health information needs. The typical profile of an Internet user searching for health information is a healthy, younger, male, from an urban area and educated into their twenties, which suggests that the use of internet might be driven by prevention besides curative reasons. Findings with regards to health status are the opposite of those found in Bundorf et al. (2004) where those with poor health status were more likely to use the Internet for health information. However, results regarding the impact of education on Internet use as a health resource are similar to those of Bundorf et al. (2004).

Our findings are not surprising given more familiarity among populations under 60 years with the Internet, those living in an urban area having more readily available Internet access, especially at high speeds, those in countries with a higher percentage of households with Internet access being more likely to have Internet access, and those with at least some higher education being more experience with the Internet both from their education and the type of employment in which they are more likely to be involved. Therefore, these characteristics appear to lower the transaction costs associated with using the Internet as a resource for health matters. This same group of individuals are also more likely to be familiar with the Internet and computer use in general, and thus more comfortable getting online and manoeuvring around the Internet.

The likelihood of the Internet becoming the main source of health information for the general population is small given the traditional value placed on the doctor–patient relationship, as well as the doctor's ability to discuss a patient's individual situation. However, as health resources available on the Internet become more tailored to specific disease groups and patient characteristics, our finding regarding how patients elect other sources as their main source of information, rather than the Internet, may no longer hold true. Increased uptake of quality health information being gathered through the Internet could also alter the way health systems disseminate information as with the increasing use of disease management and patient self-management care programmes monitored and designed by medical professionals, the doctor's role as a direct information source could be diminished without jeopardizing patient care.

This study meets several limitations, largely driven by the use of a secondary data source. Having information about whether respondents owned or had access to a computer, and the Internet would have better controlled for a significant transaction cost related to using the Internet as an information source. We were able to (roughly) proxy for this kind of effect using country level data about the percentage of households with Internet access in a respondent's country, but a question in the survey about individual respondents' access to the Internet would have better captured this transaction costs. Additionally, although education could act as a socioeconomic proxy, a more direct income variable would have allowed this study to answer questions about the use of the Internet for more economically disadvantaged population sub-groups.

Conclusions

This chapter has revisited some of the existing conceptualization of how individuals learn and update their knowledge for health purposes drawing from the example of the Internet as an information technology.

One of the main problems in garnering health information through the Internet is that of potentially unobservable levels of quality (Jaddad and Galiardi 1998). Therefore, in addition to the time and search costs resulting from using the Internet to gather specific information, one might include credibility costs in the bundle of potential limitations of information search. In order to provide a guarantee that information is trustworthy, efforts should increasingly be made to ease collaboration with those agents with a specific interest, such as a certain disease group. To an even greater extent, medical professionals who wish to reduce 'information visits' could collaborate to offer an effective Internet-based substitute for these visits. The current model of specific disease and condition-focused sites enables interactions of patients and medical professionals within each group and across the patient–doctor divide. Hundreds of sufferers of a condition reporting symptoms and treatment experiences provide a helpful resource to the medical community. In this way, health information on the Internet can aid both patients and the medical professionals who treat them.

If health information is a collective good that can be individualized through the intervention of a health care professional or through Internet search, then some of the costs attached to using the Internet for health information can be diminished. As more individuals use the Internet to access health information, transaction costs will drop across all population groups as traffic will flow more towards credible, useful sites and away from those deemed of little or no value. In this way, individuals can rely on the internal Internet market for traffic to help establish appropriateness of content.

The Internet offers a tool for changing the way the general population, medical profession, health policy makers, and health system managers approach the delivery and consumption of health care. While the current state of the general population's usage of the Internet for health information remains fairly weak, concerted efforts to lower the costs faced by patients when trying to access information online will improve the likelihood of this source ever being used effectively. The Internet provides a means to gather research about and better understand patient experience and medical practice through the volumes of information catalogued by online users. Efforts on the part of all health system actors, including patients to offer timely and accurate, as well as easily accessible information online can open up health information to individuals who may not find going to the doctor difficult or do not need to be going to the doctor and thus save health system funds.

References

Bundorf MK, Baker L, Singuer S and Wagner T (2004). *Consumer demand for health information on the Internet.* NBER Working Paper 10.386.

Cauley SD (1987). The time price of medical care. *Review of Economics & Statistics*, **69**, 59–66.

Cline R and Haynes K (2001). Consumer health information seeking on the internet: the state of the art. *Health Education Research*, **16**, 671–92.

Coffey RM (1983). The effect of time price on the demand for medical care services. *Journal of Human Resources*, **18**, 407–24.

Cotton S and Gupta SS (2004). Characteristics of online and offline health information seekers and factors that discriminate between them. *Social Science and Medicine*, **59**, 1795–806.

Fuchs D, Guidorossi G and Svensson P (1995). Support for the democratic system. In: H Klingemann and D Fuchs, eds. *Citizens and the state*, pp. 323–54. Oxford, Oxford University Press.

Goldsmith J (2000). How will internet change our health system? *Health Affairs*, **19**, 148–56.

Grossman M (1972). On the concept of health capital and the demand for health. *Journal of Political Economy*, **80**, 223–55.

Haas-Wilson D (2001). Arrow and the information market failure in health care: the changing content and sources of health care information. *Journal of Health Politics, Policy and Law*, **26**, 1031–42.

Hayek F (1937). Economics of Knowledge. *Economica*, **4**, 33–54.

Helmstädler E (2003). *The economics of knowledge sharing. A new institutional approach*. Cheltenham, Edward Elgar.

Hsieh CR and Lin SJ (1997). Health information and the demand for preventive care among the elderly in Taiwan. *Journal of Human Resources*, **32**, 308–33.

Impiciatore P and Pandolfini C (1997). Reliability of health information for the public on the World Wide Web: systematic survey of advice on managing fever in children at home. *British Medical Journal*, **314**, 1875–9.

Inglehart R (1990). *Cultural shift in advanced industrial society*. Princeton, Princeton University Press.

Jadad AR and Gagliardi A (1998). Rating health information on the Internet to knowledge or to Babel? *Journal of the American Medical Association* **279**, 611–14.

Kenkel D (1990). Consumer health information and the demand for medical care. *Review of Economics & Statistics*, **72**, 587–95.

Lester J, Prady S, Finegan Y and Hoch D. (2004). Learning from e-patients at Massachusetts General Hospital. *British Medical Journal*, **328**, 1188–90.

Lleras-Muney A (2005). The relationship between education and adult mortality in the US. *Review of Economic Studies*, **72**, 189–221.

McGuire TG (2000). Physician agency. In: AJ Culyer and JP Newhouse, eds. *Handbook of health economics*, Vol. 1A, pp. 461–528. Amsterdam, Elsevier Science, BV.

Patrick K (2000). Information technology and the future of preventive medicine: potential, pitfalls and policy. *American Journal of Preventive Medicine*, **19**, 132–5.

Schmitt H and Holmberg S (1995). Political parties in decline? In: H Klingemann and D Fuchs, eds. *Citizens and the state*, pp. 95–134. Oxford, Oxford University Press.

Shackley P and Ryan M (1994). What is the role of the consumer in health care? *Journal of Social Policy*, **23**, 517–36.

Smihily M (2007). *Internet usage in 2007: households and individuals*, Eurostat stat in focus. Available at: http://epp.eurostat.ec.europa.eu/cache/ITY_OFFPUB/KS-QA-07-023/EN/KS-QA-07-023-EN.PDF

Tu HT and Hargraves JL (2003). Seeking health care information: most consumers still on the sidelines. *Center for Studying Health Systems Change*, 1–4.

Wagner TH and Greenlick MR (2001). When parents have access to health information, does it affect pediatric utilization? *Medical Care*, **39**, 848–55.

Wagner T, Hu T and Hibbard JH (2001a). The demand for consumer health information. *Journal of Health Economics*, **20**, 1059–75.

Wagner TH, Hibbard JH, Greenlick MR and Kunkel L (2001b). Does providing health information affect self-reported utilization? Evidence from the Communities Project. *Medical Care*, 836–47.

Waldfogel J. (2003). Preference externalities: an empirical study of who benefits whom in differentiated product markets. *RAND Journal of Economics*.

Weyland K (2002). *The diffusion of innovations: a theoretical analysis*, paper presented at the Annual Meeting of the American Political Science Association, August 28. Boston, Massachusetts. Available at: http://www.allacademic.com/meta/p65140_index.html

Williams RL (2000). A note on robust variance estimation for cluster-correlated data. *Biometrics*, **56**, 645–6.

Zarcadoolas C, Blanco M, Boyer JF and Pleasant A (2002). Unweaving the Web: an exploratory studyofflow-literateadults'navigationskillsConclusionsontheWorldWideWeb.*JournalofHealth Communication*, 7, 309–25.

Chapter 17

Institutional pathways for integrating genetic testing into mainstream health care

Hristina Petkova

Introduction

This chapter considers how new knowledge generated by advances in science can be assimilated into public health care systems, allowing quicker integration of new technology into routine care. An example is drawn from the treatment of diabetes in two very different health care systems: Germany and the UK.

Diabetes is a disorder caused by deficiency in the pancreatic production of insulin, a hormone needed to transfer glucose from the bloodstream into the body's cells, where it can be stocked and converted into energy when necessary. Low levels of the insulin hormone results in increased levels of sugar in the blood, which can damage many of the body's systems, in particular the blood vessels and nerves (Department of Noncommunicable Disease Surveillance, World Health Organization, 1999). Chronic elevation of blood glucose, even when no symptoms are present to alert the individual to the presence of the disorder, eventually leads to tissue damage, with consequent, often serious disease. Complications are often devastating, and affect the kidneys, eyes, heart, brain, and lower limbs. While ill health is a major aspect to patients of the burden associated with diabetes, ensuing financial cost puts additional strain on health systems around the world, particularly as a consequence of stable increase in occurrence, with type two diabetes being the most prevalent group, which constitutes from 85 to 95 per cent of all diabetes cases (Department of Noncommunicable Disease Surveillance, World Health Organization 1999). Estimations of the cost incurred by diabetes report 5–9 per cent of the total healthcare budget in the UK (McGuire 1996), with projections that by 2025 this could reach 25 per cent of total NHS expenditure (Currie *et al.* 1997).

In an attempt to address the problem through possible early detection, and thus improve prevention and treatment, scientists worldwide have been involved in an intensive research effort to understand the underlying causes of diabetes. A significant step forward in this direction has been made over the past 15 years, with the identification of single genes, mutations that are responsible for monogenic types of diabetes (such as MODY), associated with a defect in insulin production, but where the pancreas has kept a limited capacity to produce its own insulin (Fajans 1990; Malecki 2005).

This has meant that people with the condition who have remained undetected, misdiagnosed as having a different type of diabetes, or treated on insulin prior to the scientific discovery, have recently been shown to be highly sensitive to alternative forms of treatment, such as tablets, or healthy diet and exercise alone, enabling many of them to achieve excellent glycaemic control with less insulin injections or none at all (Pearson *et al.* 2003; Shepherd *et al.* 2004). As research suggests, changes in clinical management permitted by the awareness of monogenic diabetes has led to better quality of life for patients (Shepherd *et al.* 2001, 2004), as well as to considerable cost savings from a public health system perspective (Anderson *et al.* 2006). Therefore, diagnosis for MODY can be conceptualized as a clear example of how newly generated knowledge of disease aetiology can influence treatment in a positive way. Before the discussion continues to explore the ways in which healthcare institutions make sense of innovation in diabetes diagnostics, it is important to explain why testing for MODY is so important.

Maturity-onset diabetes of the young (MODY) is often classed as a monogenetic subtype of type 2 diabetes, characterized by a young age of onset, typically under 25, non-insulin dependence, and family history of the condition (Shepherd *et al.* 2001; Stride and Hattersley 2002; http://www.projects.ex.ac.uk/diabetesgenes/gdn/index. htm 2005). MODY is estimated to represent between 1 and 2 per cent of people with diabetes[1] (http://www.projects.ex.ac.uk/diabetesgenes/gdn/index.htm 2005). Since 1992, mutations in six genes have been identified and linked to the condition, each of which is expressed in a different clinical picture. People with glucokinase mutations, for instance, have mildly raised blood sugar levels from birth, with little complications in later life and, generally, no need for insulin injections or drug treatment (Pearson *et al.* 2003). While this particular subtype is often viewed as a mild form of diabetes and rarely requires treatment, in children it may be misdiagnosed as type 1 diabetes, which is why a genetic diagnosis plays a crucial role in confirming the sub-group, in avoiding mistakes and in enabling doctors to choose the best regimen for the individual.

Another example of the importance to define the exact type of MODY through molecular analysis is the case of patients with a mutation in the hepatocyte nuclear factor 1 alpha gene (HNF1a). They are usually born with normal blood glucose, but develop diabetes between the ages of 10 and 25, and can often be misdiagnosed as having type 1 diabetes, due to similarity in the phenotypic pictures between the two conditions—slim, young age of onset, and high blood glucose levels (Stride and Hattersley 2002). Patients with this subtype of MODY are known to be particularly sensitive to the effect of sulphonylurea tablets with implications for their treatment (Pearson *et al.* 2003). As a result, they often achieve better glycaemic control on a very small dose of tablets compared with insulin injections (Shepherd *et al.* 2001).

Genetic testing as a case study

With such deeper insight into the genetics of diabetes as science has gained, a new, highly differential molecular test has become possible, which is able to distinguish between subtle nuances of one conditions and to recognize one out of six genetic

---

[1] In the UK this equals 20,000 people

mutations, each with a specific clinical expression and prone to benefit a different treatment formula. An opportunity emerges for medicine to use this sharpened diagnostic lens and to offer case-adjusted, improved diabetes care for patients. It also presents scientists and doctors with a tool for re-classification of a disorder conceptualized until very recently broadly as either Type 1 or Type 2 diabetes, which now has accurate subdivisions into narrow sub-types with different outcomes in each case, knowledge of which permits changes in clinical management, improved quality of life at the individual level and reductions in health care costs.

Bringing science out of the laboratory and into the clinic to the patient's benefit seems far from straightforward. Transformation of a new procedure into daily medical use is not a linear process. Whether and exactly how a diagnostic test is practically implemented, its potential fully realized depends largely upon the response it receives from the health care institutions of its emergence. They provide the setting, where genomic knowledge interacts with daily clinical care through unique structures of professional networks and power relations.

One part of the diffusion equation is constituted by the clear realization of the benefits to be had from differential diagnosis of MODY. The opposite end, however, appears to be occupied by a complex integral of institutional, socio-economic, and ethical factors, among which the general sensitivity around genetics associated with fear about breach of confidentiality, privacy, and possible discrimination and stigmatization in the areas of insurance and employment. While there are good reasons to assume unobstructed translation into practice of a molecular test for monogenic diabetes as it can only establish correct diagnosis with the intention to facilitate better treatment, and therefore is unlikely to cause further harm, policies of clinical implementation appear to apply a generally cautious approach regardless. This has an audible, albeit remote effect on the speed and degree of routine test implementation in Germany, for example, where the 'Gene Diagnostics Bill' has been held on pause by several governments and still is, largely because of seemingly little willingness to deal with ethically charged issues or to commit to long-term decisions on extremely dynamic fields of research.

These considerations constituting just one facet of genetics, abundant further evidence comes to suggest that medical innovation cannot remain a neutral zone. There are multiple interests involved in it, from individual actors, such as senior scientists, doctors, and patients, to governments, state institutions, commercial companies, and insurers, all with significant parts to play in decisions about which genetic technologies get developed and which do not, which receive funding, and which are not automatically reimbursed, how tests are regulated, monitored, and implemented clinically or not at all offered to patients.

The interplay among these and other factors takes place within different healthcare contexts and is therefore determined by each system's organizational set-up, funding mechanisms, value foundations, and principles, on its established routes for service implementation, its core aims. A snapshot of the extent to which innovation in medicine is interwoven into the institutional fabric of healthcare can be presented through the example of the UK with its centralized health care system, where money can be re-allocated from the general budget to genetic medicine with relative ease, should the evidence support this. This is in contrast to the case in Germany, where government and health ministry oversee, rather than manage healthcare and leave the provision of services, including fund distribution, to self-regulating non-governmental associations of physicians and insurers, as the actors directly involved in health care, and placed in the best position to deal with its delivery. Within a setting such as this, based on 'corporatist' principles, matters are better described as market-driven, rather than centrally determined, where patient groups are broadly opposed to genetic testing for fear of misuse of genetic data by government and insurers, and where private genetics laboratories operate in a competitive, rather than collaborative environment.

This line of thinking encourages the hypothesis that an identical technology, such as MODY diagnosis is likely to be adopted along diverging trajectories in two different environments, the UK and Germany. One is facilitated by the presence of a central authority under the NHS, the UK Genetic testing network (GTN), well situated to govern the process of innovation diffusion into practice through robust entry requirements, e.g. 'gene dossier', commissioning arrangements with the Genetics Commissioning Advisory Group (GenCAG), catalogue listing, etc. (http://www.ukgtn.nhs.uk/gtn/UKGTN-information/What-is-the-UKGTN.html). Management of MODY testing through a single referral centre for the whole of Britain, with close links between the laboratory and the diabetes clinic, can also be viewed in direct correlation to the centralized mode of national care, transposed on to the process of technology diffusion. The same diagnostic procedure is operationalized in a delegated manner in Germany, distributed among a number of independent laboratories offering genetic tests for MODY with clear lines of separation from each other and from clinical care. The dispersed model of service provision reflects both the federal structure of the German state, and the principle of corporatism (delegating powers to professional non-government actors).

In recapitulation, MODY is a monogenic sub-group of type 2 diabetes, caused by mutations in six identified genes. Genetic analysis of the precise type of the condition carries important implications for treatment due to the unique clinical outcomes of each underlying genetic factor. Laboratory testing allows the detection of the specific gene involved, providing thus an opportunity for alternative medical regimen to be administered by discontinuation of insulin in favour of tablets or simply by dietary alterations. The ways in which this new knowledge becomes integrated in mainstream care for patients hinges upon a variety of factors, such as regulatory requirements for genetic testing, funding mechanism of services, referral pattern, to name, but a few. They constitute the operating environment within which a medical innovation materializes in clinical use. In view of the fact that each such environment is knitted into a specific institutional structure of health care provision, pre-determined by a nation's political and legal system, historical background, traditional values, power distribution between actors, etc., the question arises as to how it is exactly that all these factors create two different contexts for the functioning of an identical new technology. To re-define the problem, advances in genetics achieved as a uniform effort to counter the burden of diabetes, appear to translate into medical use through distinct mechanisms of healthcare delivery.

Thus described, the picture gives only a flavour of the ways, in which two different health institutions adopt a novel genetic technology. The discussion now turns to a more exhaustive overview of the subject.

Different healthcare structures: different response to medical innovation

Although it is difficult to strictly isolate different types of healthcare systems, since most institutions adopt a combined approach to funding, organization, and delivery of services, three general categories emerge (Lee 1994):

- National health systems (Beveridge model).
- Sickness fund/social insurance systems (Bismarck model).
- Private insurance systems.

As the paper focuses on the health care institutions in the UK and Germany, which belong to the national and social insurance category respectively, some main features of the first two general types are presented in Table 17.1(Rothgang et al. 2005).

The British healthcare institution, with its largely centralized structure, vertical lines of accountability and state funding through budgetary distribution, belongs to the National Health Service model (Beveridge). It is also characterized by universal coverage, general tax-based mechanism of financing, and national ownership and control of the factor of production. A summary of the main points is presented below.

National Health Service (NHS), Britain: main principles

- Beveridge model.
- Universal coverage.
- General tax-based funding.
- National ownership and control of the factors of production.
- Vertical lines of accountability (managed by the Department of Health, which sets overall policy on health issues).

Table 17.1

	Financing	Service provision	Regulation	Country examples
National Health Service	Public: taxes according to income (direct taxes) and consumption	Public providers	Dominating regulation mechanism: hierarchical, planning, and tight control by the state	Finland, Italy, Portugal, Spain, Sweden, UK, Serbia/Montenegro
Social Insurance System	Public: contributions according to income	Private and public providers	Dominating regulation mechanism: collective bargaining, legal framework and some control by the state	Czech Republic, France, Germany, Lithuania

Source: Rothgang et al. (2005).

With a more balanced approach in terms of power sharing between central and local authorities, and with mixed service delivery between private and public providers, public healthcare in Germany belongs to the statutory insurance model (Bismarck model). Some further features comprise compulsory coverage of the major part of the population (90%), mandatory contributions paid jointly by the insured person and the employer, and collected by self-regulating insurance funds, which purchase care on behalf of their members. Healthcare provision is delegated almost entirely to self-administered professional associations of doctors at the local Länder [2] level, and ownership of the factors of production combines private and public sources.

Statutory Health Insurance (SHI), Germany: main principles

- Bismarck model.
- Compulsory universal coverage.
- Mandatory contributions (paid jointly by the insured and the employer and collected by self-regulating insurance funds, which purchase care on behalf of their members).
- Public/private ownership of factors of production.
- Federalism (sharing of powers between the Federal government, the Lander and the corporatist bodies).
- Corporatism (decision-making powers delegated to non-governmental corporatist bodies)
- Multiple self-regulated actors (insurers, physicians, hospitals).
- Clear separation between inpatient (hospital) and outpatient (office-based physicians) sector
- Sideline position of government.

Two important features of the German political system are worth noting, which are reflected in healthcare as well, namely (1) federalism, or sharing of powers between the Federal government, the 16 states, and the professional associations; and (2) corporatism, i.e. decision-making is delegated largely to non-governmental corporatist bodies of physicians, as providers, and insurers, as purchasers. Within this context, the government has a relatively marginal position to issue regulations and guidance, as well as to oversee compliance. It is detached from immediate involvement in healthcare in terms of funding, budget negotiation, allocation, and service delivery, all of which are managed by sickness funds and physician associations. As self-governing bodies of actors directly concerned with the provision of patient care, insurance companies and doctors are considered best equipped to operate the health system.

The British and the German institutions thus described, each finds its roots in the particular circumstances of the country's social and political past, with values, such as equality, solidarity, individual or communal responsibility, firmly interconnected in a

---

[2] Land (singular), Länder (plural), translation from German 'State', i.e. each of 16 Federal States.

'stable, recurring pattern of behaviour' (Huntington 1968; Malecki 1995). Created in 1948 in the wake of World War II, the NHS, for example, strongly upheld the principles of equity and fairness and institutionalized collective responsibility for health by establishing a central structure in charge [European Observatory on Health Care Systems (EOHCS) Copenhagen 1999].

Founded over half a century earlier, in 1883, the German health care system was a product of different circumstances. It came into existence as a result of the two-fold political aspirations of Chancellor Otto von Bismark, first, to provide the growing economy with a healthy workforce and, secondly, to ensure employees' loyalty to the state. Similarly to the NHS, it was based on the principles of collective responsibility and solidarity, but it also mirrored features of the pre-existing mutual aid societies[3] (sickness funds), with the clear assertion from the start, that the government should be allocated a marginal role, and that health care management should be left mainly to the professional associations of doctors and insurers (EOHCS Copenhagen 2000). The corporatist principle has been strongly maintained to date.

Thus embedded in history on the one hand, and as environments where new medical technologies emerge on the other, health institutions face a challenge—to continue already long-standing traditions and structures, while accommodating, at the same time, changes in medicine through flexible response mechanisms. The balance between these two strategies, between 'old' institutions (health care system) and 'new' demands (genetic testing), depends on the individual circumstances of each structure, on the level of government involvement in genetics research, funding policy and support, on the distribution of service provision between private and public actors, on the referral procedure, on the quality assurance mechanisms, etc. Just like healthcare systems are built around markedly different agendas in Britain and Germany in terms of funding, organizational pattern and delivery despite exposure to similar economic, demographic, and technological pressures, so would decisions about the transfer of bioscience from the laboratory to the clinic diverge in analogous ways between the two countries, reiterating once again the underlying principles of health care provision and perpetuating the discreteness in national models of managing health care.

The two public institutions characterized above, form the scaffolding for new diagnostic methods to diffuse through structures, where consolidated communities of practice (e.g. scientific expert networks, self-regulated bodies of physicians, and insurers) intersect with current challenges (e.g. growing pressure for cost containment, advances in technology, etc.), as well as with the political commitment by governments to contain health expenditure, while maintaining patient access to latest medical equipment within a robust, but accommodating regulatory framework. Any attempt to balance between these competing priorities creates a country-specific locus for the development of new knowledge. As a result, innovation co-develops with social, economic, and political networks at the meso-level of health-care structures (Vaughan 1999).

---

[3] Created prior to the establishment of the national health insurance, the mutual aid societies were run by employers, employees or both. The so called 'dues' were collected form members, and access to medical services was provided in return.

Results

Table 17.2 gives a brief illustration of some of the ways in which the outlined features of each healthcare system has implications for the institutional uptake of genetic testing for MODY.

The table above presents preliminary results from a doctoral study, which will not be expanded upon here due to volume limitations. Instead, several finings are selected and described in more detail, with the aim of illustrating how the production and utilization in mainstream care of a novel diagnostic procedure in diabetes is enacted in the British and the German health care systems, and based onw the routes that the technology takes in these systems, to understand how innovation is shaped by features of each institution.

Table 17.2 Implications of individual characteristics of health systems for genetic testing

Parameters for comparison	United Kingdom National Health Service	Germany Statutory Health Insurance
Research expertise	Concentrated	Spread across several teams
Structure of MODY test provision	Public NHS single referral centre (1 laboratory) Centralized	Private practices (16 laboratories), some university clinics and institutes of human genetics Dispersed
Interaction between clinical and laboratory services	Close relationship, constant flow of information between laboratory scientists and clinicians	Less direct association between laboratory staff and clinicians (competition)
Referral for testing and patient access	'Gate-keeping' through GP and geneticist (testing is done selectively only for suspected MODY cases which match clinical criteria)	'Gate keeping' exists to a lesser extent through bargaining for reimbursement of test Direct financial interest in greater numbers of MODY analyses by specialized private laboratories; Two-tier system of test provision (SHI- and privately insured patients)
Budgeting and reimbursement of MODY test	Cost of genetic testing for MODY calculated 'in house' by the testing laboratory Test paid by referring Primary Care Trust (PCT) Intention to move towards a tariff	Cost calculated according to a floating point value system with reference to a central unified scale (EBM) Test paid by sickness fund/ private patient Intention to move towards a tariff

Table 17.2 (continued) Implications of individual characteristics of health systems for genetic testing

Parameters for comparison	United Kingdom National Health Service	Germany Statutory Health Insurance
Quality assessment and regulation	Compulsory, specific requirements for single-gene disorders	Voluntary: general laboratory license with the German Accreditation Council (DAR)
	'Gene dossier" UK GTN	General compliance with professional guidelines (BVDH)
	CPA accreditation	
	EU initiatives (e.g. EMQN)	EU initiatives (e.g. EMQN)
Transfer of testing procedure from research project to clinical service	Upon completion of research stage test remains within the NHS and retains its integrated structure from the research stage	Upon completion of research stage test is "exported" from university clinic/institute of human genetics to office-based outpatient sector
	Genetic diabetes nurses (previously MODY link nurses), dedicated educational initiative for integration of testing in diabetes care	MODY Link Nurse analogue not feasible due to:
		Hierarchical subordination in the medical profession; different role of nurses
		Limited or no access to patient records
Readily available information from researcher's perspective	Relatively easy to access; single thread	Relatively difficult to access; multiple threads and sources
General political, historical and socio-economic environment for genetics with repercussions on genetic testing	Favourable, pro-genetic policy by government e.g. commitment through "White paper on genetics'	Historical endowment: association of genetics to eugenics practices from the past, with resulting fear which translates in reluctance for firm legislation and long-term commitments

Structure of MODY test provision

Molecular genetic diagnosis for MODY is provided within structurally different settings in the UK and Germany. In Germany, MODY testing is delivered in an economy-driven pattern with private laboratories acting as the main providers of the service. Currently there are around 16 private laboratories across Germany, which test for various subtypes of the condition. The majority offer diagnosis for the two most common mutations (HNF1a and glucokinase GCK, respectively, 11 and 10 laboratories), whereas a small number specialize in the rare types of monogenic diabetes (IPF1, 2 laboratories). Some university clinics and institutes of human genetics also provide testing for MODY (e.g. Institut für Humangenetik, Universitätsklinikum Aachen). This used to be more common practice until several years ago, during the research stage of the condition (e.g. Medizinische Klinik III, Universitätsklinikum Carl Gustav

Carus der TU Dresden, Institute of Human Genetics, University of Bonn). Provision of MODY services through university affiliated clinics and research centres faded, however, due to low demand for the test, the high cost involved in the procedure and, therefore, little return of invested resources.

Monogenic diabetes being a relatively rare condition (1–2% of diabetes) of which there is still fairly sparse awareness among physicians, diagnoses are low in frequency, i.e. 1–2 samples referred per laboratory per year (Interview data, PhD thesis unpublished, 2007). The presence of 16 laboratories and few other centres that offer testing means that due to comparatively even distribution of work load between them each receives only a small number of samples to analyse, hence, not much profit margin is achieved, resulting in little incentive to maintain high concentration of expertise. Furthermore, the relocation of test provision from research establishments, such as university clinics to private genetics centres occurs at a point at which financial flows from research grants have almost run out, while expertise in the clinical identification of the condition at the time of completed research projects is high. By this stage, diabetes specialists whose work often builds upon intensive exchange of information with clinical geneticists and scientists, or who themselves combine clinical and research roles, tend to have attained confidence in their ability to make clinical pre-diagnoses, followed by referral to relevant testing facilities, which are economically better situated to conduct diagnosis. As one study participant commented:

> GS9: Testing is being done more easily on an automatic order, when people do larger series, they also do it more efficiently.

This might partly explain why, at present, genetic diagnosis of MODY is available mainly through private laboratories in Germany, with a small proportion of tests still done in institutes for human genetics. In the course of the last 5 years or so, private diagnostic centres have gradually taken over provision from university clinics, research centres, and hospital establishments, as the former are deemed more efficient concentrations of capital. Seen from the perspective of service implementation, transferring gene testing for MODY from research clinics to private companies is a trend symptomatic of the demand-driven approach to health care in Germany. Evidence from a study conducted by the Organization for Economic Cooperation and Development in 2005 points to similar findings, and reveals that commercial laboratories generally provide the more common tests, performed in a straightforward way and which require stable technology.

In the British case, MODY analysis is conducted in a single laboratory, part of the NHS. This is the Peninsula Molecular Genetics Laboratory based at the Royal Devon and Exeter Hospital in Exeter, England. The laboratory was set up in 1995 to provide a molecular genetic testing facility for the Royal Devon & Exeter Trust and the Peninsula Clinical Genetics Service. Testing for MODY has been performed on research basis since 1996 and has been offered to patients as a diagnostic service since 2000. MODY analysis is available for individuals and their families throughout the UK as part of the UK Genetic Testing Network (UK GTN). A number of samples are also received from patients throughout the world (http://www.projects.ex.ac.uk/diabetesgenes/gdn/index.htm 2005).

Private laboratories in Britain do not offer genetic testing for MODY. It is a rare genetic condition the identification and treatment of which is delegated to a national laboratory, with the intention of providing 'high quality genetic testing services for single gene disorders to patients from across the whole of the UK' (http://www.ukgtn. nhs.uk/gtn/UKGTN-information/What-is-the-UKGTN.html). The referral centre for MODY is part of a nationally integrated clinical service, under the UK GTN, which builds on long-standing collaboration between local genetics centres. At the same time, locally, the laboratory is integrated in a regional genetics centre, which includes a clinical genetics service providing counselling and works in collaboration with the university department of human genetics.

The very infrastructure that accommodates genetic diagnosis for monogenic diabetes in the UK requires (through the UK GTN as a central admission point for new tests), and simultaneously encourages (through the presence of a single reference-diagnostic laboratory), close contact between geneticists, consultant diabetologists, counsellors, and specialist diabetes nurses. They operate within immediate physical proximity and work as part of a single entry point to an integrated network of genetics laboratories. Hub-like concentrated institutional settings of this type date back to the 1980s, and tend to foster intense collaboration between laboratory services and clinical medicine. This results in close working relationships between scientists and physicians to ensure the flow of knowledge from research to medical use, as well as relatively fast administration of treatment to patients.

Gradually, it becomes visible how one variable in the implementation process of MODY diagnostics, namely the structure of test provision, plays out differently in two separate health care environments. Within the market-led model in Germany, the procedure is offered largely by specialized private laboratories, which compete for a share of the profit from the supply of a service of limited quantity due to the rare nature of monogenic diabetes. The distribution of MODY diagnostics among multiple stakeholders with vested interests reflects the general pattern of health care delivery in statutory insurance systems, and can be seen in direct correlation to the founding principles of the Bismarck model. Corporatism, i.e. the delegation of powers to non-governmental bodies of insurers and physicians, for instance, explains the absence of intervention by state in-service provision, as well as the demand-driven dispersed mode of test delivery in Germany. A further historical factor that seems to influence the particular way in which MODY test is provided is the observed monopoly held by ambulatory sector practitioners in the provision of outpatient services, one of which genetic testing. This is partly related also to the historical fragmentation between inpatient (hospital) care and outpatient (ambulatory) service.

Federalism, i.e. sharing of powers between the federal government, the separate states (Länder), and the corporatist bodies, is another institutional factor, which affects test provision by way of questioning the existence of a central organization able to facilitate a nation-wide assimilation of MODY into routine clinical care.

Conversely, the hierarchical structure of the British NHS system has implications for the way in which genetic testing is utilized there, through a single institutional hub combining research, diagnostics, and diabetes care. The MODY clinical service was adopted into mainstream care following centrally established entry criteria to the UK GTN catalogue listing NHS molecular genetics services for single-gene disorders (http://www.ukgtn.nhs.uk/gtn/UKGTN-information/What-is-the-UKGTN.html).

These observations of the German and the British enactment of structure of MODY test provision as a parameter for comparison corroborate the hypothesis that translation into practice of MODY testing is determined to a strong degree by institutional characteristics of each health care system. In the German institutional 'ecology' (Consoli *et al.* 2009) corporatism, federalism, the 'monopoly' of the ambulatory sector in service delivery result in a market-driven, dispersed pattern of MODY test provision between multiple genetics centres.

By contrast, the single-centre nationally-integrated model of MODY diagnostics provision in the UK can be seen to reflect the underlying principle of centrality in the NHS. Supervision of genetic tests through the UK GTN furthers the claim that innovation in genetics is largely affected by the vertical structure of the UK health care system. Historical collaboration between scientific research and clinical care is another feature of the British institutional 'ecology', which influences MODY test provision in a regional 'hub' of academic and clinical genetics expertise.

MODY test provision is managed in notably different ways in Germany and in the UK, and is strongly associated with underlying features of the two systems.

Transfer of testing procedure from research project to clinical service

Another parameter of comparison for the analysis of country-specific responses to new genetics is the trajectory followed by MODY diagnostic test from the stage at which it is still a research project to its adoption as a clinical service. This is not to be confused with 'diffusion' of the innovation from research into practice altogether, which is the task of the thesis as a whole. Instead, the current variable is limited in time to the point at which research funding for the experimental phase of testing stops and the search for alternative means to sustain the service are contemplated.

The UK and Germany share some steps along this first stage of the implementation process for MODY testing. One point of convergence is at the initial phase of test development, during research, which in both countries begins at clinically-integrated public departments of human genetics, with high concentration of expertise in the UK and more dispersed knowledge-production in Germany. In both systems, funding is finite, and once it is discontinued and research concludes, diagnostics is passed over to the next level. It is at this 'transfer' stage that the innovation shifts directions between the UK and Germany. Whereas genetic testing for MODY remains within the NHS, as a service, well-integrated in its initial location, in Germany it is mostly 'exported' from the development setting to the private sector, as a commercially-viable context for more efficient service provision.

A landmark in the diffusion process of MODY testing through the NHS is a designated educational initiative proposed by the referral centre for monogenic diabetes in Exeter and funded by the Department of Health (DoH). Its purpose is to introduce the diagnostic procedure to health professionals, and to disseminate awareness, first, of the condition and, secondly, of the availability of a test able to confirm or rule out the presence of genetic mutations. Implementation in this way is secured through an ongoing MODY link nurse programme, which started 5 years ago and was renamed as 'genetic diabetes nurses' in 2007 to incorporate additional types of monogenic diabetes, i.e. neonatal diabetes (http://www.projects.ex.ac.uk/diabetesgenes/gdn/index.htm (accessed on 10 May 2005)). It involves 11 diabetes specialist nurses, who receive training about genetic sub-groups of type 2 diabetes and about methods to test for these. Each nurse is based within a different region in the UK. The aim, within the specific area of responsibility is to increase and update the knowledge of the local medical teams about the different types of monogenic diabetes, and the available diagnostic methods. This has been achieved by through presentations at diabetes centres, as well as at regional meetings. The nurses assist in identifying families who are likely to have the condition and the type of test that would be most appropriate. They can also discuss the implications of genetic testing with individuals and their families, and guide follow-up services for those affected once results are received. The project has been in operation in the UK since 2002 and has proved a successful model for the integration of molecular genetic testing into diabetes care (Shepherd and Hattersley 2004).

No similar initiative exists in Germany. Its feasibility is questionable in the context of clear role separation between medical doctors and nurses, with the prevailing perception that projects, such as a potential educational initiative in monogenic diabetes, falls within the professional remit of trained physicians, rather than nurses. This is broadly bound to 'genetic exceptionalism' and to the conviction that highly sensitive issues stemming from genetics research and diagnostics require specialized medical qualifications at the very least. Another reason for which a project such as the MODY link nurse initiative is difficult to operationalize within the German healthcare structure is the historically embedded policy boundary between federal ministry and local, state health authorities. According to the principle of federalism, the provision of health care including diagnostic procedures for diabetes, comes under the control of local states not of central authorities. This distribution of powers presents a barrier to the creation of any programme that requires single-centre management and central co-ordination.

With regards to the variable 'research-service transfer' examined here, there are clear points of divergence between the British and the German health care systems. The service for MODY in the UK remained at the same integrated regional centre, comprising a diagnostic laboratory, clinical genetics facility, and academic department where the test was first developed. It is also within the established 'hub' of expertise that the MODY link educational initiative began and which remains the training core for specialist nurses. Provision of MODY diagnostics and distribution of knowledge about the procedure from a single publicly-run 'nucleus' relates largely to the centralized NHS structure, to the principles of equity and solidarity underpinning the system as a whole, but also the organization in charge of genetics tests, namely the UK GTN. Keeping a specialized genetic test within the public domain under the purview of state regulations ensures firstly that the diagnosis is accessible as an NHS service by all patients who might need it, therefore, precluding a two-tier provision in the public and private sector, and secondly that quality is monitored in a compulsory way. Another factor that enhances specialization in MODY testing at a single locus is the close proximity and constant liaison between the diagnostic laboratory, the clinical setting, and the academic department allowing uninhibited flow of information from research to diabetes care, as well as feedback from the clinic back to the laboratory. This can be seen as an institutionally pre-conditioned influence from already established communities of research practice in the NHS.

The trajectory followed by the testing procedure from its development stage to service is different in the German context, where it 'exits' the academic domain and 'enters' the private sector as a commercially viable environment for service provision. This relates to the markedly specialized nature of outpatient care in Germany, where medical doctors of any discipline can establish office-based private practice, e.g. cardiologists, gynaecologists, geneticists, etc. Another factor that appears to facilitate the transfer of innovation to the private outpatient sector as a main delivery locus is that ambulatory care retains monopoly for the provision of outpatient services, including genetic testing, which goes back to the historical separation between in- and out-patient care in Germany.

Therefore, the second variable explored here, i.e. research-service transfer of MODY testing shows that there is an underlying association between assimilation of the innovation and structural characteristics of each health care system.

Access to data by the researcher

During the data collection stage of the study, an interesting point of difference emerged between the UK and Germany in terms of the ease of access to information. A relatively consistent body of literature in the UK, such as scientific publications and the discussions about them, as well as readily available policy documents, contrast some difficulties experienced in obtaining details about the German case. Contact with the research team in England was made almost immediately after the project started, and meeting observations and interviews followed soon after. The process of obtaining initial information about the actors involved in genetic testing for MODY in Germany was much slower. This is partly due to the presence of several scientific teams, diabetologists, and university departments working on monogenic diabetes, as opposed to more concentrated expertise on MODY in the UK case.

Another reason for the difference in research data availability between the two countries could be ascribed to the dispersed structure of test provision in Germany, where it is shared between a number of private laboratories and other centres, in contrast to a single referral point for MODY diagnosis in the UK. Responses from a few study participants concurred with this conclusion. Interviewees, themselves insiders to diabetes research were hardly able to come up with an exhaustive list of names and projects on MODY in Germany. When asked 'could you point me in further directions?', or 'is there a research team in diabetes which works exclusively on MODY' each respondent reported a different name, a different project, and a different testing centre.

Conclusions

Following advances in the scientific understanding of some major underlying genetic factors of diabetes, molecular analysis of monogenic diabetes has emerged as a new diagnostic tool in medicine. It enables physicians to distinguish between six subtypes of MODY, and to change the treatment of patients according to the specific clinical outcomes of each mutation from insulin interruption after years of injections, to diet alterations, with ensuing benefits for patients in terms of better quality of life, and for health care systems in terms of the opportunity to avoid complications and reduce the cost of treating those.

The way in which this innovation is operationalized by health care systems and integrated in mainstream care depends upon the interplay among various actors, such as geneticists, general physicians, and specialists, commissioners, insurers, private and public laboratories, and policy-making figures. The patterns of interaction between these stakeholders have implications for the varying routes of MODY test provision in the UK and Germany. The two countries are interesting examples of distinctly separate healthcare contexts (centralized, single-centre led approach in the UK versus delegated, multi-provider distributed method in Germany) despite shared values and exposure to similar socio-economic challenges (ageing populations, rising health care costs, higher expectations, and growing demands for the latest state-of-the-art medical technology).

Differences in the organization, funding, and delivery of care generally, is seen to persist in the area of genetic innovation. The institutional take-up of testing for MODY as a single gene disorder with highly differential diagnosis and established clinical implications for alternative treatment, shows strong association with the general pattern of the healthcare structures (top-down in UK versus horizontal in Germany). The implementation trajectories for MODY diagnosis in the two countries diverge at several points, from research expertise (concentrated, UK versus dispersed, Germany), pattern of provision (public versus private; centralized versus dispersed), to diffusion channels in mainstream service (testing remains within initial NHS research setting in the UK, with added designated model MLN initiative; testing moves from university based research to commercial setting in Germany).

References

Anderson R, Hattersley A, Shepherd M, Ellard S (2006). *Screening infants with permanent neo-natal diabetes for Kir6.2 mutations: life-time cost savings and preliminary analysis of the MODY Link Nurse scheme within the NHS*. Economics of Genetic Technologies (ESRC seminar), Manchester, May 2006.

Consoli D, McMeekin A, Metcalfe JS, Mina A and Ramlogan R (2009) The process of health care innovation: problem sequences, systems and symbiosis, Chapter 2, this volume.

Currie CJ, Kraus D, Mogan C. LI, Gill L, Stott NCH, Peters JR (1997). NHS acute sector expenditure for diabetes: the present, future and excess in-patient cost of care. *Diabetic Medicine*, **14**, 686–92.

Department of Noncommunicable Disease Surveillance, World Health Organization (1999). *Definition, diagnosis and classification of diabetes mellitus and its complications*, WHO/NCD/NCS/99.2. Geneva, WHO. Available at: http://www.diabetes.com.au/pdf/who_report.pdf (accessed 7 April 2005).

Diabetes Atlas Executive Summary, International Diabetes Federation IDF. (2006). Available at: http://www.idf.org/e-atlas (accessed on 13 March 2006).

European Observatory on Health Care Systems EOHCS Copenhagen (1999). *Health care systems in transition: United Kingdom*, AMS 5001890 Target 19. Available at: http://www.euro.who.int/document/e68283.pdf (accessed on 14 June 2003).

European Observatory on Health Care Systems EOHCS Copenhagen (2000). *Health care systems in transition: Germany*, AMS 5012667 (DEU) Target 19. Available at: http://www.euro.who.int/document/e68952.pdf (accessed on 3 July 2003).

Fajans SS (1990). Scope and heterogeneous nature of MODY. *Diabetes Care*, **13**, 49–64.

Genetic Diabetes Nurses (previously known as MODY Link Nurses), Peninsula Molecular Genetics Laboratory http:/projects.exeter.ac.uk/diabetesgenes/gdn/index.htm (accessed on 10 May 2007).

Huntington SP (1968). *Political order in changing societies*. New Haven, Yale University Press.

Lee K (1994). *Health care systems in Canada & the United Kingdom: can they deliver?* Keele, Keele University Press.

Malecki M (2005). Genetics of type 2 diabetes mellitus. *Diabetes Research and Clinical Practice*, **68**, S10–21.

McCarthy M (2004).Progress in defining the molecular basis of type 2 diabetes mellitus through susceptibility-gene identification. *Human Molecular Genetics*, **13**, Review Issue 1 R33–41.

McGuire A (1996). Economic analysis of diabetes. *Journal of Diabetes and its Complications* **10**, 149–50.

Organization for Economic Co-operation and Development (OECD) (2005). *Quality assurance and proficiency testing for molecular genetic testing: summary results of a survey of 18 OECD member countries*. Available at: http://www.oecd.org/dataoecd/25/12/34779945.pdf (accessed on 3 Sep 2006).

Pearson ER *et al.* (2003). Genetic aetiology of hyperglycaemia determines response to treatment in diabetes. *Lancet*; **362**(9392), 1275–81.

Rothgang H, Cacace M, Grimmeisen S and Wendt C (2005). The changing role of the state in healthcare systems. *European Review*, **13**, 187–212.

Schnyder S, Mullis PE, Ellard S, Hattersley AT and Flück CE (2005). Genetic testing for glucokinase mutations in clinically selected patients with MODY: a worthwhile investment. *Swiss Medical Weekly*, **135**, 352–6.

Shepherd M and Hattersley AT (2004). 'I don't feel like a diabetic any more': the impact of stopping insulin in patients with maturity onset diabetes of the young following genetic testing. *Clinical Medicine*, **4**, 144–7.

Shepherd M, Sparkes AC and Hattersley AT (2001). Genetic testing in Maturity Onset Diabetes of the Young (MODY): a new challenge for the diabetes clinic. *Practical Diabetes International*, **18**, 16–21.

Stride A and Hattersley AT (2002). Different genes, different diabetes: lessons from maturity-onset diabetes of the young. *Annals of Medicine*, **34**, 207–16.

UK Genetic Testing Network http://www.ukgtn.nhs.uk/gtn/UKGTN-informaion/What-is-the-UKGTN.htm (accessed on 1 October 2007)

Vaughan D (1999). The role of the organization in the production of techno-scientific knowledge. *Social Studies of Science*, **29**, 913–43.

Index

Note: Emboldened page numbers indicate chapters